Primary Dermatologic Care

Primary Dermatologic Care

BONNIE J. HOOPER, RN, MSN, ANP
Dermatology Associates
La Jolla, CA

Mitchel P. Goldman, MD
Dermatology Associates
La Jolla, CA

With 138 illustrations

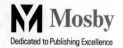
Mosby
Dedicated to Publishing Excellence

A Times Mirror
Company

Publisher: Nancy Coon
Editor: Barry Bowlus
Developmental Editor: Cynthia Anderson
Project Manager: Patricia Tannian
Senior Production Editor: Melissa Mraz Lastarria
Book Design Manager: Judi Lang
Manufacturing Supervisor: Don Carlisle
Interior and Cover Design: Brian Salisbury

Composition by Graphic World, Inc.
Printing/binding by World Color Book Group

Mosby, Inc.
11830 Westline Industrial Drive
St. Louis, Missouri 63146

Library of Congress Cataloging in Publication Data

Hooper, Bonnie J.
    Primary dermatologic care / Bonnie J. Hooper, Mitchel P. Goldman.
        p.   cm.
    Includes bibliographical references and index.
    ISBN 1-55664-412-4
    1. Skin—Diseases—Diagnosis—Handbooks, manuals, etc.   2. Skin—
Diseases—Diagnosis—Atlases.   I. Goldman, Mitchel P.   II. Title.
    [DNLM: 1. Skin Diseases—diagnosis.   2. Skin Diseases—therapy.
WR 141H785p   1999]
RL105.H66   1999
616.5—dc21
DNLM/DLC
for Library of Congress   98-29425
                                                                                  CIP

98 99 00 01 02/9 8 7 6 5 4 3 2 1

*To my husband Wayne, whose encouragement, optimism, and
belief in my potential have always been an
invaluable source of inspiration.*

*To my sons, Alex and Collin, without whose love, support, and
tolerance this book could never have been written.*

Bonnie Hooper

■

To my supportive wife, Dianne.

Mitchel Goldman

A Note to the Reader

The authors and publisher have made every attempt to check dosages and nursing content for accuracy. Because the science of pharmacology is continually advancing, our knowledge base continues to expand. Therefore we recommend that the reader always check product information for changes in dosage or administration before administering any medication. This is particularly important with new or rarely used drugs.

Foreword

With the challenges in the health care environment today it is refreshing to see that two professionals have collaborated to enhance the delivery of quality of patient care. As health care has proceeded along a continuum from generalization to specialization, providers have had to expand their knowledge base to meet the needs of their patients. That specialty knowledge base is larger then ever because of ongoing research in the medical, nursing, and pharmaceutical fields. Staying abreast of information in one specialty is a full-time commitment. Now with managed care policies delaying, or limiting, access to specialists the need for sharing information among health care providers is more important than ever.

Though there are a few life-threatening dermatologic disorders, there can be serious implications and significant morbidity associated with cutaneous disease. This fact alone is important enough that practitioners need to be able to accurately assess and diagnosis skin disease. The skin is the largest organ of the body and is an individual's presentation to the world. In the skin-conscious society in which we live, even the smallest blemish may be a source of considerable body image alteration or social stigma. But skin disorders, particularly minor ones, are often not considered to be of any significance. Bonnie Hooper, MSN, ANP, and Mitchel P. Goldman, MD, have written a wonderful clinical resource for the nondermatologic clinician. *Primary Dermatologic Care* leads the reader through an intellectual process beginning with principles of diagnosis, moving through specific disorders of the skin and its appendages, and culminating with chapters on dermatopharmacology and dermatologic therapy. Chapters are formatted in a logical manner leading the reader through evaluation, differential diagnosis, and treatment of many common cutaneous disorders in an easily readable format.

The chapter on patient education will definitely be an asset for any clinician because it provides well-organized material that will be an addition to any practice. The fact that the authors had the foresight to include a chapter with a listing of support groups makes this text even more valuable to the delivery of quality care.

This text gives the clinician valuable information that emphasizes the importance of understanding the need for accurate assessment, diagnosis, treatment, and follow-up evaluation. It is a text that should be in every clinician's library.

Marcia J. Hill, MSN, RN
Editor
Dermatology Nursing

While the number of dermatology textbooks is quite plentiful, most are based on the supposition that an accurate diagnosis has been reached. Although one advantage of dermatology is that the diagnosis is quite literally "right before your eyes," the challenge is still to attach the correct name to the signs and symptoms that bring patients to our offices.

This book is based on the premise that texts organized by pathology, although essential for research and study, are impractical to the busy clinician. It is not intended as a comprehensive review of dermatologic disorders, but rather as an **aid to making a diagnosis** and to providing **guidelines for treatment** and the patient focus we all need to provide the *best* patient care.

Contents

Part III:
Patient Education Materials 445

Part IV:
Directory of Support Groups 471

Part V:
Dermatopharmacology 475

Part VI:
Dermatologic Surgery Techniques 485

General Principles of Diagnosis

Dermatology is a highly objective specialty, depending first and foremost on the power of observation. The novice trains himself or herself in making diagnoses through examination and questioning. In no other way can true expertise in this field be attained.

A thorough and accurate history is essential. The job of the clinician is to ask appropriate questions, the answers to which may piece together the puzzle. The following questions should be committed to memory and asked routinely of every patient:

- When did the condition begin?
- What part of the body was affected first?
- Is the condition getting better or worse? (If it is getting better, what brought the patient to the office today?)
- What treatment has already been tried (including over-the-counter [OTC] remedies), and how successful was it?

- Has there been any recent systemic illness?
- What are the local symptoms, if any—itching, burning, tingling?
- What medications are currently being taken or have been taken within the past few weeks, including both prescription and OTC?
- Are there any medication allergies?
- Is there a personal or family history of asthma or any dermatologic condition such as allergy, eczema, atopic dermatitis, or skin cancer?
- What is the occupational history, specifically regarding chemical exposure?
- Has there been any recent travel?
- What are the leisure time activities, including hobbies and gardening, and has any new activity been adopted recently?
- Are there pets in the home environment?
- Are others in the household similarly affected?

The essentials of the objective approach are the following:

The use of any necessary aid to clear vision. The skin must be examined carefully and methodically using both observation and palpation. Magnification should be readily available in all examination rooms. The lighting in many offices greatly interferes with diagnostic accuracy. Daylight should enter (preferably) through a north window or large skylight uncolored by reflection from the walls, trees, or buildings. Artificial, inadequate, or colored light creates deceptive reflections, obscures fine detail, and reduces the interpretation of color changes to guesswork.

The undressed patient. Piecemeal examination is less satisfactory.

Systematic and orderly notation and description:

General description of the patient, that is, age, sex, color, build, general state of health.

Distribution of the lesions, that is, generalized, localized, bilaterally symmetric, and/or patchy. This observation is a highly important clinical feature of all eruptions. There are many characteristic distributions in dermatology, the recognition of which may be tantamount to making the diagnosis.

Arrangement of the lesions: Are they discrete? confluent? grouped in a characteristic manner? well or poorly defined?

Configuration, or shape and outline of the individual lesion or group of lesions: The clinician should learn to recognize the arciform, polycyclic, annular, linear, and serpiginous configurations, as well as those that follow natural skin lines.

The primary lesion should be identified: Ask the patient to point out the most recent lesion to erupt and follow it through the evolutionary process. For instance, does the lesion begin as a macule and develop into a papule?

Characteristics of the lesion should be described.

- Is it dry, greasy, oozing, or bleeding?
- What color is it?
- Is it indurated? (Determined by touch.)
- Is the border rolled or advancing?
- Is there central clearing?
- Are blisters present?
- What is the size of the lesion? (Measured to the nearest millimeter, for later comparison.)
- Is there any tenderness?
- Are atrophic changes present?

Involvement of the mucus membranes, hair, and nails should be noted: Certain conditions never appear on the mucus membranes; in others, the involvement is characteristic.

Primary Dermatologic Lesions

Abcess: A nodule containing pus.

Bulla: A large vesicle or blister at least 5 mm in diameter. The average bulla is 1 to 2 cm in diameter. **Bullae** is the plural form of *bulla.* (See Figure P1-1.)

Cyst: An enclosed subcutaneous sac that contains fluid or solid material. (See Figure P1-1.)

Furuncle: A lesion containing pus that is greater than 0.5 cm in diameter. (See *Pustule.*)

Macule: A spot without elevation or depression. If there is any visible or palpable elevation or depression, the lesion is not a macule. Examples: freckles, purpura. (See Figure P1-1.)

Nodule: A sharly circumscribed lesion larger than a papule and firmer than normal surrounding tissue. Examples: fibroma, epithelioma, sarcoma. (See Figure P1-1.)

Papule: An elevated lesion of the skin, produced by tissue infiltration, whether with fluid or cells, or by a localized proliferation in the epidermis. A papule has definite mass, no matter how little. It has "feel." Example: goose bumps. (See Figure P1-1.)

Patch: A macule larger than 1 cm.

Plaque: A large flat-topped papule. (See Figure P1-1.)

Pustule: A lesion containing pus. It may be papular or vesicular at onset. The solid papule undergoes central softening with pus formation, or the vesicle contents become purulent. The term is restricted to lesions less than 0.5 cm in diameter. Examples: acne, variola, folliculitis. (See Figure P1-1.)

Figure PI-I

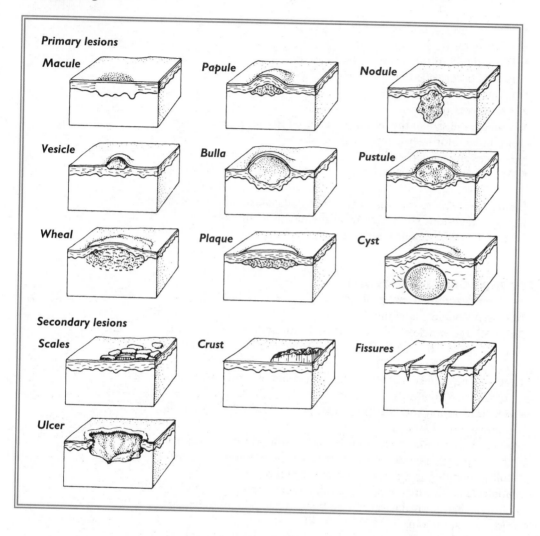

Primary lesions

Macule Papule Nodule

Vesicle Bulla Pustule

Wheal Plaque Cyst

Secondary lesions

Scales Crust Fissures

Ulcer

Telangiectasia: Groups of dilated superficial capillaries.

Tumor: A new growth of varying size. It may be composed of any of the structures of the skin or subcutaneous tissue.

Wheal: A distinctive modification of a papule. A wheal is an edematous, superficial lesion that appears and disappears rapidly, leaving no permanent changes. It is usually sharply circumscribed and slightly elevated. Morphologically, it is a papule produced by acute edema. (See Figure P1-1.)

Every wheal passes through a definite characteristic cycle. It begins as a slight blanching, with elevation of the skin producing "orange-peel" pitting of the surface as a result of intense inter-follicular edema. The stage of pallor passes into a stage of erythema in which the wheal takes on a rose-colored tinge. As the wheal involutes, it loses its pink color, but the elevation persists for a considerable period.

Wheals may be surmounted by vesicles or bullae. They may also be hemorrhagic. The tendency to wheal formation may be latent and appear only on irritation of papules or macules. **Dermographism** is the production of a wheal by scratching or stroking the skin.

Secondary Dermatologic Lesions

Atrophy: Thinning of the skin with loss of hair and sweat glands, resulting from wasting of the dermis. Relaxation of the subepidermal tissues results from loss of elastic tissue. The skin is whitened, and there is a depression of the epidermis into the deeper layer of the cutis.

Cicatrix: A scar, formed of fibrous tissue, replacing normal dermis that has been destroyed by illness or injury.

Crust: A "scab" composed of dried exudate, serum, pus, and/or blood. It is often mingled with hair, scales, and/or medicinal applications. Crust does not form on mucus membranes. (See Figure P1-1.)

Erosion: A superficial, denuded lesion of the epidermis.

Excoriation: The loss of superficial tissue produced by scratching. Excoriations occur on accessible surfaces and are parallel, linear abrasions.

Fissure: Deep linear crack or defect in the continuity of the epidermis. It is frequently painful and may be a portal of entry for infection. (See Figure P1-1.)

Hyperkeratosis: Abnormal thickening of the outermost layer of the skin. It appears rough, dry, and sometimes cracked.

Hyperpigmentation:
   Extrinsic: Originating from outside the skin. Example: tattoo.
   Intrinsic: Developing in the skin from the activity of cutaneous structures; the formation of melanin in the basal layer of the epidermis. Example: melasma.

Hypopigmentation: Lightening of the normal skin tone caused by either a destruction of melanocytes or an inability of the melanocytes to produce melanin.

Lichenification: Increased visibility of the superficial skin markings, associated with thickening and induration. In appearance it may resemble aggregated papules. Often there is an increase of pigment in lichenified areas.

Scale: A dry or greasy flake of epidermis; an exfoliation. Scale is the normal end product of the keratinization cycle of the epidermis. (See Figure P1-1.)

Ulcer: Destruction of the skin extending beneath the epidermis. It always leaves a scar. (See Figure P1-1.)

Anatomy of the Skin

The skin is the largest and most visible organ of the body and mirrors the patient's general condition. It is the body's first line of defense. There are two types of skin:

Glabrous: Characterized by the lack of hair follicles and sebaceous glands, and the presence of encapsulated sense organs. It is found on palms and soles.

Hairy: Characterized by not having encapsulated sense organs. Present everywhere but on the palms, soles, and lips.

The skin is composed of two layers (see Figure P1-2).

The **epidermis** is the outermost layer, composing 5% of the entire skin depth. The epidermal cells pass through an evolutionary cycle (keratinization) as they move toward the outer surface of the skin, where they are eventually sloughed. There are five stages or layers of the epidermis through which the cells pass. In order, from innermost outward, they are stratum basalis (basal layer), stratum spinosum (prickle layer), stratum granulosum (granules of keratohyaline), stratum lucidum (cells containing eleidin), and stratum corneum (horny layer). Total renewal time is 3 to 4 weeks. The pigment of the skin is determined by the number and type of melanocytes, located in the basal layer.

The **dermis** or **cutis** is the inner layer, comprising 95% of the total skin thickness. It is composed largely of connective tissue, including collagen and elastic fibers, that together provide strength and elasticity to the skin. The dermis supports a profuse vascular network, nerve fibers, the pilosebaceous system, and sweat glands. The surface has fingerlike projections (papillae) supporting and nourishing the epidermis.

The **adnexa** is composed of eccrine and apocrine glands and pilosebaceous units, including:

Figure PI-2

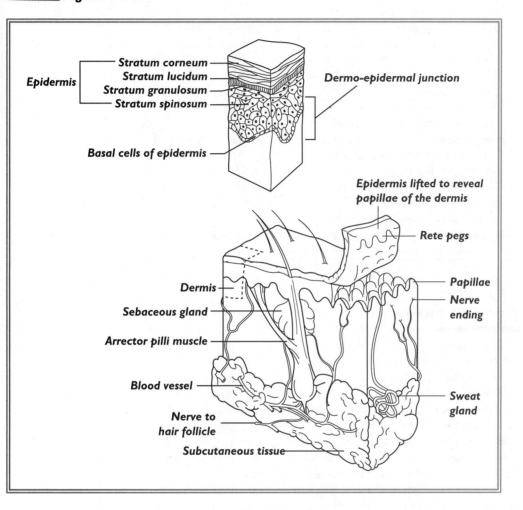

Hair: A projection of epidermis at the bottom of a deep pit (follicle). It is a solid structure with a keratin core. The pigment is derived from the basal layer. There is hair everywhere except on the palms, soles, and lips.

Sebaceous gland: An offshoot of the hair follicle that opens into the upper third of the follicle wall. The sebaceous gland produces sebum, an oily secretion that maintains skin flexibility and tensile strength of the hair.

Arrector piloris muscle: A muscle that is under autonomic innervation and helps to control body temperature by raising body hairs. This raising traps a cushion of air near the skin surface and acts as an insulating space.

Eccrine (sweat) gland: A simple coiled gland that opens to the skin surface through a spiral duct. Located throughout the body, they are most numerous on the palms, soles, forehead, and axillae. The primary function of these glands is to produce sweat, thereby regulating body temperature. Eccrine glands are under cholinergic innervation, with heat and psychologic factors (e.g., emotional stress) as primary stimuli.

Apocrine gland: An outgrowth of the upper portion of the hair follicle. Apocrine secretion is under adrenergic innervation. It is odorless until it reaches the skin surface, where it is altered by bacteria and becomes odoriferous. Apocrine glands are located primarily on the axillae, areolae, anogenital area, external auditory canal, and eyelids.

Nerve supply: An exceedingly complicated and elaborate nervous system located primarily in the dermal layer. There are, however, many terminal fibers in the epidermis.

Physiology of the Skin

The primary function of the skin is to serve as a cutaneous defense mechanism. It has several components:

The outermost layer of the epidermis is the **stratum corneum,** which forms an anatomic barrier between the internal and external environments. The intercellular spaces are filled with a lipid, which acts as the principal route of penetration for many substances. Permeability is increased by changes in the water content through hydration or dehydration of the keratinocytes. The acid mantle gives the skin a natural buffering action against alkalinity.

The **dermis** forms a physical barrier against mechanical friction and trauma with its tough fibrous and elastic components.

The **vascular bed** plays a thermoregulatory role to keep the body temperature within the homeothermic range.

The **sebaceous gland lipid** is enzymatically degraded to produce free fatty acids, which have both antifungal and antibacterial actions.

Part II

Specific Dermatologic Disorders

Acneiform Lesions and Pustules

Figure 1-1   ACNE

A, Teenage male with both open and closed comedones. *B,* Teenage male presenting with nodular cystic acne, inflammatory lesions, and open and closed comedones.

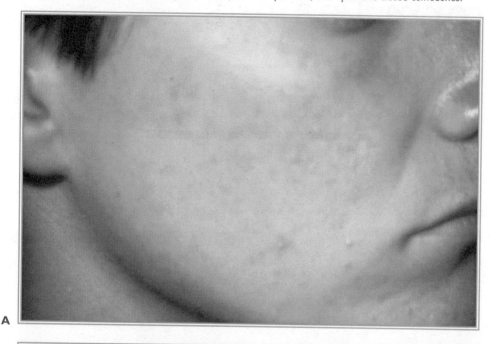

A

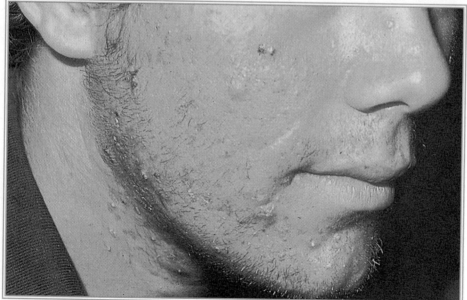

B

Figure 1-2 Acute Candida Intertrigo

Note peripheral fringe of scale and satellite lesions.

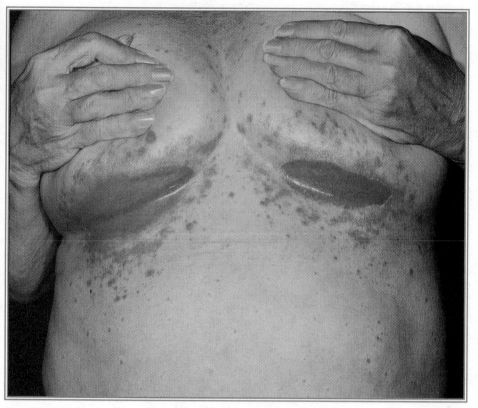

(From Habif TP: *Clinical dermatology,* ed 3, St Louis, 1996, Mosby.)

Figure 1-3   CHICKENPOX

Small vesicles on an erythematous macular base, in a generalized distribution on the back. Lesions vary in size from (early) papular lesions to (later) macular lesions.

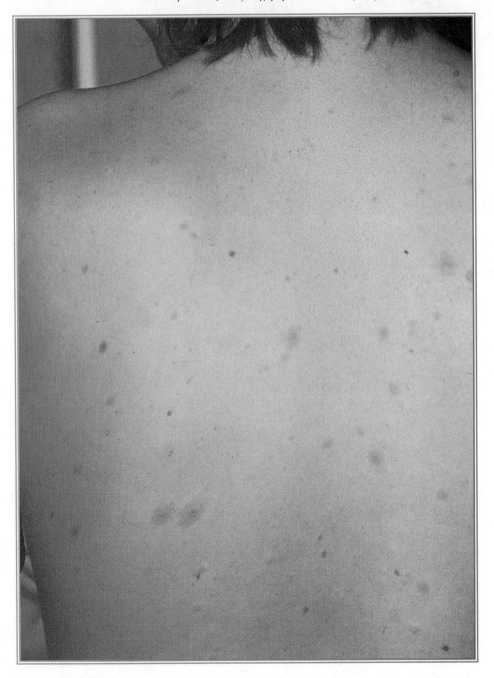

Figure 1-4   EPIDERMAL CYST

The posterior auricular fold is a common location of many epidermal cysts.

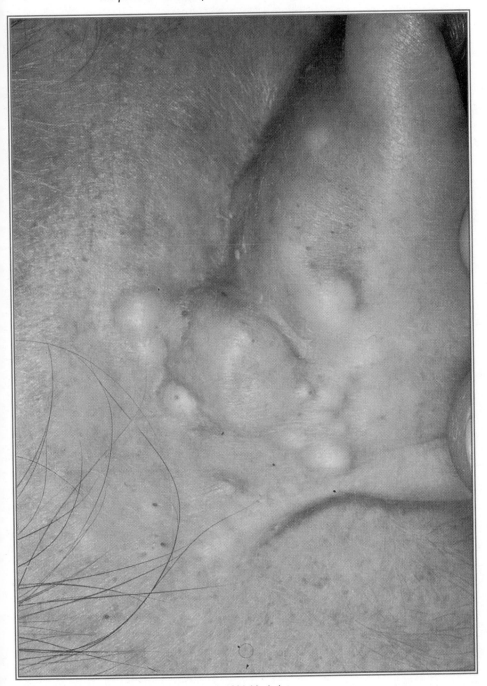

(From Habif TP: *Clinical dermatology,* ed 3, St Louis, 1996, Mosby.)

Figure 1-5 ERYTHEMA INFECTIOSUM

Facial erythema ("slapped cheek"), sparing the nasolabial fold and circumoral region.

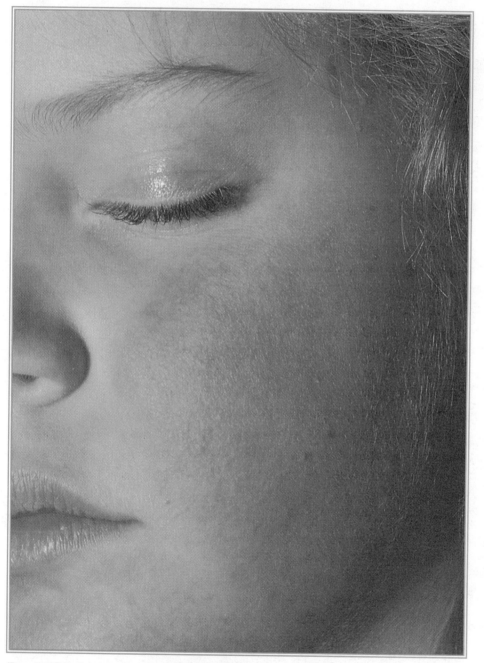

(From Habif TP: *Clinical dermatology,* ed 3, St Louis, 1996, Mosby.)

Figure 1-6   **FOLLICULITIS**

Extensive inflammatory closed comedones centered around hair follicles on the cheek of a male electrical worker exposed to fluorocarbons.

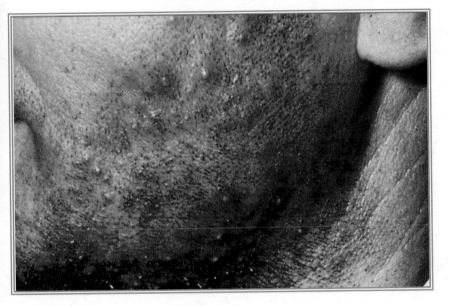

Figure 1-7   **FURUNCLE**

Pustular deep nodule on the posterior aspect of the right neck.

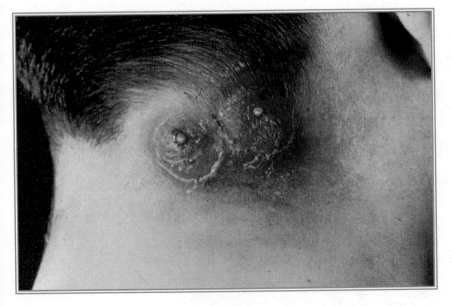

Figure 1-8   CARBUNCLE

Multiple pustular nodules on the posterior aspect of the neck. Many of the nodules have a confluent nature and exude pus.

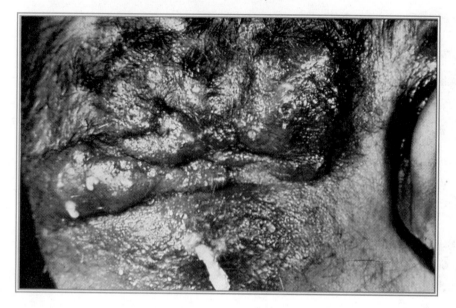

Figure 1-9   HIDRADENITIS SUPPURATIVA

Inflammatory dermatitis of the axilla with multiple sinus tracts, some of which are draining pustular fluid. Note presence of scarring.

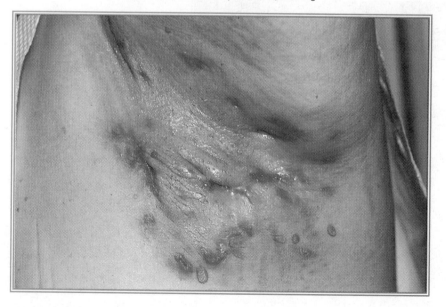

Figure 1-10   IMPETIGO

Erythematous lesions with honey-colored crust on the posterior thigh and buttocks region.

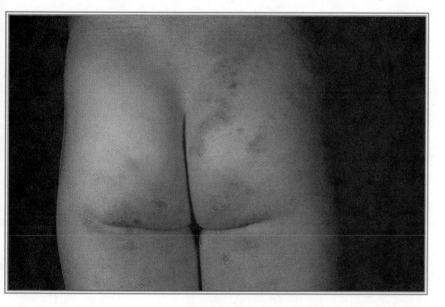

Figure 1-11   INSECT BITES

Insect bites with characteristic purpuric spots in the center of the papule. A central punctum is typical.

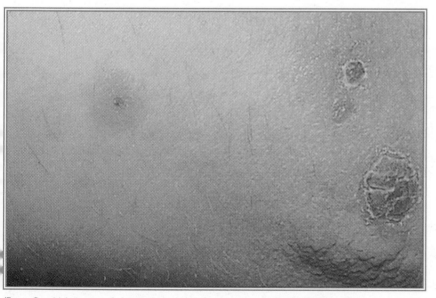

(From Cox N, Lawrence C: *Diagnostic problems in dermatology,* St Louis, 1998, Mosby.)

Figure 1-12 **KERATOSIS PILARIS**

Lateral aspect of the arm in a teenage girl, showing erythematous hyperkeratotic papules overlying hair follicles.

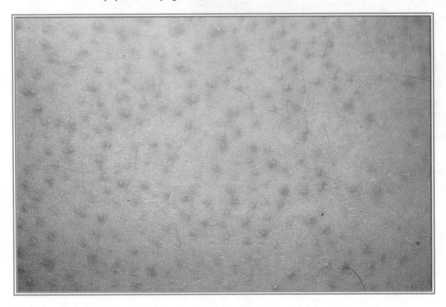

Figure 1-13 **MOLLUSCUM CONTAGIOSUM**

Pearly, dome-shaped papule in the pubic region of a teenager.

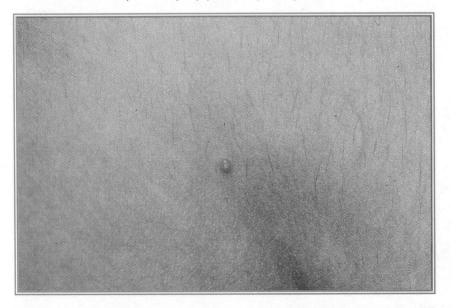

Figure 1-14   PERIORAL DERMATITIS

Inflammatory closed comedones and generalized inflammation in a perioral distribution.

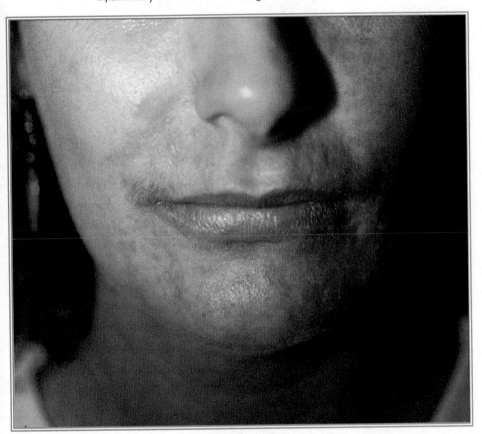

Figure 1-15 PSEUDOFOLLICULITIS

Inflammatory lesions with some pustules in the mandibular angle. Note curled hairs, some of which are embedding back into the skin.

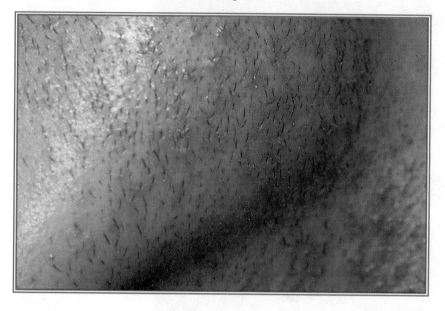

Figure 1-16 PUSTULAR PSORIASIS

Erythematous, plaquelike lesion on the anterior aspect of the scalp extending to the forehead, with overlying hyperkeratosis and lichenlike scales.

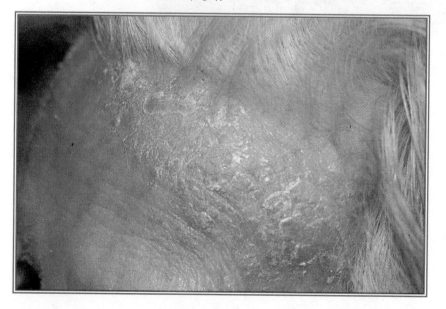

Figure 1-17   ROSACEA

Generalized inflammation with multiple inflammatory papules and pustules, predominantly located on the central aspect of the face and nose.

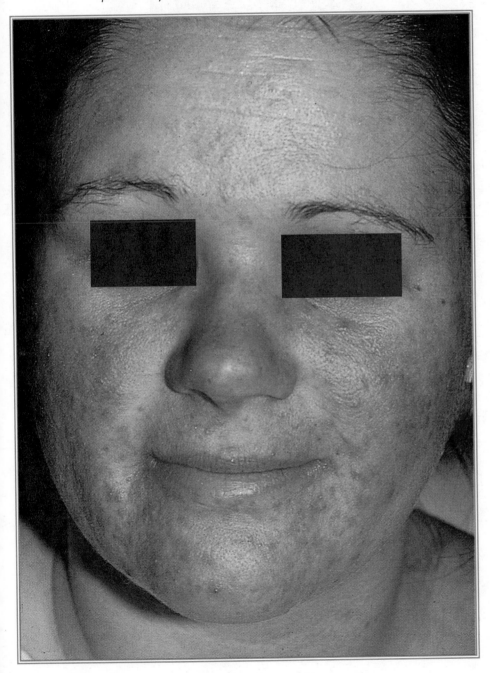

Figure 1-18 **SEBORRHEIC DERMATITIS**

Erythematous patches with some evidence of scale in the usual facial distribution.

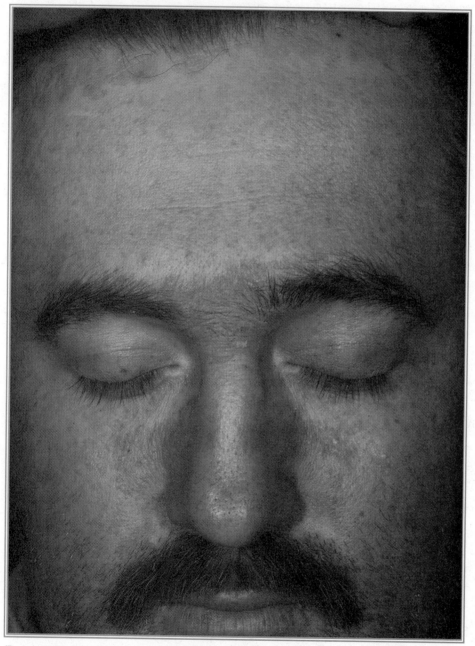

(From Habif TP: *Clinical dermatology,* ed 3, St Louis, 1996, Mosby.)

Figure 1-19 **Tinea Corporis**

Annular lesion with a sharply marginated, erythematous border.

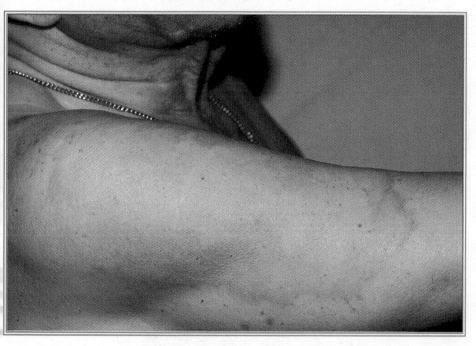

Figure 1-20 VIRAL EXANTHEM

Maculopapular eruption without follicular orientation.

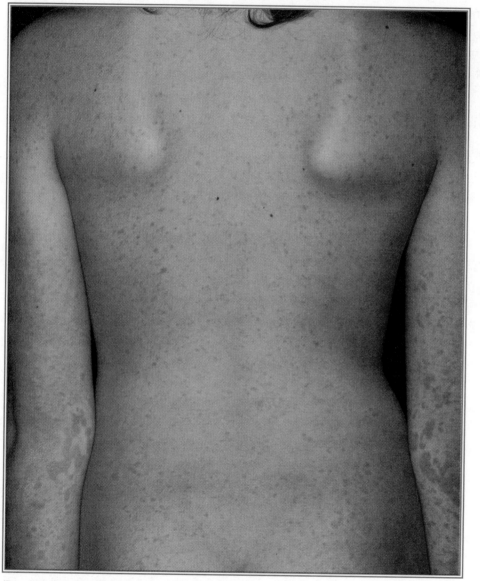

(From Habif TP: *Clinical dermatology,* ed 3, St Louis, 1996, Mosby.)

▓ *Table 1-1*

Differential Diagnosis of Acneiform Lesions and Pustules

DISORDER	TEXT	KEYS TO DIAGNOSIS
Acne vulgaris	Ch. 1, p. 29 (Figure 1-1)	Comedones, papules, pustules, cysts are present on face, neck, shoulders, chest, back; peak age 14 to 15 for females, age 16 to 17 for males.
Candidiasis	Ch. 1, p. 33 (Figure 1-2)	Satellite pustules; sharp, scaling border; erythematous, macerated patches; favors warm, moist environment; may be pruritic or tender.
Chickenpox (varicella)	Ch. 2, p.64 (Figure 1-3)	Maculopapular rash that begins on chest and back, then forms small superficial vesicles on an erythematous base ("dewdrop on a rose petal"); intensely pruritic.
Epidermal cyst	Ch. 5, p. 243 (Figure 1-4)	Subcutaneous, fluctuant swelling. Central opening may exude pasty, odoriferous material. Usually on scalp, face, neck, or trunk.
Erythema infectiosum	Ch. 4, p. 183 (Figure 1-5)	Erythematous, bright red macules and papules occur suddenly on the cheeks. Lacy rash on trunk, buttocks, and upper arms. Generally known as "slapped cheek" appearance.
Folliculitis	Ch. 1, p. 36 (Figure 1-6)	Follicular, erythematous papules and pustules on any hair-bearing surface; *Pseudomonas* folliculitis occurs 1 to 3 days after use of a hot tub.
Furuncles and carbuncles	Ch. 1, p. 38 (Figs. 1-7 and 1-8)	Furuncles: 1 to 5 cm tender nodules with surrounding erythema. May become fluctuant. Carbuncles: 3 to 10 cm tender erythematous nodules that drain pus from multiple follicular orifices.
Hidradenitis suppurativa	Ch. 1, p. 41 (Figure 1-9)	Double comedone, foul-smelling discharge. Subcutaneous sinus tracts. Adenopathy. Axillae, groin, perineum.
Impetigo	Ch. 2, p. 73 (Figure 1-10)	Vesicles on an erythematous base that rupture to form honey-colored crusts, usually around mouth. Regional adenopathy and pruritus are common.
Insect bites	(Figure 1-11)	Erythematous papule with central punctum. Usually pruritic.
Keratosis pilaris	Ch. 1, p. 43 (Figure 1-12)	Small, discrete follicular papules on posterior pilaris, upper arms, and anterior thighs. May be erythematous.
Molluscum contagiosum	Ch. 5, p. 253 (Figure 1-13)	Multiple flesh-colored, firm, domed umbilicated papules. Asymptomatic.
Perioral dermatitis	Ch. 1, p. 44 (Figure 1-14)	Pruritic, burning, discrete erythematous or flesh-colored papules and pustules around mouth and in nasolabial folds.
Pseudo-folliculitis	Ch. 1, p. 46 (Figure 1-15)	Erythematous papules and pustules on shaved areas, especially beards of men with coarse, curly hair. May be asymptomatic or painful and pruritic.
Pustular psoriasis	Ch. 3, p. 135 (Figure 1-16)	Discrete pustules and scaly plaques on palms and soles or erythema with sheets of pustules over much of the body, usually with fever, polyarthralgias, chills, and malaise.

continued

Table 1-1 *continued*

Disorder	Text	Keys to Diagnosis
Rosacea	Ch. 1, p. 48 (Figure 1-17)	Facial papules and pustules but no comedones; flushing, telangiectasias, rhinophyma; triggered by hot foods, emotional stress.
Seborrheic dermatitis	Ch. 3, p. 138 (Figure 1-18)	Sharply marginated yellowish-red patches with sharp borders and greasy scales. Scalp, central face, eyebrows, eyelids, nasolabial folds, and external ear are most commonly affected. May be pruritic.
Tinea corporis	Ch. 3, p. 118 (Figure 1-19)	Erythematous, ring-shaped patches with central clearing and advancing, scaling border.
Viral exanthem	(Figure 1-20)	Maculopapular eruption without follicular orientation.

Acne Vulgaris

Overview

Pathophysiology

Anatomic
Retention hyperkeratosis occurs when keratin in the hair follicle forms a plug above the level of the sebaceous duct, instead of shedding normally. This blockage leads to the formation of both open and closed comedones (blackheads and whiteheads, respectively) (see Figure 1-1, *A*). The eventual rupture of the follicle into the dermis sets up a foreign body inflammatory reaction (see Figure 1-1, *B*). The dark color of closed comedones is related to bacteria and bacterial breakdown products mixed with sebaceous material and densely packed horny cells. The actual causes of comedogenesis are unknown. Comedones only form in sebaceous follicles. Sebum is a necessary but not the sole component of acne production. Heat, humidity, and ultraviolet radiation may also produce follicular hyperkeratosis.

Endocrine
Circulating androgens are always present (acne does not occur in male castrates) and act to stimulate the production of sebum. The active androgen is dihydrotestosterone (DHT). Patients with severe acne usually have high circulating levels of androgens (usually free testosterone and/or dehydroepiandrosterone sulfate [DHEA-S]). Estrogens, on the other hand, can suppress sebum formation and help reduce acne. Oral contraceptives containing norgestrel, norethindrone, and norethindrone acetate may provoke acne eruptions, whereas those containing higher levels of estrogen suppress them.

Bacterial
Propionibacterium acnes (P. acnes), found in normal skin flora, produces an enzyme, lipase, that breaks down triglycerides in sebum to free fatty acids, which can provoke a severe inflammatory reaction. Colonization with P. *acnes* occurs around puberty under the influence of increased sebum production.

Epidemiology
Acne vulgaris affects about 70% of the U.S. population and 25% of people between the ages of 12 and 25. Up to 30% of all teenagers require treatment. It may begin as early as ages 5 to 8 with small comedones first appearing on the nasal bridge. Rapid progression

appears at puberty, with a peak in severity at ages 14 and 15 for girls and ages 16 and 17 for boys. For 10% of patients, eruptions may persist into the thirties. Severe eruptions occur 10 times more frequently in males. Transient relapses may occur before menstrual periods and during periods of stress. A positive family history is present in 70% of patients. There is 100% concordance between identical twins. Scarring, both physical and psychologic, may result if left untreated.

Assessment

Clinical Presentation
Lesions occur primarily on the **face,** but the **neck, shoulders, chest,** and **back** may also be involved. Skin, scalp, and hair are frequently oily. Inflammatory lesions may itch as they erupt and be painful to pressure.

> Grade I: Comedones without inflammation
> Grade II: Comedones with superficial papules, and pustules
> Grade III: Comedones, papules, pustules, and some cysts
> Grade IV: Severe cystic and destructive lesions that heal with scarring (uncommon in women)

Diagnostics
Diagnosis is made by clinical presentation. **Comedones are a hallmark** of acne vulgaris and must be present to support the diagnosis. **DHEA-S levels are elevated** in 80% of patients with cystic or severe acne. **Free testosterone levels may be elevated** in up to 50% of women over 18 years of age who have severe acne. Increased DHEA-S levels are therefore more clinically relevant in female acne.

Differential Diagnosis
- Hidradenitis suppurativa (lesions occur in groin and axillae and have sinus tracts) (see Figure 1-9)
- Rosacea (comedones are not present; lesions appear on a telangiectatic background) (see Figure 1-17)
- Pyoderma faciale (lesions are more cystic in number)
- Steroid acne (lesions are usually at the same stage of development with multiple, prominent, and extensive closed comedones; there is a history of steroid use)
- Erythema infectiosum (bright red macules and papules occur suddenly on the cheeks, with a lacy rash on the trunk, buttocks, and upper arms) (see Figure 1-5)

ACNE

- Begins under the skin surface when hair follicles become blocked with sebum and keratin
- Becomes inflammatory (papules and pustules develop) if the blocked follicles rupture into the dermis
- Is not caused by dirtiness, diet, or stress
- Is affected by hormones

Treatment

Nonpharmacologic

Acne Surgery

Remove comedones either manually or with a suction device and incise and drain cysts. The treatment is less painful and more effective if the patient has been using topical keratolytic agents for at least 2 weeks before treatment, and if the area is moistened with a humidifier before extraction.

Pharmacologic

Topical Agents

Apply **benzoyl peroxide** to affected areas qid or bid. Benzoyl peroxide has various strengths; higher percentages require a prescription. Benzoyl peroxide serves as a keratolytic and antibacterial agent. Gels are more effective than creams, although more drying. The agent may be combined with alpha-hydroxyacids or antibiotics to increase efficacy.

Apply **clindamycin (Cleocin-T)** or **erythromycin (Aknemycin, Erygel, T-stat)** to affected areas bid. These agents are less effective than systemic agents. Resistance to one topical antibiotic may occur; such a reaction does not preclude a therapeutic response to another agent.

Sulfacetamide (Klaron) is a less irritating keratolytic, antibacterial gel that is very effective for patients with sensitive skin.

Apply **tretinoin cream or gel (Retin-A, Avita)** sparingly at night only (it is inactivated by sunlight). Begin use on an alternate-day schedule to prevent or minimize irritation. Microcomedones may be converted to pustules during the first few weeks of therapy, after which the inflammation subsides. Slight and reversible hypopigmentation may occur in darkly pigmented patients. Irritation may result from overuse or hydration of the skin before application or in cold or dry climates. Improvement may require as much as 2 months. Photosensitivity occurs, and use of sunscreens is advised.

Adapalene (Differin) 0.01% gel is a comedolytic agent with less irritation potential than **Retin-A.** It should be applied daily, either morning or night.

Azelaic acid (Azelex) 20% cream is a pore declogger and antibacterial agent with mild depigmentation properties. It is ideal for use once daily (in the morning) in patients who experience postacne hyperpigmentation (common in blacks and those with darker skin tones).

Intralesional Corticosteroids

Shake **triamcinolone (Kenalog)** 2.5 mg/ml thoroughly before injection. It is useful in the treatment of inflammatory or painful cysts. Inject enough steroid to blanch the cyst (not more than 0.1 ml). It may produce a temporary (up to 6 months) steroid-induced localized atrophy if injected too deeply. Resolution of the lesion usually occurs within 24 hours.

Systemic Agents

Tetracycline is the drug of choice for inflammatory acne lesions. Typical dosage is 1 g per day in divided doses, either 250 mg PO qid or 500 mg PO bid (depending on gastrointestinal [GI] tolerance), taken on an empty stomach to increase absorption, until clear improvement is noted. The dosage may then be decreased to a maintenance level of 250 to 500 mg per day. Dosage may be increased to 2 to 3 g per day for several weeks to induce remission in an otherwise unresponsive patient. It is the least expensive of oral antibiotic therapies. Photosensitivity may occur. It should not be given to children less than 12 years old as it may cause a permanent staining of teeth.

Erythromycin 250 mg PO qid or 333 mg PO tid may be used if tetracycline is ineffective or is not tolerated; it is almost as effective. The enteric-coated form may be taken with food since its absorption is not affected.

Dosage of **minocycline** is 50 to 100 mg PO bid. Minocycline is more effective than tetracycline or erythromycin but is also more expensive. It should be taken on an empty stomach, but 85% absorption occurs even when taken with meals. Dizziness may rarely occur during initial stages of therapy. Photosensitivity is less common than with tetracycline.

> ■ NOTE: *With all oral antibiotic medications, therapy is continued until a therapeutic response occurs. At that time, dosages can be lowered or the medication switched to a topical product.*

Estrogens are effective in women with severe acne. An estrogen-dominant birth control pill with 80 to 100 μg of mestranol or ethinyl estradiol such as **Demulen, Ortho Tri-Cyclen,** or **Desogen** is used.

For recalcitrant acne:

Spironolactone, an androgen blocker, reduces sebum production by 45%. Begin dosage at 25 to 50 mg PO bid. The dosage may be increased to 100 mg bid, but **breakthrough vaginal bleeding** can occur at doses over 100 mg qd. **Check potassium levels at 2-month intervals** since spironolactone is a potassium-sparing diuretic and may cause hyperkalemia. Continue therapy for 9 to 12 months. Patients should be informed that it has been known to cause breast cysts in laboratory animals, and mammography every 2 years is therefore recommended.

Isotretinoin (Accutane) is used in a dosage of 0.5 to 2 mg/kg/day for 20 weeks. It is highly effective in preventing scarring, and for antibiotic-resistant cystic acne. Prolonged remissions and cures are reported. Multiple side effects include chelitis; dryness; increase in liver function test results (LFTs) and lipid levels; photosensitivity; joint pain; nosebleeds; visual changes (tunnel vision); depression; and headache (pseudotumor cerebri). It is an absolute teratogen, making it **completely contraindicated during pregnancy.** Check complete blood count (CBC), chemistry panel, and human chorionic gonadotropin (HCG) level before treatment and every month during treatment.

Indications for Referral

- Hormonal abnormalities suspected as cause of acne, as detailed by blood test results and recalcitrance to treatment.

For Acne Vulgaris Patient Teaching information and materials, turn to p. 447.

Candidiasis (Moniliasis)

Overview

Pathophysiology

The most common species of *Candida* that infects humans is *Candida albicans.* It is a normal inhabitant of the gastrointestinal tract in 70% of people and is a normal organism on mucus membranes. It is capable of infecting only the outer layer of the epithelium. Factors responsible for promoting this disorder are many and include the following:

1. Any form of local tissue damage causes a disturbance of the integument and/or an alteration in skin pH, which in turn causes increased susceptibility to a yeast infection.
2. Removal of competing organisms (usually removal of bacteria by antibiotic treatment) leads to an increase in yeast numbers.

3. An increase in the amount of glucose (as in the saliva, sweat, and urine of diabetics) will prevent bacteria from inhibiting yeast growth.
4. A warm, moist environment (such as that found in intertriginous areas, inside shoes, etc.) provides an excellent medium for yeast growth.

Epidemiology

Infection is most common in the very young and very old. Patients who are pregnant, have iron deficiency anemia, take birth control pills, have high plasma cortisol levels, or have various systemic and debilitating illnesses are also at increased risk for development of candidiasis.

Assessment

Clinical Presentation

Intertriginous Areas

The primary lesion is a pustule, the contents of which peel away the stratum corneum, leaving erythematous macerated patches covered by a gray-white membranous plaque with a **sharp, scaling border. Satellite erythematous papules** and **pustules** are common (see Figure 1-2). Chronic lesions may appear psoriatic. **Soreness and pruritus** are usual and may be severe. It may occur on large body areas or may be present only under a ring or piece of tight-fitting jewelry.

Perlèche (Angular Cheilitis)

Appears as erythematous, macerated, fissuring inflammation at the corners of the mouth. Usually seen in the elderly with dentures and in children and individuals with orthodontic devices.

Vulvovaginitis

Presents with itching and soreness, frequently with a thick, creamy white vaginal discharge. Vaginal mucosa is beefy red with curdy white flecks of discharge on the vulvar skin. Perianal area is also frequently affected.

Candida Balanitis

Infection of the glans penis, especially prevalent in the uncircumcised. May present with either tiny, transient papules that develop into white pustules or with vesicles that rupture, leaving a peeling border.

Interdigital Candidiasis
An erosive, chronic inflammation with white macerated tissue and fissuring between the fingers, especially the third interspace. Occurs chiefly in housekeepers, launderers and barbers. May be superinfected with gram-negative bacteria.

Paronychia
See Nail Disorders, Chapter 9, p. 366.

Thrush (Oral Candidiasis)
See Oral Lesions, Chapter 11, p. 405.

Diagnostics
KOH scraping of the satellite pustules reveals budding spores and elongated pseudohyphae.

Differential Diagnosis
- Pustular psoriasis (discrete pustules and scaly plaques on palms and soles, or erythema with sheets of pustules over much of the body, usually associated with malaise) (see Figure 1-16)
- Tinea corporis (erythematous, ring-shaped patches with central clearing and advancing scaling border) (see Figure 1-19)
- Seborrheic dermatitis (lesions are usually on the central face and scalp) (see Figure 1-18)

Treatment

Nonpharmacologic
Reduce predisposing factors (humidity, antibiotics, hyperglycemia, obesity). Wearing loose-fitting cotton clothing is helpful.

Pharmacologic

Topical Agents
Cool water or **Burow's solution** soaks, followed by air drying several times a day, is both soothing and beneficial. Body powders such as **Zeasorb-AF** help to reduce moisture in intertriginous areas and help prevent the condition.

For cutaneous infections, the topical antifungals **ketoconazole (Nystatin), clotrimazole (Lotrimin, Mycelex), miconazole (Monistat-Derm),** and **econazole (Spectazole)** applied bid are effective. The last three are effective against both dermatophyte and *Candida albicans* infections.

CANDIDIASIS

- Patients should wear loose-fitting clothing and cotton underwear, change out of wet clothing as soon as possible, and keep skin dry
- Frequently develops in skinfolds, where conditions are warm, dark, and moist; obesity should therefore be reduced

Hydrocortisone cream 1% is helpful in providing symptomatic relief. Combination therapy of a topical corticosteroid plus an antifungal (**Mycolog, Lotrisone**) is sometimes helpful, but its use should be limited to 1 week because of the higher potency of the steroid. (If it is used at all, prescribe only a 15 g tube with no refills.)

Miconazole (Monistat) vaginal suppository 200 mg qhs for 3 days is effective in the treatment of vulvovaginitis.

Systemic Agents

For vulvovaginitis or persistent and/or extensive lesions **ketoconazole (Nizoral)** 200 to 400 mg qd is taken with food for 2 weeks. Weekly therapy of a single 400 mg oral dose may prevent recurrences and prolong remissions. Check liver enzyme levels after 2 weeks of treatment if prolonged therapy is indicated. Alternatively, **fluconazole (Diflucan)** can be given as a single oral dose of 150 mg, plus once monthly for prophylaxis.

Indications for Referral

- Development of concomitant disseminated candidiasis lesions in more than one anatomic location, that is, mouth and genital area.
- Ineffective response to treatment (recurrence within a few weeks after cessation of treatment).

For Candidiasis Patient Teaching information and materials, turn to p. 449.

Folliculitis

Overview

Pathophysiology

A superficial inflammation of hair follicles, chronic folliculitis may lead to follicle destruction and consequent permanent alopecia. The majority of patients have a **history of seborrheic dermatitis.** The condition may result from many different factors (friction or chemicals), but most commonly from an infection by *Staphylococcus aureus*.

Pseudomonas folliculitis **(hot tub dermatitis)** invades the open hair follicle pores after superhydration of the stratum corneum. *Pseudomonas aeruginosa* (the causative agent) is able to withstand temperatures of up to 107° F (42° C) and chlorine levels of up to

3 mg/l. Occlusion of the skin with tight-fitting or nylon clothing promotes infection. Symptoms occur abruptly within 1 to 3 days after use of a contaminated hot tub or pool.

Epidemiology
Most commonly occurs in middle-aged persons (ages 40 to 60).

Assessment

Clinical Presentation
Papules and **pustules** associated with hair follicles surrounded by a 1 to 2 mm area of erythema present a hallmark of diagnosis (see Figure 1-6). Folliculitis may develop on any hair-bearing surface. Pustules resolve into red macules, which fade to leave postinflammatory hyperpigmented scars in susceptible individuals. The condition is usually asymptomatic but may be pruritic.

    Pseudomonas folliculitis presents as follicular erythematous papules, pustules, or vesicles over the back, buttocks, and upper arms. Associated features include pruritus, malaise, low-grade fever, sore throat and eyes, and axillary lymphadenopathy. It resolves spontaneously within 10 days.

Diagnostics
- Culture pustular material to evaluate antibiotic sensitivities.

Differential Diagnosis
- Pseudofolliculitis (close inspection reveals ingrown hairs) (see Figure 1-15)
- Acne vulgaris (various stages of papules and pustules are present) (see Figure 1-1, *B*)
- Impetigo (lesions are crusted) (see Figure 1-10)
- Pustular psoriasis (pustules on a background of psoriatic plaques) (see Figure 1-16)
- Insect bites (lesions are larger and more erythematous without follicular orientation) (see Figure 1-11)
- Varicella (lesions occur in crops, rapidly changing from papules to pustules to crusted lesions) (see Figure 1-3)
- Viral exanthem (maculopapular eruption without follicular orientation) (see Figure 1-20)

FOLLICULITIS

- Is usually caused by a bacterial infection in hair follicles
- May worsen as a result of friction or irritation
- May be treated by the use of antibiotics (topical or systemic), antibacterial soaps, use of fresh razor blades daily, and laundering of soiled items to prevent contamination

Treatment

Nonpharmacologic
Wash the area bid with antibacterial soap **(Lever 2000, Safeguard, Dial).** Avoid chemicals that are known to cause irritation. Decrease friction from clothing. Use a fresh razor blade daily when shaving

infected areas. Use a brushless shaving cream. Launder towels, washcloths, sheets, and clothing daily to prevent contamination.

Pharmacologic

Topical Agents

Topical **benzoyl peroxide** solution or gel may be applied to lesions qhs or bid (if not irritating).

Clindamycin (Cleocin-T 1%) is used bid after bathing.

Apply **erythromycin solution (Em-gel, T-Stat)** are applied bid after bathing.

Hydrocortisone 1% cream applied over the antibiotic may provide symptomatic relief of pruritus and/or excoriation.

Benzoyl peroxide cleansers 2.5% to 10% **(Triaz cleanser, Benzac Desquam X)** may be used bid. Patients who do not respond to therapy should be evaluated for possible status as chronic nasal carriers of *Staphylococcus aureus* (with a culture of the nares). These patients require a 6-month course of **mupirocin (Bactroban)** intranasally bid.

Systemic Agents

Erythromycin or dicloxacillin 250 mg PO q6h is prescribed for 10 days if lesions do not respond to topical therapy. For *Pseudomonas folliculitis*, **ciprofloxacin (Cipro)** 500 mg PO bid is ingested for 5 days.

Indications for Referral

- Recurrent or persistent infections that do not respond to the above treatment regimen.

For Folliculitis Patient Teaching information and materials, turn to p. 451.

Furuncles and Carbuncles

Overview

Pathophysiology

A furuncle, or boil, is a small perifollicular abscess that develops as the body attempts to "wall off" a follicular infection. The hair follicle is destroyed. The lesion represents a deep inflammatory reaction caused by *Staphylococcus aureus*, usually incited by obstruction of a sebaceous gland or ingrown hair.

A carbuncle is a more extensive and inflammatory infection of a group of contiguous (connecting) follicles, caused by *Staphylococcus aureus*. A resulting abscess commonly forms in the subcutaneous tissue.

Epidemiology

Furuncles are most common in adolescence and early adulthood. Their peak incidence parallels that of acne vulgaris. Increased frequency is seen in patients with seborrheic dermatitis, anemia, alcoholism, diabetes, hypogammaglobulinemia, and malnutrition.

Carbuncles occur predominantly in men, usually in middle or old age. They are more common in the presence of diabetes, malnutrition, cardiac failure, prolonged steroid therapy, or severe generalized dermatoses.

Assessment

Clinical Presentation

Furuncles are usually 1 to 5 cm nodules, most frequently found on hair-bearing skin subject to friction and maceration (see Figure 1-7). The face, scalp, buttocks, and axillae are common sites. A furuncle presents initially as a small follicular inflammatory nodule, which becomes fluctuant within a few days. Lesions become pustular and necrotic, resolving into a purple macule and ultimately a permanent scar. The surrounding skin is erythematous and tender. Furuncles can be quite painful when they occur in the nose or external ear canal. Lesions may be single or multiple and tend to appear in crops.

A *sty* is a furuncle that involves a sebaceous gland of the eyelid margin.

Carbuncles begin as painful, hard, smooth, red nodules that increase in size to 3 to 10 cm or more (see Figure 1-8). After 5 to 7 days, pus drains from *multiple* follicular orifices, leaving a crateriform nodule. Most lesions are on the back, neck, intertriginous areas, shoulders, or hips. Patients may have a high fever and malaise accompanying or preceding the carbuncle's development. There may be regional lymphadenopathy. Lesions heal with scarring.

Diagnostics

The diagnosis is made on the basis of clinical presentation, although a culture of the pustular material will help in defining appropriate antibiotic therapy. The purulent fluid can also be used to eliminate other bacterial and fungal infections, as well as epidermal and pilar cysts (which are sterile).

Differential Diagnosis
- Acne vulgaris (usually there are many lesions in various stages of development and involution) (see Figure 1-1, *B*)
- Folliculitis (lesions are all associated with hair follicles) (see Figure 1-6)
- Hidradenitis suppurativa (extensive lesions in tracts under the skin) (see Figure 1-9)
- Epidermal cyst (subcutaneous, fluctuant swelling; central opening may exude pasty, odoriferous material) (see Figure 1-4)

Treatment

Nonpharmacologic
Incision and drainage of the abscess are appropriate when the lesion is fluctuant. Warm compresses will help relieve discomfort.

Pharmacologic

Topical Agents
Antibiotic *ointments* such as **bacitracin-polymixin-neomycin (Neosporin)** or **mupirocin (Bactroban)** or antibiotic *solutions* such as **clindamycin (Cleocin-T 1%)** all applied bid may be helpful, although oral antibiotic therapy is preferred. Patients with recurrent furuncles or carbuncles may be chronic carriers of *Staphylococcus aureus* and may benefit from the application of **Bactroban** intranasally bid indefinitely to reduce the population of the bacteria where it lives and breeds.

Systemic Agents
Dicloxacillin 250 mg PO q6h is preferred. **Erythromycin** (same dosage schedule) is appropriate for patients allergic to penicillin. Continue treatment for at least 4 weeks or until lesions have resolved.

Often lesions may be mixed with both gram-positive and gram-negative organisms. If so, **amoxicillin** and **clavulanate potassium (Augmentin)** 875 mg bid or **azithromycin (Zithromax)** 250 mg, 2 capsules on day 1, and 1 capsule daily for the next 4 days, may be a more appropriate antibiotic.

FURUNCLES AND CARBUNCLES

- Are more severe forms of folliculitis: a furuncle is an abscess in a hair follicle, whereas a carbuncle is a more extensive abscess, which occurs in connecting follicles and lies deeper in the subcutaneous tissue
- May be eased with warm, moist compresses
- May continue to drain for several days after they have been incised

Indications for Referral

- Lesions unresponsive to treatment.
- Deep, difficult anatomic location, or cosmetically disfiguring abscesses requiring incision and drainage and/or excision.

For Furuncles and Carbuncles Patient Teaching information and materials, turn to p. 451.

Hidradenitis Suppurativa

Overview

Pathophysiology

Occlusion of apocrine sweat glands whose cause is unknown leads to secondary bacterial infection in genetically predisposed individuals. Dilatation of the glands and severe inflammation follow the localized infection, which in turn is followed by healing with fibrosis.

Epidemiology

The onset occurs solely after puberty. Predisposing factors include obesity and acne vulgaris. Blacks and young women are affected most often.

Assessment

Clinical Presentation

A hallmark is the **double comedone,** a blackhead with two surface openings that communicate under the skin. A **painful follicular pustule** may develop; it in turn progresses into a sinus tract that ruptures and expels a **purulent, foul-smelling discharge.** Lesions are recurrent and may involve any apocrine gland–bearing area. The disorder is most common in the **axillae** (see Figure 1-9) but may also occur in the groin and perineum. (Axillary involvement is more frequent in women; perianal involvement is more frequent in men.) Eventually scar formation occurs. **Adenopathy** is usually a prominent finding.

Diagnostics

- Bacterial culture usually demonstrates gram-negative aerobic organisms, but almost any organism may be cultured.

Differential Diagnosis

- Furuncles and carbuncles (single or multiple cutaneous nodular cysts without sinus tracts) (see Figures 1-7 and 1-8)
- Folliculitis (lesions are usually associated with a hair follicle; no evidence of a "double comedone") (see Figure 1-6)

Treatment

Nonpharmacologic

Culture the drainage frequently to monitor changing antibiotic sensitivities. Minimize friction on the skin through weight control, wearing of loose-fitting clothing, gentle cleansing, and dusting with cornstarch powder. Incision and drainage of fistulas should be done only rarely, as they may predispose to sinus tract infection.

Surgical excision of the affected areas is curative.

Pharmacologic

Systemic Agents

Cephalexin (Keflex) 500 mg PO bid, **trimethoprim** and **sulfamethoxazole (Bactrim, Septra)** 1 to 2 tablets PO bid for 10 days are most useful.

Isotretinoin (Accutane) 0.5 mg/kg/day is prescribed for 20 weeks. Higher doses may cause inflammatory flares. It is helpful in preventing new lesions but does not treat existing sinus tract inflammation. Contraindicated in pregnancy.

Intralesional Agents

Triamcinolone (Kenalog) 10 mg/ml IL, 0.1 to 0.2 ml in a single dose, will help to control inflammation but should be administered when there is no infection.

Indications for Referral

- Surgical excision of the sinus tract may be desired.
- Any underlying infection should be treated before referral by a course of antibiotics and/or incision and drainage.

HIDRADENITIS SUPPURATIVA

- Is a bacterial infection caused by the occlusion, dilatation, and inflammation of sweat glands
- Can be reduced by wearing loose-fitting clothing and not shaving or otherwise irritating affected areas

Keratosis Pilaris

Overview

Pathophysiology
An autosomal dominant inherited condition in which a keratotic plug forms in each affected hair follicle.

Epidemiology
The condition is usually first apparent in early childhood (ages 2 to 3 years). It becomes more noticeable in adolescence and may persist until spontaneous regression occurs in adulthood. Those with atopic or severely dry (xerotic) skin are most often affected.

Assessment

Clinical Presentation
The most common sites of predilection are the posterior lateral upper arms, with the anterior thighs second. In severe cases the condition may become widespread, extending to the face, forearms, and legs. Discrete lesions are small, pointed follicular papules, which may or may not be erythematous. They usually appear gray as a result of the superimposed keratotic plug but may present as punctate erythematous papules (see Figure 1-12).

Diagnostics
- Diagnosis is made by clinical presentation and can be confirmed by skin biopsy if necessary.

Differential Diagnosis
- Acne vulgaris (comedones are present) (see Figure 1-1, A)
- Folliculitis (lesions are usually pustular) (see Figure 1-6)
- Molluscum contagiosum (flesh-colored, firm, domed, umbilicated papules) (see Figure 1-13)

Treatment

Nonpharmacologic
Lubrication with body lotions several times daily, especially after bathing, is essential. Avoidance of tight-fitting clothing and scratching of the affected areas may help prevent infection of the papules. Use of a buff-puff or loofah sponge in the bath or shower is helpful in removing the keratotic plugs.

KERATOSIS PILARIS

- Occurs when a keratinous plug forms in a hair follicle, but does not develop into an infection
- Is a chronic condition that cannot be cured
- Can be controlled through consistent exfoliation and lubrication

Pharmacologic

Topical Agents

Topical agents should be applied to damp skin to enhance penetration of the medication. **Lac-Hydrin 12%** lotion or cream (or other glycolic acid lotion) applied bid to qid is the most effective treatment. **Retinoic acid (Retin-A) 0.1%** cream applied bid may also be helpful. Group V steroid creams **(Aclovate 0.05%, Westcort 0.2%)** applied bid will minimize inflamed lesions.

Systemic Agents

None are indicated.

Indications for Referral

- Generally unnecessary because of the benign nature of the disorder.

Perioral Dermatitis

Overview

Pathophysiology

Perioral dermatitis is an eczematous condition affecting the lower half of the face, often with pinpoint pustules clustered around the mouth. The exact cause is largely unknown, but it may be precipitated by the prolonged use of fluorinated topical corticosteroids or irritation from contact with saliva (caused by poorly fitting dentures or orthodontic devices, as well as atrophic changes in the gums) or cosmetics. The disorder may also be related to a low-grade irritant or allergic contact dermatitis from tartar control toothpastes or cinnamon flavoring in toothpastes or chewing gum. It may also represent a variant of either seborrheic dermatitis or rosacea.

Epidemiology

Occurs most often in **females of childbearing age.**

Assessment

Clinical Presentation

Pruritic, sometimes burning, **discrete erythematous,** or flesh-colored **papules** and/or **pustules,** singly or in clusters located

around the mouth, bilaterally or symmetrically (see Figure 1-14). The vermilion border is spared. **Nasolabial folds** are often erythematous. The lateral aspect of the upper and lower eyelids, as well as the glabella, may rarely be involved. Lesions become confluent and scaly with time and may become superinfected with gram-negative bacteria. Patients may report intolerance to heat, wind, hot water, soaps, and cosmetics.

Diagnostics
- The diagnosis is usually made on the basis of clinical presentation.
- Bacterial, fungal, and/or viral cultures may be helpful in determining other causes of this clinical appearance.

Differential Diagnosis
- Acne vulgaris (lesions occur outside the perioral area) (see Figure 1-1)
- Rosacea (lesions occur with telangiectasias and diffuse erythema) (see Figure 1-17)
- Seborrheic dermatitis (greasy scales with distribution common in perinasal area, eyebrows and frontal scalp) (see Figure 1-18)

PERIORAL DERMATITIS
- Is not contagious
- May be worsened by constant contact of the skin with saliva, cosmetics, tartar control toothpastes or cinnamon-flavored toothpastes

Treatment

Nonpharmacologic
Wash gently with a mild soap **(Dove, Cetaphil, Basis)** and avoid known irritants.

Pharmacologic

Topical Agents
Metronidazole (MetroGel, Metrocreme, or **Noritate)** is used qhs or bid. **Sodium sulfacetamide (Sulfacet-R)** lotion applied qAM is also effective. Shake well before using. Patients may alter the basic shade of the lotion to match the skin color exactly. It contains both an antibacterial and a keratolytic agent. For those with very sensitive skin, sodium sulfacetamide in the form of **Klaron 10%** may be preferred. **Hydrocortisone 1%** cream may be used for symptomatic relief on a temporary basis but may be ineffective if used alone. Higher potency steroids may aggravate the condition.

Systemic Agents
Tetracycline 500 mg bid until clear, followed by slow tapering, is an effective and inexpensive treatment. **Minocycline (Minocin, Dynacin)** 50 to100 mg bid can be used if tetracycline is not tolerated.

> ## Indications for Referral
>
> - Unsatisfactory response to treatment as outlined.
> - Patch testing to determine or eliminate an allergic cause.

Pseudofolliculitis

Overview

Pathophysiology
A papulopustular eruption, pseudofolliculitis is caused by a hair's curving back and penetrating the skin outside the hair follicle. Shaving leaves cut hairs with a sharp tip at the surface. The penetration of the cut hair back into the skin initiates a foreign body reaction with resultant inflammation.

Epidemiology
The disorder can occur on any hair-bearing surface, but most commonly presents on the **anterior** and **posterior neck** of men with coarse, curly hair. There is a predilection for **black men.**

Assessment

Clinical Presentation
Pseudofolliculitis is characterized by erythematous papules or acneiform pustules that occur on **shaved areas** (see Figure 1-15). Involvement may be mild to severe with hundreds of papules and pustules. Secondary bacterial infection, usually caused by *Staphylococcus aureus*, with abscess formation may occur. Lesions may be asymptomatic or painful and pruritic. Patients may be more concerned with the cosmetic appearance than the physical discomfort.

Diagnostics
- Diagnosis is made by clinical examination. If the diagnosis is unclear, the result of a skin biopsy will demonstrate a foreign body reaction to the ingrown hair.

Differential Diagnosis
- Folliculitis (close examination does not reveal ingrown hairs) (see Figure 1-6)
- Acne vulgaris (presents with various stages of papules, pustules, and comedones and does not have a follicular orientation) (see Figure 1-1, *B*)

PSEUDOFOLLICULITIS

- Is caused by cut hairs curling around and growing back into the skin, causing inflammation
- Can be reduced by using an electric razor or *single-edged blade* with shaving *gel*
- Can be prevented by growing a beard

Treatment

Nonpharmacologic

Shave only every few days and avoid close shaving. Electric razors are preferable to straight edge blades. Do not resume shaving until inflammation is gone. Growing a beard is preventative. (In 3 to 5 weeks the external loop of hair reaches about 1 cm in length, at which time the hair's spring action causes the embedded tip to dislodge itself.)

Shaving should be done on well-hydrated hair and skin, using shaving gel instead of cream and a single-edged razor. A double-blade system will cut the hair below the skin surface, increasing the chance for internal growth.

Warm compresses with saline solution, tap water, or Burow's solution will remove crust, soothe the lesions, and soften the epidermis to allow easier release of ingrown hairs.

Hair loops should be released with a sterile needle but not plucked.

Depilatory creams may be helpful in treatment but can be irritating to the skin.

Pharmacologic

Topical Agents

Hydrocortisone 1% cream is applied bid to decrease inflammation.

Erythromycin solution (Em-gel, T-Stat, A/T/S) applied bid may help to prevent a secondary bacterial infection.

Retinoic acid (Retin-A) 0.05% cream applied qhs may be helpful in preventing ingrown hairs.

Systemic Agents

Erythromycin or **dicloxacillin** 250 mg PO q6h for 10 days should be reserved for treatment of a secondary bacterial infection.

Indications for Referral

- Unsatisfactory response to treatment as described previously may indicate referral to a physician trained in laser therapy. Treatment with various lasers of high-intensity pulsed light sources (Epilyte, ESC Medical Inc., Needham, MA) will eliminate hair with near-permanent results.
- Electrolysis, although less effective and more tedious than laser hair removal, can also be performed. Refer to an electrologist.

For Pseudofolliculitis Patient Teaching information and materials, turn to p. 459.

Rosacea

Overview

Pathophysiology
The exact mechanism of causation is unknown but is probably a re-action pattern to many different stimuli in predisposed individuals. Precipitating factors may include **hot food and drinks, alcoholic beverages, sunlight** (which will always aggravate the clinical appearance to some degree), emotional **stress,** and **vasodilating drugs.** There is no correlation between skin sebum secretion rate and severity of disease. The mechanism responsible for thickening of the skin is not known.

Epidemiology
Onset most often occurs between **ages 30 and 50. Women** are three times as likely as men to have rosacea. It is more common in **light-skinned, fair-complexioned** individuals. In 30% of patients there is a familial tendency.

Assessment

Clinical Presentation
May be divided into four stages:

Stage I: Flushing
Stage II: Persistent erythema and telangiectasias
Stage III: Papules and pustules
Stage IV: Rhinophyma

Rosacea begins with **recurrent erythema of the central face,** progressing to a persistent flush with **telangiectasias.** Patients report that they **flush easily** in response to both emotional stimuli and hot foods and alcohol. The skin tends to become thickened and coarse. Erythema blanches with diascopy (pressure on the skin with a glass slide). Transient facial edema may also be present after intense flushing reactions. Acneiform papules, pustules, and cysts may occur (see Figure 1-17), especially with long-standing disease. A hallmark of diagnosis, however, is that **comedones** and **scarring are absent. Rhinophyma** usually presents in men as hypertrophic soft masses on the nose tip, forehead, and chin.

Diagnostics

- Diagnosis is made on the basis of clinical presentation. No laboratory studies are indicated.

Differential Diagnosis

- Acne vulgaris (comedones are present) (see Figure 1-1, *A*)
- Perioral dermatitis (distribution is not on cheeks) (see Figure 1-14)
- Seborrheic dermatitis (characterized by greasy scales) (see Figure 1-18)
- Lupus erythematosus (skin is atrophic and photosensitive; telangiectasias are prominent)
- Steroid acne (lesions are of uniform size and symmetric distribution; comedones occur on normal skin; there is a history of steroid use)

ROSACEA

- Is a chronic condition, but is controllable with medication (taken indefinitely)
- Can be reduced by avoiding precipitating factors such as hot foods and drinks, alcohol, sunlight, stress, and vasodilating drugs

Treatment

Nonpharmacologic

Avoid hot, spicy foods and drinks; caffeinated beverages; and sun exposure.

Pharmacologic

Topical Agents

Metronidazole (MetroGel 0.75%, Metrocreme 1.0%, or **Noritate 1% cream)** may be applied bid. May require 4 to 8 weeks for optimal response. When it is used in conjunction with oral antibiotics, the resolution of lesions may occur more rapidly.

Hydrocortisone 1% cream may be helpful for reducing erythema when used bid. More potent corticosteroids should be avoided as they may exacerbate the disease.

Sodium sulfacetamide (Sulfacet-R) lotion applied bid helps to decrease inflammation in addition to decreasing acneiform lesions.

Sunscreens should be used consistently.

Systemic Agents

Although improvement in the control of rosacea may be noted within 2 to 3 weeks of the initiation of antibiotic therapy, 6 to 8 weeks is required to evaluate the antibiotic's effectiveness accurately. Dosage schedules should therefore not be adjusted any more frequently than at 6- to 8-week intervals.

Tetracycline 250 to 500 mg PO bid to tid is prescribed until a response occurs; then the dose is tapered slowly by 250 to 500 mg per day to the lowest level that will maintain control. Chronic antibiotic therapy may be indicated or used as needed for disease control.

Erythromycin 250 to 500 mg PO bid or **minocycline** 50 to 100 mg PO bid should be tried if tetracycline is ineffective.

Isotretinoin (Accutane) 1 to 2 mg/kg/day may induce long-term remission when used for 3 to 6 months. Precautions and contraindications are as described in the section on acne vulgaris. Low-dose therapy of 10 mg qod may suppress the extent of disease when used over a long period (years) and may also be helpful in the treatment of rhinophyma.

Nonsteroidal antiinflammatory agents may be helpful.

Indications for Referral

- Pronounced telangiectatic vessels and rhinophyma with fibrosis may be significantly reduced or eliminated through laser surgery, which has also been found to decrease the need for oral or topical antibiotics. Referral to a laser surgeon is appropriate.

Chapter 2

Blistering (Vesiculobullous) Lesions

Figure 2-1 **ACUTE NUMMULAR ECZEMA**

Multiple coinlike, hyperkeratotic erythematous lesions on the medial aspect of the thigh, with surrounding erythematous papules.

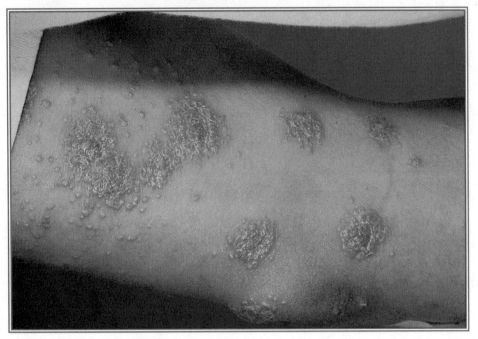

(Courtesy of Stacy R. Smith, MD.)

Figure 2-2 ALLERGIC CONTACT DERMATITIS

A, Well-demarcated, erythematous macule caused by contact with the undersurface of a nickel-plated watch. **B,** Rhus variety: Linear vesicular lesions on the thigh and knees are characteristic of poison ivy exposure.

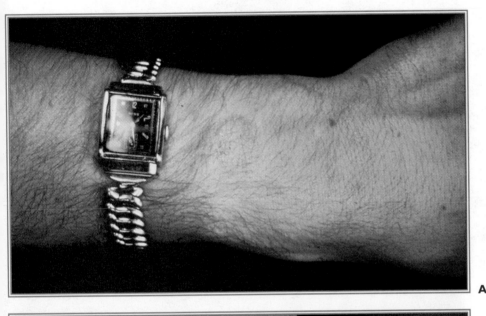

A

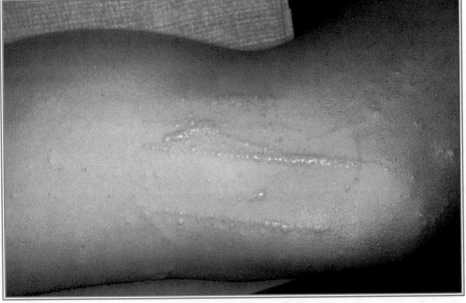

B

Figure 2-3   APHTHOUS STOMATITIS

Multiple small round, shallow ulcerations of grayish white appearance with surrounding erythema.

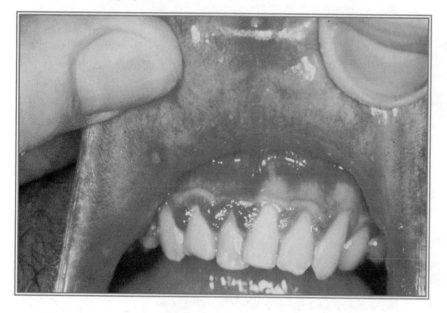

Figure 2-4   ACUTE CANDIDA INTERTRIGO

Note peripheral fringe of scale and satellite lesions.

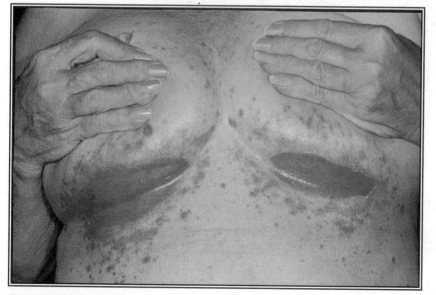

(From Habif TP: *Clinical dermatology,* ed 3, St Louis, 1996, Mosby.)

Figure 2-5 CHICKENPOX

Small vesicles on an erythematous macular base, in a generalized distribution on the back. Lesions vary in size from (early) papular lesions to (later) macular lesions.

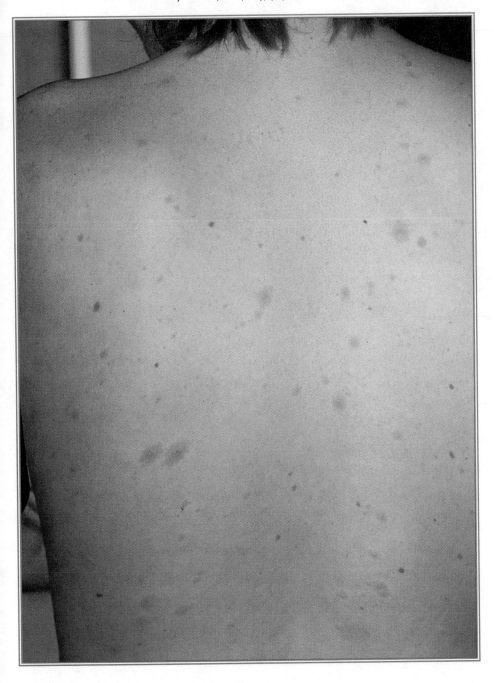

Figure 2-6   ERYTHEMA MULTIFORME

Erythematous, macular, targetlike lesions on the palms.

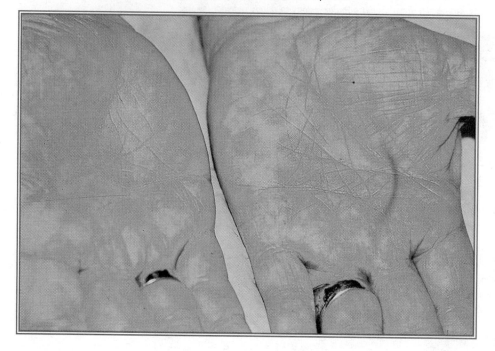

Figure 2-7 GERMAN MEASLES (RUBELLA)

Faint pink maculopapules, paler than the lesions characteristic of measles.

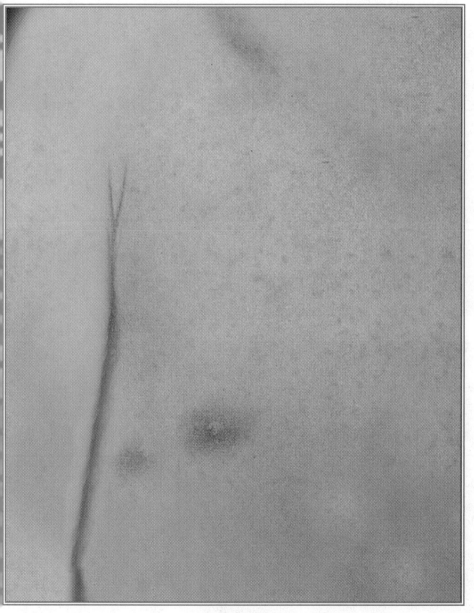

(From Habif TP: *Clinical dermatology*, ed 3, St Louis, 1996, Mosby.)

Figure 2-8 HERPES SIMPLEX

A, Oral: Slightly crusted vesicular lesion on the upper lip. *B,* Genital: A small group of vesicles on an erythematous base.

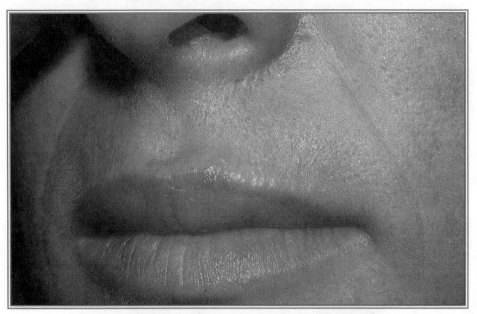

A

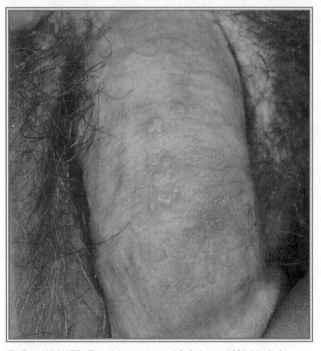

B

(**B,** From Habif TP: *Clinical dermatology,* ed 3, St Louis, 1996, Mosby.)

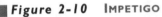**Figure 2-9**   HERPES ZOSTER

Vesicular lesion on an erythematous base in a dermatomal pattern, extending from the right midback across the anterior and lateral aspects of the nipple line.

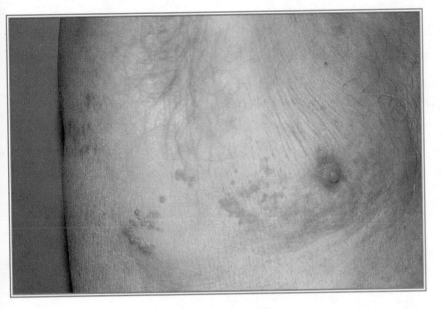

Figure 2-10   IMPETIGO

Erythematous lesions with honey-colored crust on the posterior thigh and buttocks region.

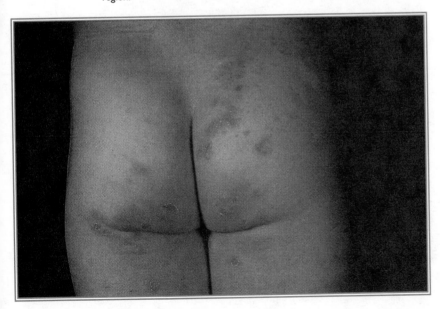

Figure 2-11   **INSECT BITES**

A, *Papular flea-bite reaction at typical site above the top of the sock. Note grouping of lesions.* **B,** *Insect bites with characteristic purpuric spots in center of papule. A central punctum is typical.*

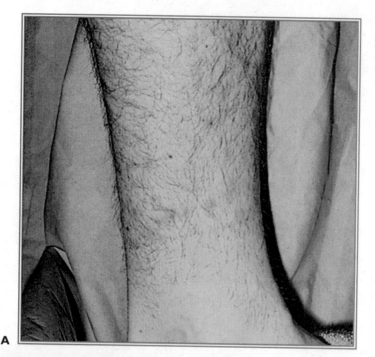

A

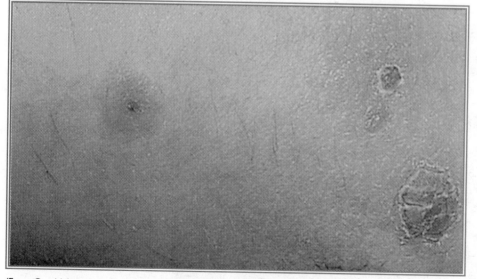

B

(From Cox N, Lawrence C: *Diagnostic problems in dermatology,* St Louis, 1997, Mosby.)

Figure 2-12 SYPHILIC CHANCRE

Well-dermarcated primary chancre with clean base.

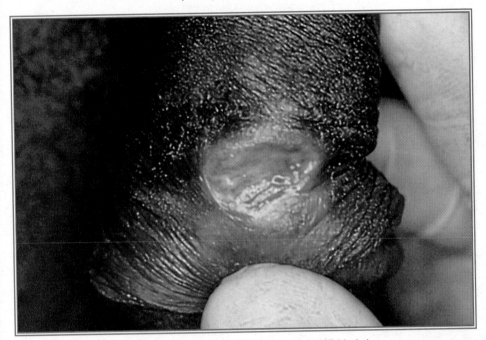

(From Goldstein BG, Goldstein AO: *Practical dermatology,* ed 2, St Louis, 1997, Mosby.)

Figure 2-13

A, Urticaria: Typical urticarial lesions, showing edematous macules over slightly erythematous skin. **B,** Dermatographism: Erythematous urticarial lesions that appeared within 1 to 2 minutes after drawing on the patient's back with a blunt object.

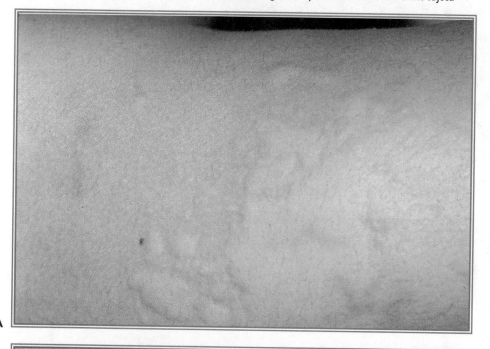

A

B

Table 2-1

Differential Diagnosis of Blistering (Vesiculobullous) Lesions

DISORDER	TEXT	KEYS TO DIAGNOSIS
Acute nummular eczema	Ch. 7, p. 332 (Figure 2-1)	Pruritic, coin-shaped plaques or papulovesicles on an erythematous base, which may become exudative and crusted.
Allergic Contact dermatitis	Ch. 7, p. 333 (Figure 2-2)	Intensely inflammatory, pruritic, papulovesicular eruption in distribution of contact with allergen.
Aphthous stomatitis	Ch. 11, p. 412 (Figure 2-3)	Ulcers in the movable oral mucosa; yellowish-gray base and erythematous margins.
Candidiasis	Ch. 1, p. 33 (Figure 2-4)	Satellite pustules; sharp, scaling border; erythematous, macerated patches; warm, moist environment; pruritus, soreness.
Chickenpox (varicella)	Ch. 2, p. 64 (Figure 2-5)	Maculopapular rash that begins on chest and back, then forms small superficial vesicles on an erythematous base ("dewdrop on a rose petal"). Intensely pruritic.
Erythema multiforme	Ch. 4, p. 185 (Figure 2-6)	Macules, papules, vesicles, and bullae all may be present ("multiform"). Hallmark is the iris or target lesion, usually on extensor surfaces, palms, and soles. Some may appear urticarial.
German measles (rubella)	Ch. 4, p. 187 (Figure 2-7)	Mild prodromal headache, malaise, low-grade fever. Rash begins on face or neck as dusky red, blotchy macules. Extends to trunk and extremities as maculopapular eruption.
Herpes simplex	Ch. 2, p. 66 (Figure 2-8)	Grouped vesicles with clear to cloudy fluid, on an erythematous and edematous base. May be preceded by a prodrome of burning and tingling before the eruption occurs.
Herpes zoster	Ch. 2, p. 70 (Figure 2-9)	Grouped vesicles on an erythematous, tender base along a sensory nerve (dermatome). Lesions usually unilateral and painful. Thoracic, trigeminal, and cervical distributions are most common.
Impetigo	Ch. 2, p. 73 (Figure 2-10)	Vesicles on an erythematous base that rupture to form honey-colored crusts, usually around mouth. Regional adenopathy and pruritus are common.
Insect bites	(Figure 2-11)	Erythematous papule with central punctum. Usually pruritic.
Syphilic chancre	Ch. 10, p. 395 (Figure 2-12)	Base of lesion is clean and smooth; edges are raised and well-circumscribed. Usually occurs in genital region or on lips.
Urticaria	Ch. 4, p. 198 (Figure 2-13)	Intense pruritus. Primary lesion is the wheal. Characteristics include: migration of lesions, angioedema, and dermatographism.

Chickenpox (Varicella)

Overview

Pathophysiology

Primary infection occurs through transmission of the varicella zoster virus (VZV) (herpes family) by droplet infection from the nasopharynx. Vesicular fluid is also contagious. During an incubation period of 14 to 16 days VZV multiplies in the respiratory tract and regional lymph nodes. It is released into the bloodstream and is disseminated throughout the body. The varicella virus is highly transmissible, with contagion rates of 70% to 90%. The virus may be transmitted from between 2 days before to 6 days after the eruption of the first skin lesions. Infection usually confers lifelong immunity. Persons who have not been immunized may contract a typical case of chickenpox if exposed to herpes zoster (shingles).

Epidemiology

Chickenpox may occur in an individual of any age who is not immune, although 50% of cases occur in children younger than age 5, and 85% occur in children 2 to 10 years old. Most cases occur during the months of February through June, with the highest incidence in March. With the development of the varicella vaccine, it is anticipated that the incidence will be greatly reduced.

Assessment

Clinical Presentation

After a 2-week incubation period mild **prodromal symptoms of fever, headache, and malaise** develop; they last 24 hours in children, longer and more intensely in adolescents and adults. The skin eruption appears as a **maculopapular rash that rapidly develops into small, superficial vesicles on an erythematous base ("dewdrop on a rose petal")** (see Figure 2-5). Vesicles at first are clear and become turbid and crusted by the fourth day. New lesions continue to appear in crops for the first 3 days. **Lesions first form on the chest and back** and may extend to the face, scalp, sclera, palate, oral cavity, and vagina. They are usually intensely **pruritic.** Minimal involvement occurs on the distal aspect of the extremities. Scarring is rare except when lesions occur on the forehead or upper face or in the case of a secondary bacterial infection.

Continued eruption after 5 days may indicate an underlying immunosuppressive disease. If varicella develops in a person taking steroids, the course may be severe, with possible dissemination to the central nervous system (CNS) and viscera.

The major complication is **bacterial skin infection;** the second is **varicella pneumonia,** which occurs in up to 50% of adults with chickenpox and develops within a week after the eruption appears.

Diagnostics
- Diagnosis is usually made by clinical impression and history.

Differential Diagnosis
- Disseminated herpes zoster (primary site is usually a linear eruption along a sensory nerve) (see Figure 2-9)
- Disseminated herpes simplex (most lesions occur as grouped vesicles; lesions are usually at the same stage of development) (see Figure 2-8)
- Enterovirus vesicular eruptions (noncrusted, smaller vesicles that occur chiefly during the summer; usually do not occur in crops; lesions are maculopapular, rarely vesicular)
- Insect bites (erythematous papules with central punctum; distribution of lesions may differentiate disorder) (see Figure 2-11)
- Urticaria (primary lesion is the wheal; lesions migrate; dermatographism is common (see Figure 2-13)

Treatment

Nonpharmacologic
Tepid baths and cool compresses help relieve pruritus. After the bath pat gently, rather than rubbing skin dry. Oatmeal baths are also soothing, since they leave a film on the skin.

Pharmacologic

Topical Agents
Zinc oxide or **calamine lotion** may provide temporary relief from pruritus and may be used as needed. **Bacitracin-polymixin (Poly-sporin)** or **mupirocin (Bactroban)** may be applied tid to qid to infected lesions.

Systemic Agents
Oral antihistamines such as **hydroxyzine (Atarax, Vistaril)** or **diphenhydramine (Benadryl)** are helpful in relieving pruritus. **Dosage** for children below age 6 is 25 mg bid; for children ages 6 to 12, 25 mg bid to tid. Dosage for adults is 25 to 50 mg tid to qid. Benadryl is safe for use during pregnancy. **Acetaminophen (Tylenol)** may be used for relief of malaise, fever, or headache, but **salicylates (Aspirin) should be strictly avoided** since they

---

CHICKENPOX

- Is extremely contagious for up to 6 days after the eruption of the first skin lesions
- Is spread by droplet infection
- Is related to the herpes simplex and herpes zoster viruses
- Lesions may become infected and/or leave permanent scars if they are scratched
- Symptoms of fever, malaise, and headache should NOT be relieved with aspirin or aspirin-containing products, as they increase the risk of Reye's syndrome

increase the risk of Reye's syndrome. **Acyclovir (Zovirax)** 800 mg PO qid for five days for adults and children over 40kg, **valacyclovir (Valtrex)** 500 mg PO tid, or **famciclovir (Famvir)** 500 mg PO bid will rapidly stop further development of lesions and produce a resolution of symptoms within hours. For children over 2 years of age or older, dose **acyclovir (Zovirax)** at 80 mg/kg/day in four divided doses, for five days. The safety of valacyclovir and famiclovir in children under 18 years has not been established.

Indications for Referral

- Chickenpox in high-risk patients (neonates, immunocompromised, hematologic malignancies).
- Development of Reye's syndrome.
- Development of viral pneumonia (common in adults).
- Varicella during pregnancy (congenital varicella syndrome).
- Development of hepatitis (common complication in immunosuppressed patients).

Herpes Simplex (Cold Sore, Fever Blister)

Overview

Pathophysiology

Seven types of herpes virus are known to infect humans and can be differentiated into two antigenic types: herpes simplex virus I (HSV-I), which is nongenital, and herpes simplex virus II (HSV-II), which is mostly genital (venereally transmitted). Because multiple strains of HSV-I and HSV-II exist, reinfection can occur with a different strain, but the new primary infection will be much more benign. The herpes virus survives up to $3\frac{1}{2}$ days on moist gauze, up to 3 days on toilet seats, and up to 12 hours on spa benches. It is not able to survive in super-chlorinated water. The disease begins after an incubation period of 2 to 12 days.

The virus is transmitted from person to person by close contact during the vesicular stage, by penetration of the viral particles through mucus membranes or traumatized epithelia. Viral replication occurs to permit infection of either sensory or autonomic nerve endings.

Persons with recurrent HSV may shed virus when no lesions or symptoms are present. This asymptomatic shedding is undoubtedly responsible for much of viral transmission. It is essential for patients to realize that the disease is highly contagious with or without the presence of symptoms.

Recurrences can be initiated by stress, trauma, sunlight, fever, or menses, with the latent virus conducted to the epidermis via peripheral nerve fibers 2 to 4 days after viral replication occurs.

Epidemiology

Herpes simplex is one of the most common infections throughout the world. Thirty-five to fifty percent of adults in higher socioeconomic groups and up to 90% in poorer or more densely populated communities have antibodies to HSV-I by age 40. Twenty to forty-five percent of the population have recurrent disease at some time. Genital herpes has recently surpassed gonorrhea and syphilis as the most common venereal disease in the United States. Recent studies indicate HSV-I accounts for up to 50% of genital herpes, an occurrence attributed to an increase in oral sex. HSV-I results in a much lower incidence of recurrence than HSV-II.

The risk of development of HSV is less than 5% for infants delivered vaginally from mothers who have a history of recurrent HSV infection. Reports have shown that elective cesarean section does not always eliminate the risk of neonatal infection but should be performed if lesions are present in the birth canal 1 week before labor or if the cervical culture result is positive for HSV and the membranes have not been ruptured for over 4 hours. Fifty to seventy percent of neonatal HSV cases are associated with mothers who have no history of peripartum genital HSV. Forty-three percent of pregnant women infected with HSV manifest no clinical signs or symptoms.

Assessment

Clinical Presentation

In *primary herpes simplex infection,* the **small, multiple papules or vesicles** (see Figure 2-8, *A*) coalesce into large pustular or ulcerative lesions. A painful acute gingivostomatitis in which the gums become red and swollen may also occur. Cervical adenopathy, malaise, headache, sore throat, and a nonspecific febrile episode run a course of 1 to 2 weeks in 50% of patients.

In females a vulvovaginitis is invariably seen with widespread vesicles, erosions, and edema of the vulva, labia, and surrounding skin. There is exquisite tenderness. Pain on the average lasts at least 2 weeks, and lesions may continue to appear for a month.

In *recurrent herpes simplex infection* most patients experience five to eight episodes per year. The recurrent lesion consists of **grouped vesicles with clear to cloudy fluid, on an erythema-**

tous and edematous base, associated with a moderate degree of pruritus and a variable covering of crusted serous fluid. Regional, often tender, **adenopathy** is almost always present and may preceed the actual eruption. The eruption tends to occur at the same site periodically and heals in 5 to 15 days. Lips, cheeks, and genitalia are most frequently affected, but the lesions may occur anywhere by autoinoculation. Recurrent lesions are preceded several hours by **a burning or tingling** sensation **(prodrome).** Recurrent genital lesions appear to be symptomatic longer in women (6 to 8 days) than in men (3 to 4 days).

Herpetic whitlow indicates HSV infection of the finger. It appears abruptly with edema, erythema, and localized tenderness of the infected finger. Vesicular or pustular lesions are present. Fever, lymphadenitis, and epitrochlear, as well as axillary lymphadenopathy, are common. The frequency of recurrence is less than for oral or genital infections.

Over 50% of neonates infected by *neonatal herpes simplex* show cutaneous involvement. Incubation time until clinical symptoms appear is between 2 and 21 days, with an average of 6 days. The scalp is a common site for the development of initial herpetic vesicles, as are the buttocks when infants are delivered in the breech position. Skin lesions in the newborn may rapidly become bullous and denuded or pustular. Constitutional symptoms such as fever, hypothermia, poor feeding, irritability, lethargy, and vomiting appear soon after birth. Seventy percent of cases lead to disseminated or CNS infection, including refractory grand mal seizures associated with a bulging fontanelle, flaccidity, opisthotonos, and rapid progression to coma and death. Infection of the eye may begin as conjunctivitis and progress to keratitis. Neonatal herpes simplex is approximately 50% fatal, with the majority of survivors manifesting some neurologic sequelae.

Diagnostics
- Viral culture of the vesicular fluid.
- Tzanck test of scrapings from the base of an early vesicle demonstrates multinucleated giant cells.
- Increased levels of immunoglobulin M (IgM) and G (IgG) are found in the serum of patients with primary or recurrent lesions, respectively.

Differential Diagnosis

Primary Infection
- Aphthous stomatitis (occurs on buccal mucosa, appearing as yellowish-grayish erosions) (see Figure 2-3)

HERPES SIMPLEX

- Is easily transmitted by close personal contact
- May be contagious without the presence of symptoms, or while a person is taking suppressive therapy
- Is precipitated by stress, trauma, sunlight, fever, and menses
- Treatment should begin within the first few hours of prodrome to avoid skin eruption
- Does not readily infect infants delivered vaginally from mothers with a history of recurrent herpes simplex virus (HSV) infection, unless lesions are present in the birth canal 1 week before labor

- Mucosal erythema multiforme (large, denuded areas of mucosa)
- Pemphigus vulgaris (erosions are deeper and occur more commonly on the posterior pharynx)

Recurrent Infection
- Syphilic chancre (lesions are painless) (see Figure 2-12)
- Chancroid (large ulceration without multiple vesicles)
- Herpes zoster (dermatomal distribution) (see Figure 2-9)
- Acute nummular eczema (rarely painful, and with no evidence of vesicles) (see Figure 2-1)
- Impetigo (lack of grouped vesicles; not painful) (see Figure 2-10)

Congenital Infection
- Congenital syphilis (positive rapid plasma reagin [RPR], negative Tzanck test results)
- Bullous impetigo (lesions are singular)
- Neonatal enteroviral infections (lesions usually present in a generalized distribution)
- Rubella (lesions usually present in a generalized distribution) (see Figure 2-7)
- Candidiasis (white pustules on an erythematous base that bleeds with scraping) (see Figure 2-4)
- Cytomegalovirus infection (generalized lesions with a bluish appearance)
- Congenital varicella (clinical appearance is nearly identical to that of HSV; maternal history is key)
- Allergic contact dermatitis (lesions are more erythematous and eczematous) (see Figure 2-2)

Treatment

Prevention is the best treatment. Consistent use of sunscreen, condoms during sexual contact, and cesarean section for pregnant women with active vulvar lesions will help to reduce the incidence of infection. In recurrent herpes infections if oral antiviral medication is begun within the first few hours of the prodrome, the actual skin eruption may be aborted entirely.

Nonpharmacologic
Clinical surveillance and serial cultures, especially in the third trimester, are recommended for pregnant patients who have been identified as having HSV.

Pharmacologic

Topical Agents
Benadryl mouthwash or other topical anesthetics will help reduce discomfort. Topical acyclovir is virtually ineffective. **Penciclovir (Denavir)** cream bid has been demonstrated to minimize and shorten the course of recurrent HSV infections.

Systemic Agents
Famciclovir (Famvir) 250 mg PO qd to bid for 5 days accelerates healing time.

    Valacyclovir (Valtrex) 500 mg PO bid to tid for 7 days is also an effective treatment.

    A less expensive alternative, **acyclovir (Zovirax)** 200 mg PO five times daily for 10 days, has been the mainstay of treatment for years. It must be initiated at the first sign of lesions or prodrome and acts to stop new lesion formation. It decreases the duration of viral shedding and the viral titer but does not decrease symptoms in recurrent episodes. For patients with monthly recurrences prophylaxis with 400 mg PO bid may be warranted. Patients should be counseled that they may transmit infection even while on suppressive therapy.

Indications for Referral

- Neonatal herpes simplex
- Herpes infection of the eye
- Presence of herpes virus in the immunocompromised host

For Herpes Simplex (Fever Blisters, Cold Sores) Patient Teaching information and materials, turn to p. 453.

Herpes Zoster (Shingles)

Overview

Pathophysiology
Herpes zoster is the reactivation of latent varicella-zoster virus, usually of sensory neurons, in persons with a previous primary varicella (chickenpox) infection. Factors predisposing to zoster include an impaired immune system, therapeutic radiation, local trauma,

surgery, spinal cord tumors, emotional upsets, lymphoma, fatigue, and age. It generally occurs in the area of the body that was most densely covered with vesicles during chickenpox.

Epidemiology

Most cases occur in patients above age 50. Approximately 300,000 cases occur in the United States each year. One attack usually confers lifelong immunity. The spread of zoster by direct contact with a person having active lesions is rare.

Assessment

Clinical Presentation

Prodromal symptoms of pain, burning, itching, or a dull ache in the affected dermatome; systemic symptoms such as malaise, fever, and headache; and localized lymphadenopathy may occur 1 to 2 days before the development of vesicles. **Grouped vesicles** appear on an **erythematous, tender base** unilaterally along the distribution of a sensory nerve **(dermatome).** They regress and become crusted in 5 to 10 days. The **thoracic distribution** is most common, although the **trigeminal and cervical regions** are involved in 20% of cases. Some vesicles may be seen away from the affected dermatome, but if more than 25 vesicles are seen, disseminated herpes zoster should be considered.

The percentage of patients who subsequently experience **postherpetic neuralgia** (pain 4 weeks or more after the lesions resolve) increases dramatically with age. Whereas only 5% of patients are affected before age 40, 20% are affected between ages 40 and 50, and 60% of those above age 50 experience postherpetic neuralgia. The pain may be itching, burning, sharp and shooting, or a combination of all, and may be severe enough to warrant suicide precautions. Commonly there is exquisite pain to touch, even from wearing clothing.

Diagnostics

- Clinical presentation and history
- Tzanck test
- Viral culture from vesicular fluid
- Biopsy if necessary

Differential Diagnosis

- Herpes simplex (especially likely if the lesions are recurrent and in the same location) (see Figure 2-8)
- Dermatitis herpetiformis (lesions are symmetric, more generalized, and in a nondermatomal distribution)

HERPES ZOSTER

- Has a low contagion rate
- Is a viral disorder that affects persons who previously had chickenpox
- May result in postherpetic neuralgia, necessitating strong analgesics and emotional support

- Allergic contact dermatitis (lesions are not dermatomal in distribution; pruritus is the presenting symptom, rather than pain) (see Figure 2-2)

Treatment

Nonpharmacologic

Emotional support is essential, including referral to pain clinics and support groups as needed. Families and caregivers may experience role strain and benefit from emotional support as well.

Pharmacologic

Topical Agents

Soaks with **Burow's solution** four to five times daily will help dry and soothe wet or crusted lesions. Postherpetic neuralgia may be lessened with the liberal application of **capsaicin (Zostrix)** cream four to five times daily.

Systemic Agents

Relief of pruritus may be achieved through oral antihistamines such as **hydroxyzine (Atarax)** 25 to 50 mg PO tid.

 Indications for Referral

- Persistent hemorrhagic disseminated lesions, present for 3 to 4 weeks, should be evaluated for malignancy by a dermatologist.
- Lesions on the external ear, ear canal, or other areas of the neck and face, as well as neck, jaw, or ear pain, could indicate Ramsay Hunt syndrome (trigeminal nerve involvement with possibility of corneal infection) and should be referred to a dermatologist.
- Patients with disseminated herpes zoster should be referred to a dermatologist for evaluation of immunocompetency. High-risk groups include patients with Hodgkin's disease and acquired immunodeficiency syndrome (AIDS).
- Complications including encephalitis and pneumonitis should be referred to an appropriate specialist.
- Lesions on the tip or side of the nose, which could indicate involvement of the ophthalmic branch of the trigeminal nerve, should be referred to an ophthalmologist.

Pain may be lessened with narcotic analgesics such as **oxycodone with acetaminophen (Percocet)** 1 to 2 tablets q4-6h or **hydrocodone (Vicodin)** 1 tablet PO q4-6h.

Combining amitriptyline (Elavil) 25 mg PO tid and oral analgesics is worthy of trial in cases of recalcitrant pain.

Systemic steroids **(prednisone)** 1 mg/kg PO qd for 1 week, followed by tapering over 3 weeks in patients over 50 who present within the first week of an eruption may be helpful adjuncts in pain control and prevention of postherpetic neuralgia.

Oral antivirals such as **valacyclovir (Valtrex)** 500 mg PO tid for 10 days, **famciclovir (Famvir)** 500 mg PO tid for 7 days, or **acyclovir (Zovirax)** 800 mg five times daily may speed healing, reduce the number of new lesions, decrease pain, and lower the incidence of postherpetic neuralgia.

Impetigo

Overview

Pathophysiology

Impetigo is a bacterial skin infection produced by *Staphylococcus aureus* and/or group A beta-hemolytic *Streptococcus*, limited to the stratum corneum. When occurring together, the organisms promote the growth of each other, producing rapid spread. Biting and stinging insects, including mosquitoes and flies, may transmit the infection, which is highly contagious, especially in infants. Impetigo is commonly transferred from infected individuals through direct contact. The prognosis is more severe in adults than in children.

Bullous impetigo is caused by coagulase-positive *Staphylococcus* that causes a vesicle or bulla to form. *Nonbullous impetigo* is caused by group A beta-hemolytic *Streptococcus*, which results in a superficial pustular eruption. *Ecthyma* is a deeper infection of the dermis, usually caused by beta-hemolytic streptococci with staphylococci as secondary pathogens.

Epidemiology

True staphylococcal impetigo is relatively frequent throughout the world, with large outbreaks occurring often. True streptococcal impetigo is common in the tropics and less so in temperate climates. There is an increased incidence in lower socioeconomic groups; poor hygiene and existing skin disease may predispose to infection. Staphylococcal impetigo may be associated with immunodeficiency diseases. Both types occur predominantly in children of 5 to 7 years.

Assessment

Clinical Presentation

Pruritus is common in both staphylococcal (bullous) and strepto-coccal (nonbullous) impetigo. The lesions expand laterally with the formation of satellite lesions. Lesions are most frequently present on the face (especially around the mouth), legs, hands, genitalia, and scalp, but any site except the palms and soles may be involved (see Figure 2-10). In blacks the lesions may be followed by temporary hypopigmentation. Scarring or atrophy is rare.

Bullous impetigo presents initially as a thin-walled **vesicle** on an erythematous base that ruptures quickly. The dried serum forms a characteristic **superficial golden-brown or honey-colored crust.**

Nonbullous impetigo presents as 1 to 3 mm pustules on an erythematous base. The pustules, like the vesicles of staphylococcal impetigo, rupture quickly and form **superficial honey-colored crusts.** Untreated, it usually clears spontaneously in about 10 days. Regional **lymphadenopathy** is common.

Ecthyma presents as an **ulcerated,** rather than superficial, impetigo. It is often localized on the shins or dorsal feet. Bullae are **tender** and first seen on an erythematous base. Ecthyma is characterized by an adherent crust, beneath which ulceration occurs. Scarring is common.

Diagnostics

- A bacterial culture is helpful to assess antibiotic sensitivity.

Differential Diagnosis

- Acute nummular eczema (vesicles, if present, are smaller than the macular lesions and are sterile) (see Figure 2-1)
- Herpes simplex (grouped vesicles on an erythematous base) (see Figure 2-8)
- Candidiasis (positive KOH examination finding, white pustules on a friable base that bleeds readily) (see Figure 2-4)

Treatment

Nonpharmacologic

Removal of crusts by soaking in warm tap water three to four times a day for 10 to 15 minutes each time will hasten the healing process. Washing with gentle antibacterial soap **(Lever 2000, Dial, Hibiclens)** three to four times daily is also helpful. Prevention of contact with infected persons is essential in reducing the spread of impetigo, as is avoidance of sharing towels. Changing pillow cases daily will help prevent autoinoculation.

IMPETIGO

- Is a bacterial skin infection that is highly contagious and transmitted through direct contact
- Can be prevented by not sharing personal items and by avoiding contaminated persons
- Resolution can be enhanced by soaking and removing crusts as they form

Pharmacologic

Topical Agents
Betadine applied qid demonstrates definite effectiveness in preventing infection when applied to traumatized skin, but is not as effective in treating established infections. **Polysporin or mupirocin (Bactroban)** applied three to four times daily to maintain continuous coverage is also a helpful adjunct.

Systemic Agents
Systemic antibiotics help to decrease contagiousness. The mainstay of therapy is **dicloxacillin** 250 mg PO q6h for at least 14 days. **Duricef** 500 mg PO bid for 14 days or **erythromycin** 250 mg PO q6h for 14 days is an alternative, although many organisms may be resistant.

Indications for Referral

- Development of acute glomerulonephritis (if *Streptococcus* is the infectious agent).

Chapter 3

Papulosquamous Disorders

Figure 3-1 ACNE

A, Acne: Teenage male with both open and closed comedones. B, Acne: Teenage male with nodular cystic acne, inflammatory lesions, and open and closed comedones.

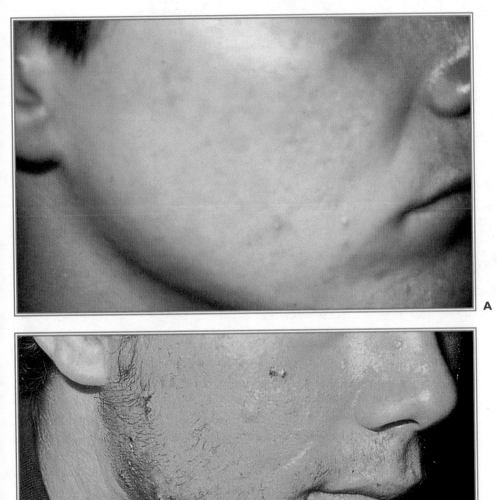

A

B

Figure 3-2   ACTINIC KERATOSIS

Slightly erythematous, rough, scaling papules and plaques on sun-damaged skin.

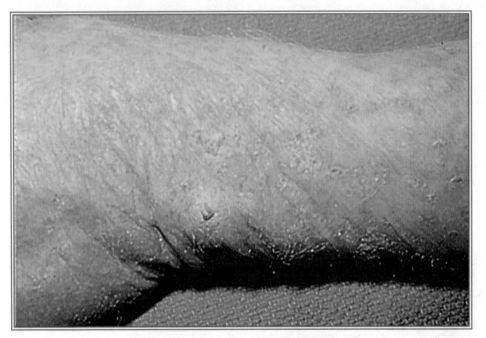

(From Goldstein BG, Goldstein AO: *Practical dermatology,* ed 2, St Louis, 1997, Mosby.)

Figure 3-3 ALLERGIC CONTACT DERMATITIS

A, Well-demarcated, erythematous macule caused by contact with the undersurface of a nickel-plated watch. *B,* Rhus variety: Linear vesicular lesions on the thigh and knees are characteristic of poison ivy exposure.

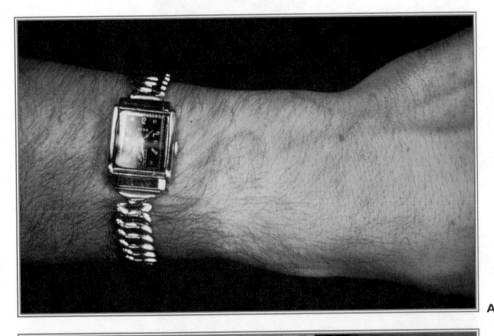

A

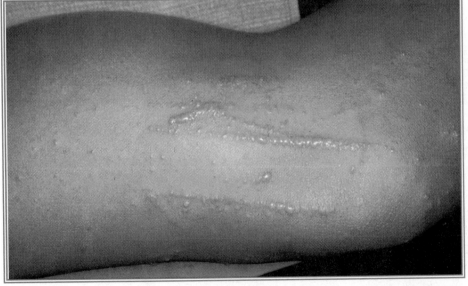

B

Figure 3-4   ATOPIC DERMATITIS

Blotchy, erythematous lesions on the face with accentuation in the central facial area.

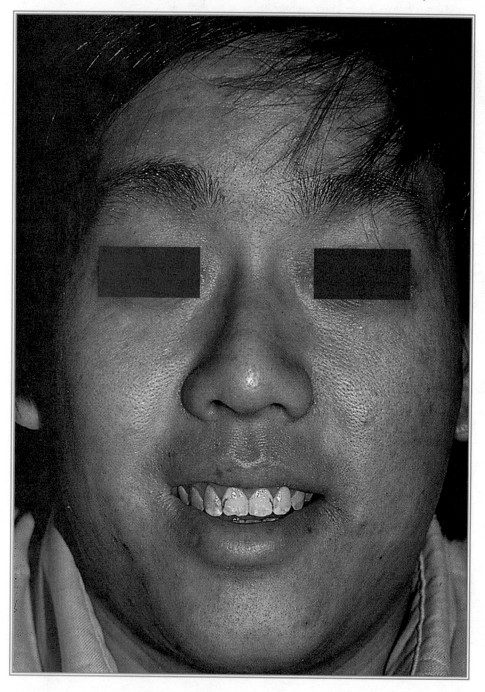

Figure 3-5 BASAL CELL CARCINOMA

Pearly papule with slight erythema.

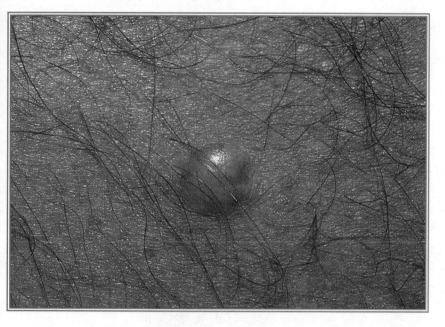

Figure 3-6 BOWEN'S DISEASE

Erythematous, keratotic, poorly marginated lesion on the arm of a 57-year-old male.

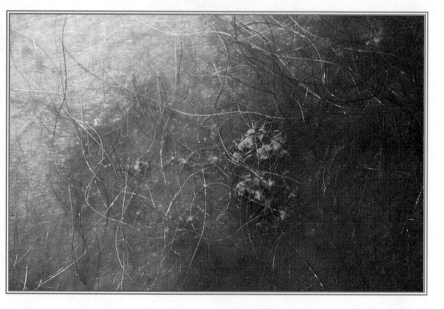

Figure 3-7   ACUTE CANDIDA INTERTRIGO

Note peripheral fringe of scale and satellite lesions.

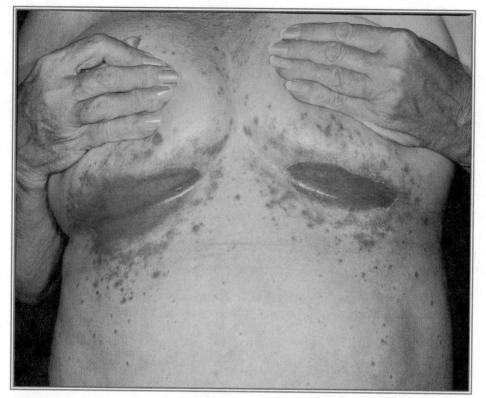

(From Habif TP: *Clinical dermatology,* ed 3, St Louis, 1996, Mosby.)

Figure 3-8   CHICKENPOX

Small vesicles on an erythematous macular base, in a generalized distribution on the back. Lesions vary in size from (early) papular lesions to (later) macular lesions.

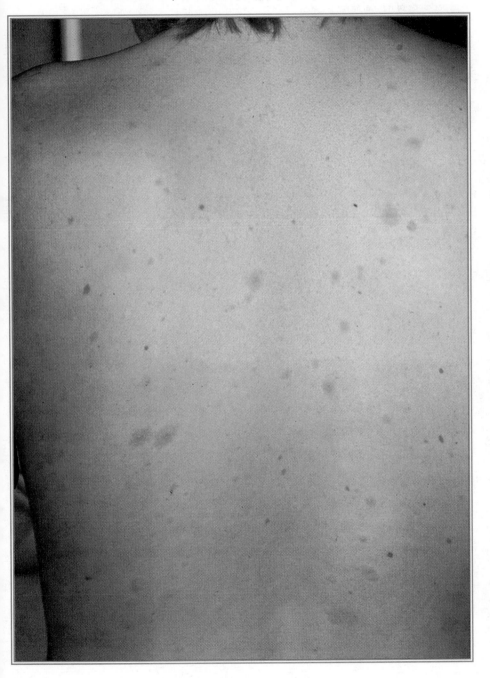

Figure 3-9

A, Tinea capitis: Thick scale and crust on the apical aspect of a child's head. **B,** Tinea corporis: Annular lesion with a sharply marginated, erythematous border. Note central clearing with appearance of normal skin.

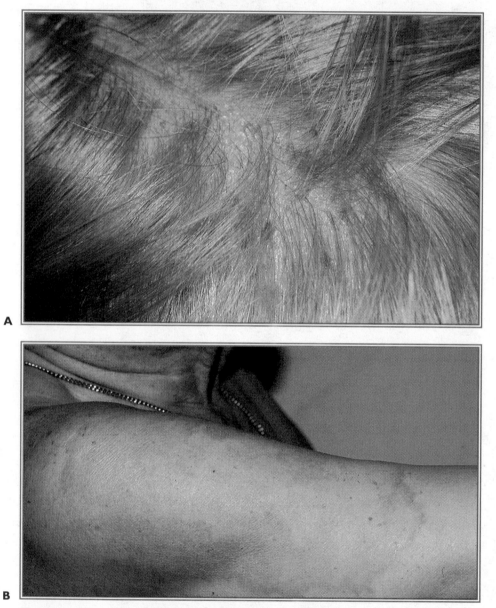

A

B

(**C through F,** From Habif TP: *Clinical dermatology*, ed 3, St Louis, 1996, Mosby)

Figure 3-9—cont'd

C, Tinea cruris: A half-moon-shaped erythematous plaque with a slightly scaling border. Note sparing of the scrotum. D, Tinea manus: Tinea of the palm. Note thickened, dry, scaly skin.

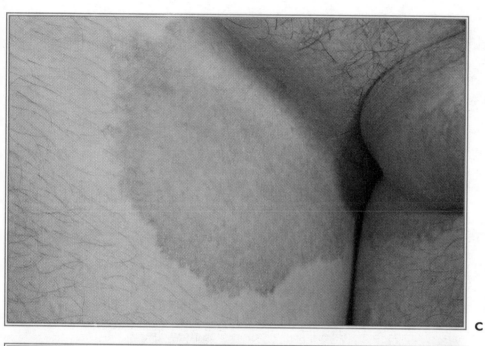

C

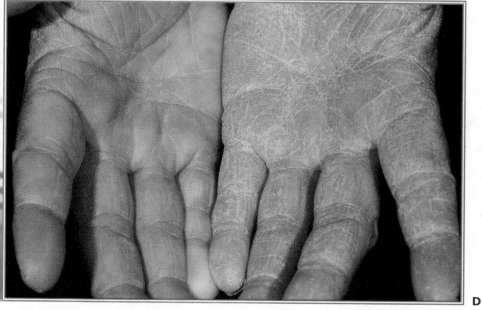

D

continued

Figure 3-9—cont'd

E, Tinea pedis: Inflammation of the soles and lateral edges of the foot give it a moccasin-like appearance. *F,* Tinea pedis: The infection has macerated the skin in the toe web. Inflammation extends to the dorsum of the foot.

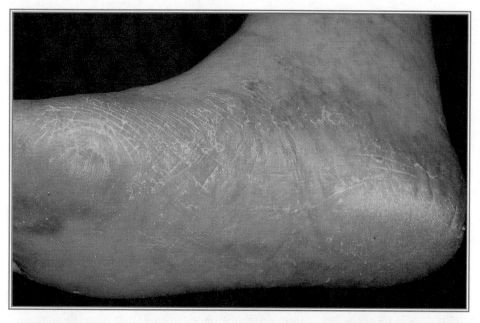

E

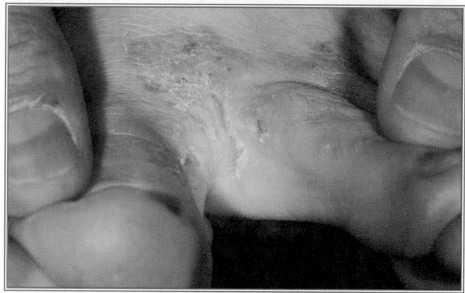

F

Figure 3-10 ERYTHEMA MULTIFORME

Erythematous, macular targetlike lesions on the palms.

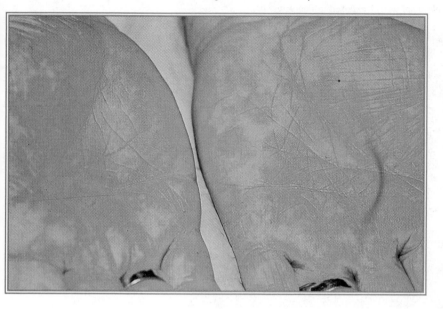

Figure 3-11 FOLLICULITIS

Extensive inflammatory closed comedones centered around hair follicles on the cheek of a male electrical worker exposed to fluorocarbons.

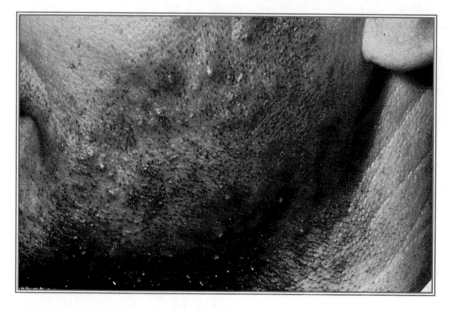

Figure 3-12 FURUNCLE

Pustular deep nodule on the posterior aspect of the right neck.

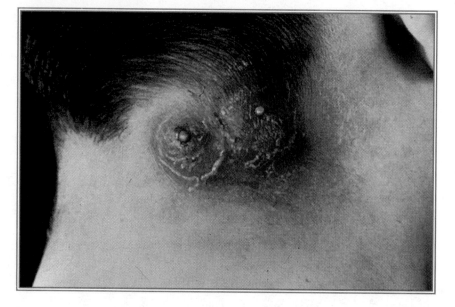

Figure 3-13 **CARBUNCLE**

Multiple pustular nodules on the posterior aspect of the neck. Many of the nodules have a confluent nature and exude pus.

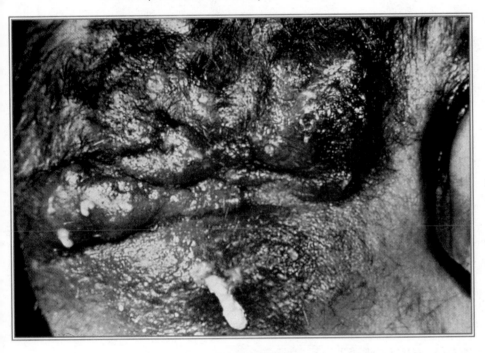

Figure 3-14   HERPES SIMPLEX

A, Herpes simplex–oral: Slightly crusted vesicular lesion on the upper lip. B, Herpes simplex–genital: A small group of vesicles on an erythematous base.

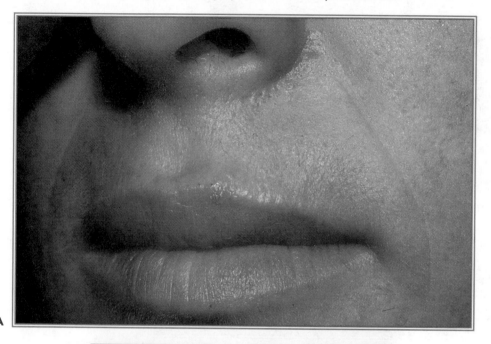

A

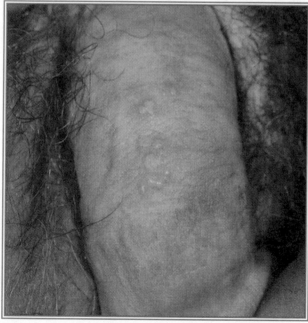

B

(**B,** From Habif TP: *Clinical dermatology,* ed 3, St Louis, 1996, Mosby.)

Figure 3-15 HERPES ZOSTER

Vesicular lesion on an erythematous base in a dermatomal pattern, extending from the right midback across the anterior and lateral aspects of the nipple line.

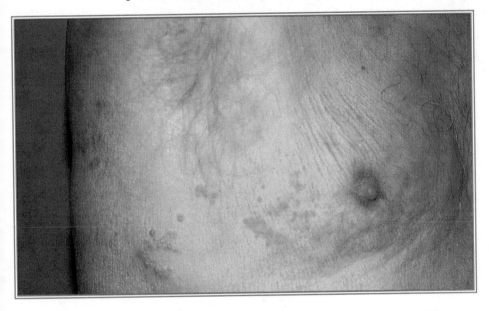

Figure 3-16 HIDRADENITIS SUPPURATIVA

Inflammatory dermatitis of the axilla with multiple sinus tracts, some of which are draining pustular fluid. Note presence of scarring.

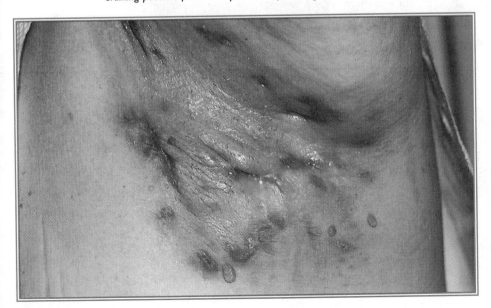

Figure 3-17 Icythyosis Vulgaris

Polygonal, scalelike lesions of brown hyperkeratotic skin of the lower extremities.

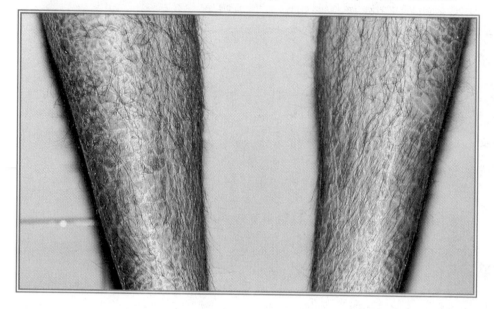

Figure 3-18 Impetigo

Erythematous lesions with honey-colored crust on the posterior thigh and buttocks region.

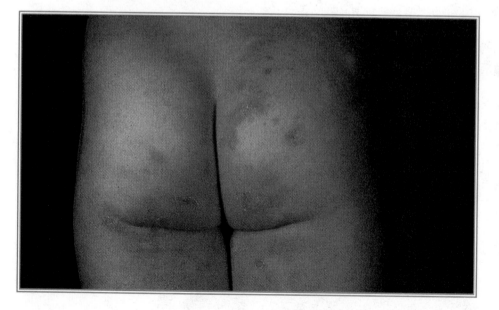

Figure 3-19 INSECT BITES

Insect bites are characteristic purpuric spots in center of papule. A central punctum is typical.

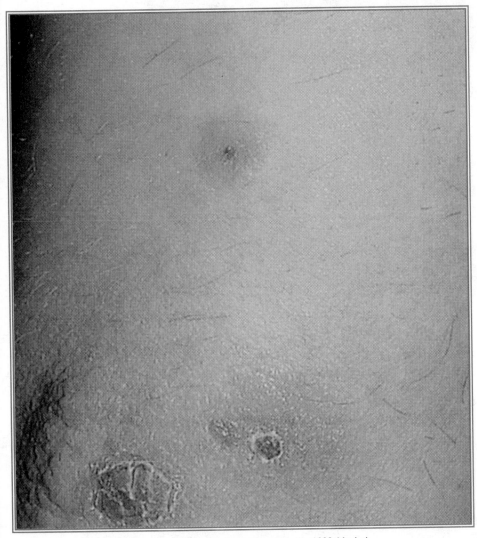

(From Cox N, Lawrence C: *Diagnostic problems in dermatology,* St Louis, 1998, Mosby.)

Figure 3-20   KERATOACANTHOMA

Rapidly enlarging nodule with a central crater-form crust.

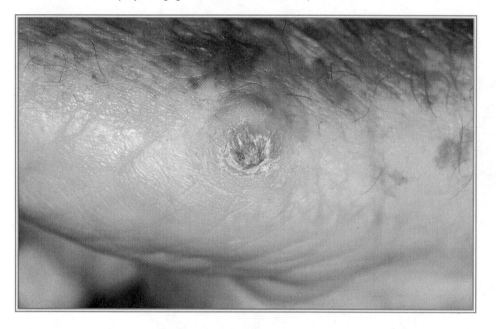

Figure 3-21   KERATOSIS PILARIS

Lateral aspect of the arm in a teenage girl, showing erythematous hyperkeratotic papules overlying hair follicles.

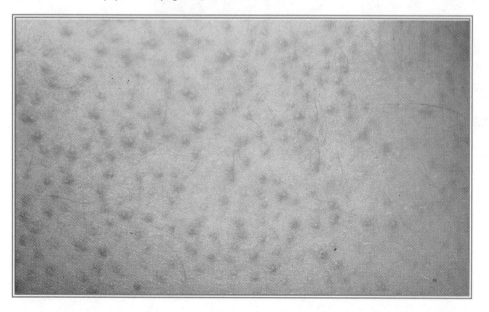

Figure 3-22 **LICHEN PLANUS**

Erythematous to violaceous, flat-topped polygonal papules on the dorsal and lateral aspects of the foot.

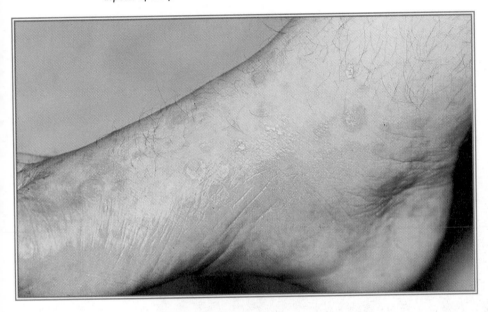

Figure 3-23 **LICHEN SIMPLEX CHRONICUS**

Thick, eczematous hyperkeratotic plaque with accentuated skin lines, created by rubbing with the opposite heel.

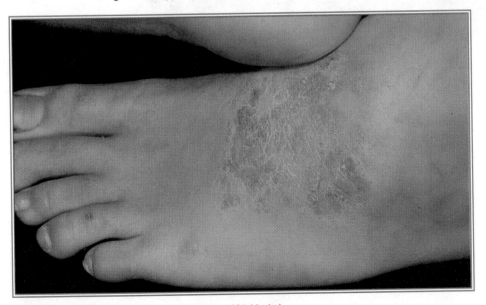

(From Habif TP: *Clinical dermatology*, ed 3, St Louis, 1996, Mosby.)

Figure 3-24   PERIORAL DERMATITIS

Inflammatory closed comedones and generalized inflammation in a perioral distribution.

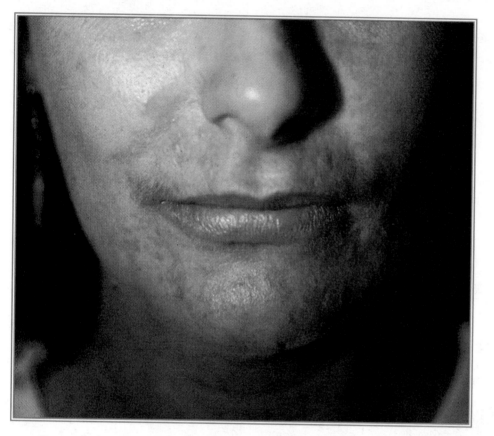

Figure 3-25 PHOTOALLERGIC REACTION

Erythematous to violaceous dermatitis on the dorsal aspect of the hand of a photographer who uses multiple chemicals to develop film.

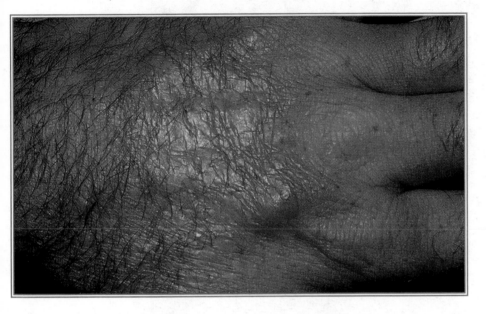

Figure 3-26 POLYMORPHOUS LIGHT ERUPTION

Diffuse, erythematous eruption, noted predominantly over sun-exposed areas.

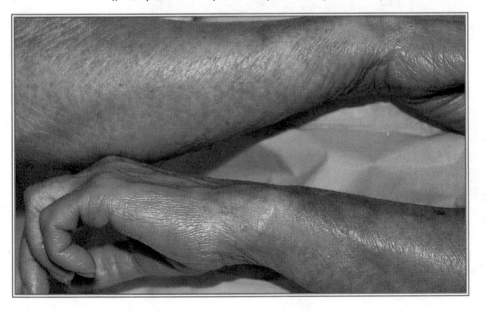

Figure 3-27   PITYRIASIS ALBA

Well-demarcated hypopigmented area on the lateral aspect of the cheek.

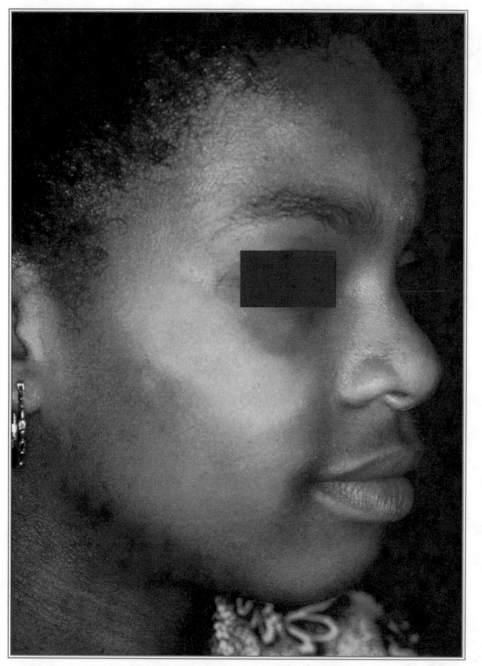

(Courtesy of Stacy R. Smith, MD.)

Figure 3-28 PITYRIASIS ROSEA

Both small erythematous papules and oval plaques with faint tissuelike scale (collarette scale) are present.

Figure 3-29 PITYROSPORUM FOLLICULITIS

Follicular papules and pustules mimicking acne.

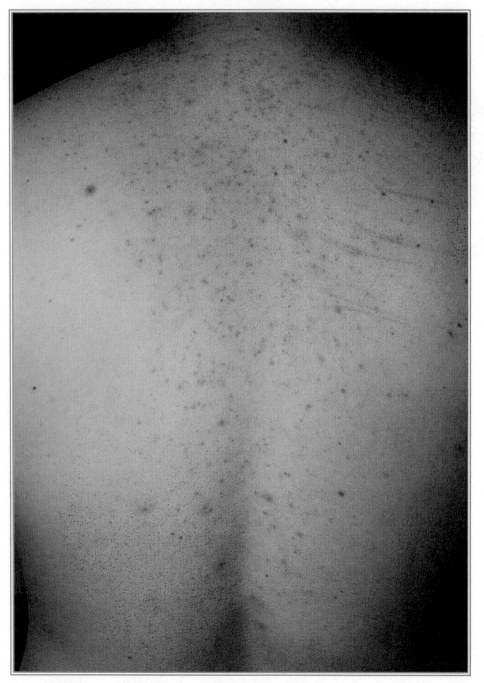

(From Habif TP: *Clinical dermatology*, ed 3, St Louis, 1996, Mosby.)

Figure 3-30 **PSEUDOFOLLICULITIS**

Inflammatory lesions with some pustules in the mandibular angle. Note curled hairs, some of which are embedding back into the skin.

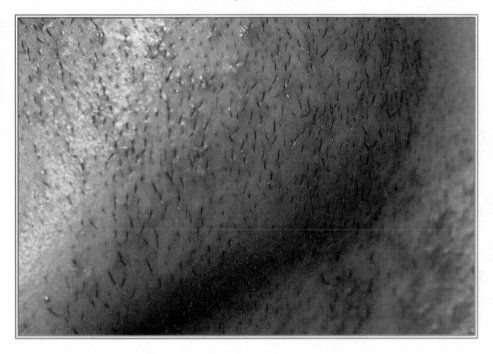

Figure 3-31 PSORIASIS

A, Psoriasis: Thick, lichenlike plaques with some erythematous excoriation on the foot. Note: hyperkeratotic nails. **B,** Guttate psoriasis: Generalized erythematous papular eruption on the trunk.

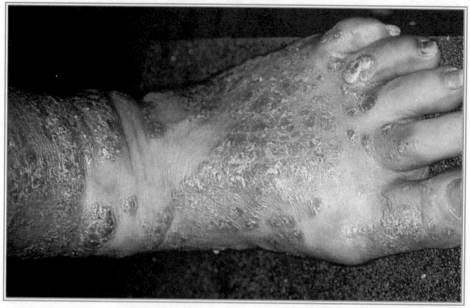

A

(**A,** Courtesy of Stacy R. Smith, MD.)

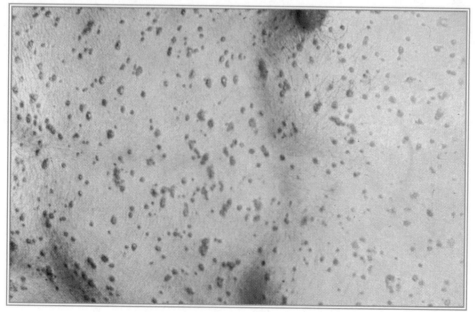

B

Figure 3-31 **Psoriasis**

C, Pustular psoriasis: An erythematous plaque with multiple pustules. *D,* Scalp psoriasis: Erythematous, plaquelike lesion on the anterior aspect of the scalp extending to the forehead, with overlying hyperkeratosis and lichenlike scales.

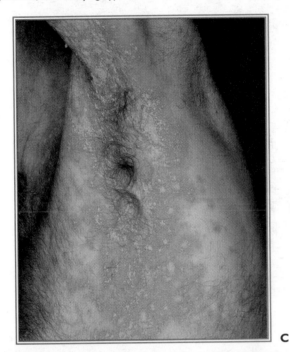

C

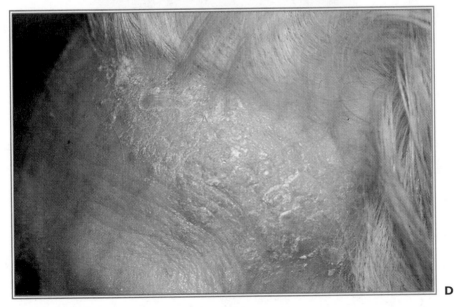

D

Figure 3-32   PYOGENIC GRANULOMA

Rapidly growing necrotic papule on the posterior aspect of the neck.

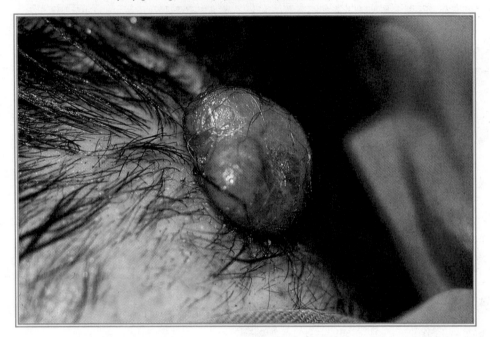

Figure 3-33   **ROSACEA**

Generalized inflammation with multiple closed comedones, predominantly located on the central aspect of the face and nose.

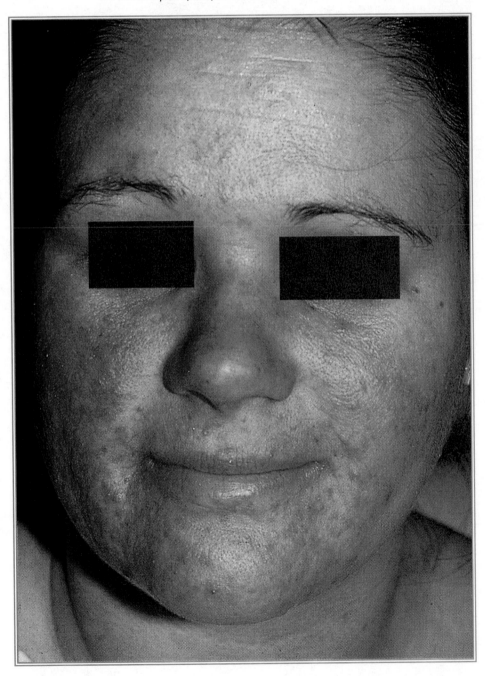

Figure 3-34   SCABIES

Black linear tract with surrounding erythema.

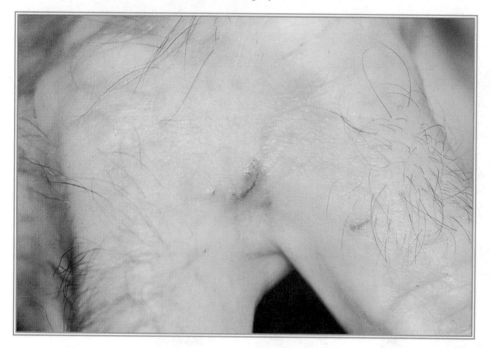

Figure 3-35 **SEBORRHEIC DERMATITIS**

Erythematous patches with some evidence of scale in the usual facial distribution.

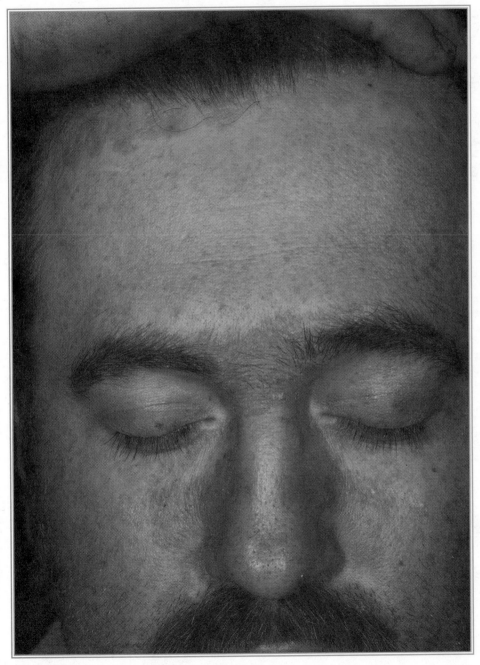

(From Habif TP: *Clinical dermatology,* ed 3, St Louis, 1996, Mosby.)

Figure 3-36 Seborrheic Keratosis

Extensive greasy, stuck-on hyperkeratotic lesions of the face.

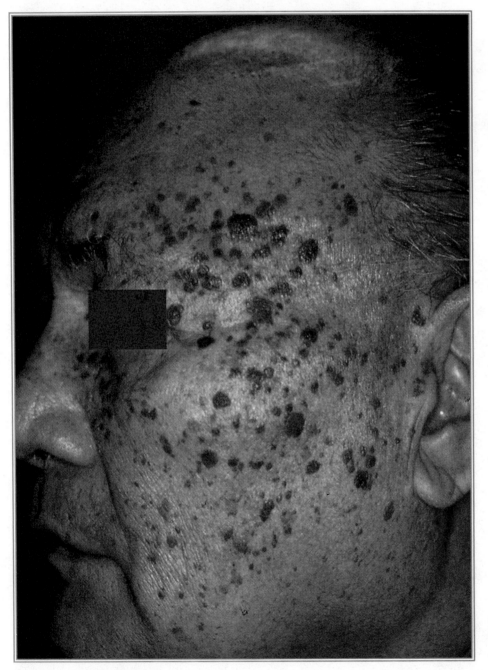

(Courtesy of Stacy R. Smith, MD.)

Figure 3-37 SQUAMOUS CELL CARCINOMA

Firm, elevated mass with central crust, occurring on sun-damaged skin of the lower lip.

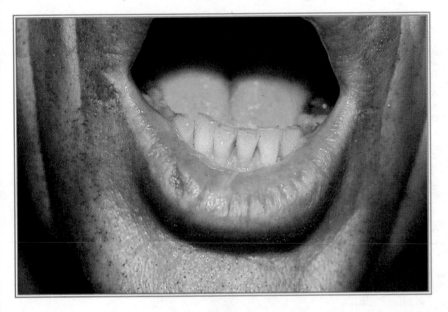

Figure 3-38 TINEA VERSICOLOR

Multiple oval tan to brown macules on the back.

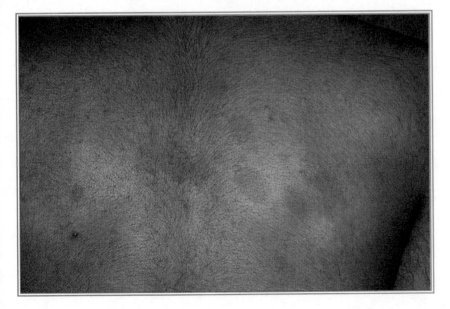

Figure 3-39   XEROSIS

Parchmentlike skin with overlying scales on a background of erythema.

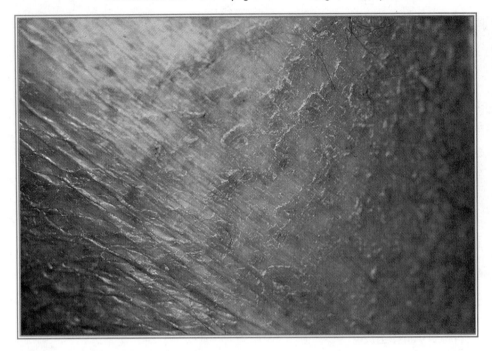

Figure 3-40 WARTS

A, *Common warts: Multiple hyperkeratotic growths with characteristic black dots.*
B, *Filiform warts: An extruding papular growth with fingerlike projections on the right cheek.*

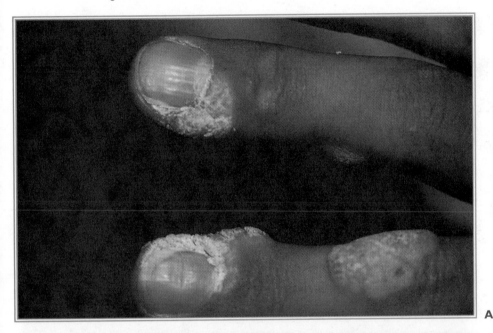

A

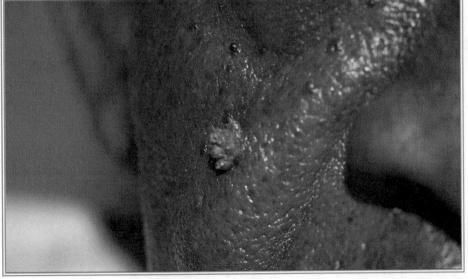

B

continued

Figure 3-40   WARTS

C, *Genital warts: Broad-based wart on the shaft of a penis. Note verrucous surface texture.* **D,** *Plantar warts: Firm, keratotic macule with multiple black dots on the plantar aspect of the great toe.*

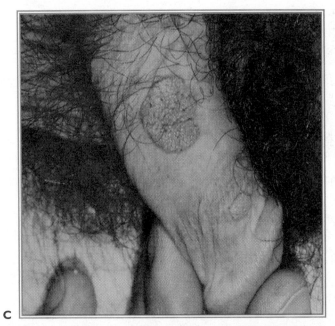

C

(**C,** From Habif TP: *Clinical dermatology,* ed 3, St Louis, 1996, Mosby.)

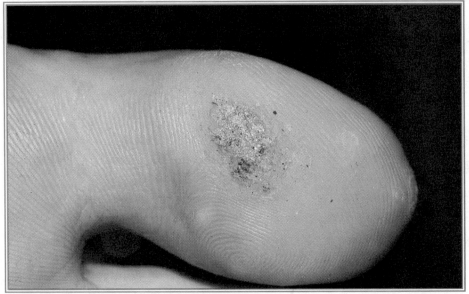

D

Table 3-1

Differential Diagnosis of Papulosquamous Disorders

DISORDER	TEXT	KEYS TO DIAGNOSIS
Acne vulgaris	Ch. 1, p. 29 (Figure 3-1)	Comedones, papules, pustules, cysts are present on face, neck, shoulders, chest, back; peak age 14 to 15 for females, age 16 to 17 for males.
Actinic keratosis	Ch. 5, p. 235 (Figure 3-2)	Skin-colored to slightly erythematous macules with dry, rough scale.
Allergic contact dermatitis	Ch. 7, p. 333 (Figure 3-3)	Intensely inflammatory, pruritic, papulovesicular eruption in distribution of contact with allergen.
Atopic dermatitis	Ch. 7, p. 336 (Figure 3-4)	Severe pruritus; dermatographism. Palmar markings and infra-orbital folds increase. Red cheeks in infancy; sides of neck and flexural surfaces most commonly affected after age 12.
Basal cell carcinoma	Ch. 5, p. 237 (Figure 3-5)	Pearly or waxy papule that may have a central depression or ulceration, often with fine telangiectasias.
Bowen's disease	Ch. 5, p. 240 (Figure 3-6)	Erythematous, flat to slightly raised, scaly plaque with erythematous and irregular surface.
Candidiasis	Ch. 1, p. 33 (Figure 3-7)	Erythematous, macerated patches with a sharp, scaling border. Satellite papules and pustules that are tender and pruritic are common.
Chickenpox (varicella)	Ch. 2, p. 64 (Figure 3-8)	Maculopapular rash that begins on chest and back, then forms small, superficial vesicles on an erythematous base ("dewdrop on a rose petal"); intensely pruritic.
Dermatophyte infections	Ch. 3, p. 116 (Figure 3-9)	Presentation depends on area of involvement: patchy loss of hair; erythematous ring-shaped patches with central clearing and advancing scaling border; fissured, macerated skin between toes. Pruritus is common.
Erythema multiforme	Ch. 4, p. 185 (Figure 3-10)	Macules, papules, vesicles, and bullae may be present ("multiform"). Hallmark is the iris or target lesion, usually on extensor surfaces, palms and soles. Some may appear urticarial.
Folliculitis	Ch. 1, p. 36 (Figure 3-11)	Follicular, erythematous papules and pustules on any hair-bearing surface; *Pseudomonas* folliculitis occurs 1 to 3 days after use of a hot tub.
Furuncles and carbuncles	Ch. 1, p. 38 (Figures 3-12 and 3-13)	*Furuncles:* 1 to 5 cm tender nodules with surrounding erythema. May become fluctuant. *Carbuncles:* 3 to 10 cm tender erythematous nodules that drain pus from multiple follicular orifices
Herpes simplex	Ch. 2, p. 66 (Figure 3-14)	Grouped vesicles with clear to cloudy fluid, on an erythematous and edematous base. May be preceded by a prodrome of burning and tingling before eruption.

continued

Table 3-1 *continued*

DISORDER	TEXT	KEYS TO DIAGNOSIS
Herpes zoster	Ch. 2, p. 70 (Figure 3-15)	Grouped vesicles on an erythematous, tender base along a sensory nerve (dermatome). Lesions usually unilateral and painful. Thoracic, trigeminal, and cervical distributions are most common.
Hidradenitis suppurativa	Ch. 1, p. 41 (Figure 3-16)	Double comedone, foul-smelling discharge; subcutaneous sinus tracts; adenopathy. Axillae, groin, perineum affected.
Icythyosis vulgaris	Ch. 3, p. 126 (Figure 3-17)	Dry, white, rectangular scales on an erythematous base, especially over extensor extremities. Accentuation of palmar and sole creases. Pruritus and rough skin are common.
Impetigo	Ch. 2, p. 73 (Figure 3-18)	Vesicles on an erythematous base that rupture to form honey-colored crusts, usually around mouth. Regional adenopathy and pruritus are common.
Insect bites	(Figure 3-19)	Erythematous papule with central punctum. Usually pruritic.
Keratoacanthoma	Ch. 5, p. 247 (Figure 3-20)	Red, dome-shaped nodule with central crater. Has raised, rolled borders; frequently covered with crust.
Keratosis pilaris	Ch. 1, p. 43 (Figure 3-21)	Small, discrete follicular papules on posterior upper arms and anterior thighs. May be erythematous.
Lichen planus	Ch. 3, p. 128 (Figure 3-22)	Pruritic, flat, irregular purple papules with fine white lines and scales. Commonly on flexor surfaces, nails, and scalp.
Lichen simplex chronicus (neurodermatitis)	Ch. 7, p. 343 (Figure 3-23)	Lichenified plaques on ankles, anterior tibial, and nuchal areas. Pruritus is severe, paroxysmal, and worse just before or during sleep.
Perioral dermatitis	Ch. 1, p. 44 (Figure 3-24)	Pruritic, burning, discrete erythematous or flesh-colored papules and pustules around mouth and in nasolabial folds.
Photoallergic reaction	Ch. 4, p. 190 (Figure 3-25)	Erythematous papular rash in sun-exposed areas; no sharp borders; pruritus. Occurs 24 hours or more after sun exposure.
Polymorphous light eruption	Ch. 4, p. 192 (Figure 3-26)	Pruritic, erythematous papules, widely scattered over sun-exposed areas. Occurs within a few hours of sun exposure.
Pityriasis alba	Ch. 6, p. 301 (Figure 3-27)	Round to oval patches with fine scale, occurring predominantly on face, upper arms, neck, and shoulders.
Pityriasis rosea	Ch. 3, p. 130 (Figure 3-28)	Single oval, well-demarcated salmon-colored patch with a fine collarette scale develops (herald patch); followed by other lesions on trunk and proximal extremities. Christmas tree distribution on non–sun-exposed areas.
Pityrosporum folliculitis	Ch. 3, p. 132 (Figure 3-29)	Follicular papules and pustules on upper back and chest, upper arms, and neck. May be slightly itchy. Frequently diagnosed as acne.
Pseudofolliculitis	Ch. 1, p. 46 (Figure 3-30)	Erythematous papules and pustules on shaved areas, especially beards of men with coarse, curly hair. May be asymptomatic or painful and pruritic.

Table 3-1 *continued*

Disorder	Text	Keys to Diagnosis
Psoriasis	Ch. 3, p. 134 (Figure 3-31)	Erythematous papules and plaques with silver-white scales. Symmetric distribution is common. Frequently on knees, elbows, scalp, back, genitalia, intergluteal folds, and nails.
Pyogenic granuloma	Ch. 12, p. 434 (Figure 3-32)	Solitary, rapidly growing dark red papule with moist or scaly surface, usually on fingers, face, shoulders, or feet; common in children, during pregnancy, or after trauma.
Rosacea	Ch. 1, p. 48 (Figure 3-33)	Facial papules and pustules but no comedones; flushing, telangiectasias, rhinophyma; triggered by hot foods, emotional stress.
Scabies	Ch. 7, p. 346 (Figure 3-34)	Crusted papules or burrows on genitals, wrists, finger webs, belt line. Intensely pruritic.
Seborrheic dermatitis	Ch. 3, p. 138 (Figure 3-35)	Sharply marginated yellowish-red patches with sharp borders and greasy scales. Scalp, central face, eyebrows, eyelids, nasolabial folds, and external ear are most commonly affected. May be pruritic.
Seborrheic keratosis	Ch. 5, p. 257 (Figure 3-36)	Warty, greasy, sharply marginated pigmented lesion. Appears "stuck-on."
Squamous cell carcinoma	Ch. 5, p. 260 (Figure 3-37)	Firm skin-colored or reddish-brown nodule on sun-damaged skin. Ulceration, scaling, and crusting are frequently present.
Tinea versicolor	Ch. 3, p. 141 (Figure 3-38)	Asymptomatic white-pink to brown macules with fine scale on back, chest, and upper arms.
Xerosis (dry skin)	Ch. 7, p. 349 (Figure 3-39)	Dry, slightly scaly skin with variable erythema and superficial fissuring. Pruritus is common. Most prominent on extremities.
Verrucae	Ch. 5, p. 262 (Figure 3-40)	Skin-colored lesions with rough surface. Normal skin lines are obscured. Multiple black dots may be visible within lesion.

Dermatophyte Infections

Tinea Capitis (Ringworm of the Scalp)

Overview

Pathophysiology

Trichophyton tonsurans is most often the causative agent in the United States. The disorder is contagious and is transmitted by personal contact. Organisms have been cultured from barbers' instruments, hairbrushes, theater seats, and hats. Occasionally infection is transmitted from animals, including pets. Once the organism becomes established on the scalp (frequently as a result of a break in the skin), the hair acts as a trapping device, allowing infection to develop and spread. Signs and symptoms are first noticeable at about 3 weeks.

Epidemiology

Children are most frequently affected, with a dramatic decrease in incidence at puberty. Infants, however, are rarely affected. Blacks seem to be more susceptible, and boys are affected five times more often than girls.

Assessment

Clinical Presentation

Tinea capitis is asymptomatic and presents with a patchy loss of hair. Numerous broken hairs, inflammation, and scaling also occur (see Figure 3-9, *A*). The presentation may vary, depending on the causative organism.

Black dot ringworm (caused by *T. tonsurans* and *T. violaceum*) presents as irregular patches of partial alopecia with broken hairs at the scalp surface, giving it the characteristic appearance of black dots. Patches are usually multiple and diffuse, with an irregular border and minimal scaling. The amount of inflammation varies. A low-grade folliculitis is commonly present. Recurrences are frequent.

Gray-patch ringworm presents with scaling. The areas of alopecia are well marginated, are often circular, and show numerous broken-off hairs. The name derives from the dull gray color resulting from a coating of the hair shafts by spores. Inflammation is minimal.

Inflammatory tinea capitis, caused by *Microsporum canis*, may present with mild to intense erythema. A kerion (a red, swollen, soft, and often purulent mass) may occur in the most severe cases.

Diagnostics
- KOH of the infected hairs will reveal spores either inside the hairs (endothrix) or outside (ectothrix), depending on the causative organism.
- Gray-patch tinea capitis fluoresces green under a Wood's light examination
- Black-dot type is nonfluorescent.

Differential Diagnosis
- Alopecia areata (sudden onset of bald patches of scalp a few cm in diameter; usually without symptoms) (see Figure 8-1)
- Traumatic alopecia (broken-off hairs with remaining hairs at various lengths)
- Lupus erythematosus (bald areas with a slight pink appearance without evidence of hair follicles)
- Seborrheic dermatitis (usually associated with facial lesions; most common in the hairline, not as a circle of hair loss) (see Figure 3-35)
- Impetigo (lesions have honey-colored crusts) (see Figure 3-18)
- Psoriasis (symmetric, erythematous lesions with gray-white scale) (see Figure 3-31, *D*)

TINEA CAPITIS

- Can be transmitted by personal contact through the sharing of hairbrushes, hats, or other personal items
- All household members should be treated simultaneously

Treatment

Nonpharmacologic
The scalp must be shampooed daily for 3 to 4 weeks, preferably with a 2% selenium sulfide shampoo **(Selsun Blue),** to wash off debris and damaged hair. A scalp oil or ointment may be applied to prevent further spread and contagiousness. Family members should be similarly treated for prophylaxis.

Pharmacologic

Topical Agents
Topical therapy with various antifungal agents is of questionable efficacy.

Systemic Agents
Terbinafine (Lamisil) 250 mg PO qd (adults) or 10 mg/kg/day (children) is prescribed for 4 weeks.

    Itraconazole (Sporanox) 100 mg PO bid (adults) or 5 mg/kg/day (children) is a safe alternative.

    Griseofulvin ultramicrosize (Gris-PEG) 250 mg PO bid for 1 to 2 months (adults) or 7 to 10 mg/kg/day for 4 to 12 weeks (children) is the treatment of choice against inflammatory tinea capitis. Ingesting it with a high-fat meal will enhance absorption.

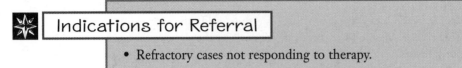

Indications for Referral

- Refractory cases not responding to therapy.

Tinea Corporis (Ringworm of the Body)

Overview

Pathophysiology

The infecting dermatophyte varies by geographic region and carrier: *Trichophyton rubrum* is most common on the West Coast of the United States; while *Trichophyton verrucosum* is most prevalent in central Canada. *Trichophyton mentagrophytes* is commonly transmitted from cats and dogs, whereas *Trichophyton rubrum* may be transmitted from human to human.

One to three weeks after the primary infection with the etiologic dermatophyte, the host tissue responds by eliminating the dermatophyte and its toxic allergenic metabolites from the center of the lesion, thus resolving the inflammatory response at that site, resulting in central clearing and the characteristic ring shape. That particular area then becomes resistant to reinfection. Subclinical infection with the dermatophyte may extend up to 8 cm from the clinically active border.

Epidemiology

Tinea corporis may occur at any age, with the highest frequency in children. It is most prevalent in hot, humid climates and in rural areas. Epidemics have been reported on geriatric wards.

Assessment

Clinical Presentation

Lesions vary from papules, pustules, vesicles, eczemas, and granulomas to an annular, scaly erythematous patch with an indurated, hyperkeratotic and at times vesicular border with a clear center (see Figure 3-9, *B*). Lesions are multiple and fairly uniform in size, usually located on exposed areas of the body. *T. rubrum* infections have central clearing whereas *T. mentagrophytes* presents as annular lesions without central clearing. The disorder may be asymptomatic or mildly pruritic and is much more extensive in immunosuppressed individuals and those with zoophilic infections.

Diagnostics
- KOH examination of scrapings taken from the **border** and lateral to the lesions.
- Fungal culture if the KOH finding is negative or if identification of the specific etiologic agent is necessary.

Differential Diagnosis
- Psoriasis vulgaris (symmetric, erythematous lesions with gray-white scale) (see Figure 3-31, *A*)
- Pityriasis rosea (salmon-colored herald patch on trunk; Christmas tree distribution of lesions) (see Figure 3-28)
- Seborrheic dermatitis (lesions usually occur on face, scalp, and central chest) (see Figure 3-35)
- Acute nummular eczema (lesions usually occur on arms, legs, and neck) (see Figure 2-1)
- Lichen simplex chronicus (usually a single, larger lesion) (see Figure 3-23)
- Mycosis fungoides (lesions are widespread, uniformly erythematous and without peripheral scale)

TINEA CORPORIS

- Is a contagious fungal disorder
- Medication should be applied to the lesion as well as the surrounding clinically normal skin, since the fungus spreads outward

Treatment

Nonpharmacologic
Avoidance of the infecting source will prevent further spread.

Pharmacologic

Topical Agents
Topical antifungal creams such as **clotrimazole (Lotrimin, Mycelex), miconazole (Monistat-Derm), ketoconazole (Nizoral), econazole (Spectazole), and ciclopirox olamine (Loprox)** may be applied bid until 3 weeks after clinical resolution.

Terbinafine (Lamisil) and **oxiconazole (Oxistat)** need only qd application, both to the lesion and to the surrounding clinically normal skin.

Systemic Agents
Griseofulvin ultramicrosize (Gris-PEG) 250 mg PO qd to bid is used; **griseofulvin microsize suspension (Grifulvin V suspension)** 125 mg/5 ml may be preferred for children above 2 years of age at a dosage of 11 mg/kg/day. Treatment should continue until there is evidence that the dermatophyte has been eradicated, usually after about 4 weeks.

Terbinafine (Lamisil) 250 mg PO qd, also for 3 to 4 weeks, is an alternative therapy.

Indications for Referral

• Widespread lesions not responding to treatment.

Tinea Cruris (Jock Itch)

Overview

Pathophysiology
Tinea cruris is commonly caused by infection with *Trichophyton rubrum*, *Trichophyton mentagrophytes*, or *Epidermophyton floccosum*. Heat, humidity, friction, tight-fitting underwear, athletic supporters, and maceration commonly predispose to infection.

Epidemiology
Most commonly found in obese men or during hot, humid summer months.

Assessment

Clinical Presentation
Tinea cruris ("jock itch") begins as a symmetric, slowly enlarging, annular erythematous lesion with peripheral scaling, usually noted on the upper inner thigh and groin (see Figure 3-9, *C*). The lesion may be unilateral and commonly spares the scrotum (an important differentiation from candidiasis, in which the scrotum is commonly severely inflamed). The penis is rarely, if ever, involved. Eruptions may be asymptomatic, but are more frequently pruritic with a superimposed lichenification. Often it is simultaneously associated with tinea pedis. Perineal and perianal skin may also be involved.

Diagnostics
• Clinical presentation and history are usually sufficient to make the diagnosis.
• KOH examination of scrapings from the border and lateral to the lesion may be used for confirmation. (However, if the patient has already tried over-the-counter antifungal treatments, the results may be negative.)

Differential Diagnosis
• Erythrasma (positive Wood's light result with coral-red fluorescence; lesions are bilateral)
• Candidiasis (lesions are beefy red; satellite lesions are present) (see Figure 3-7)

- Psoriasis vulgaris (symmetric erythematous lesions with gray-white scale) (see Figure 3-31, *A*)
- Seborrheic dermatitis (distribution occurs on scalp, face, and central chest) (see Figure 3-35)
- Intertrigo (erythematous, oozing lesions)
- Allergic contact dermatitis (lesions occur in areas that have contact with the offending agent) (see Figure 3-3)

Treatment

Nonpharmacologic

Correction of exacerbating factors may entail attention to several conditions: weight loss or liposculpture where indicated (to decrease the amount of opposing skin surface), reduction of moisture in the area (changing wet swimsuits or exercise clothing), use of cotton rather than nylon underwear (for increased absorption of perspiration), and liberal application of absorbent powder.

Pharmacologic

Topical Agents

Zeasorb-AF powder is both absorbent and fungistatic.

Lotions and/or creams such as **clotrimazole (Lotrimin), mycostatin (Nystatin), miconazole (Monistat-Derm), and ketoconazole (Nizoral)** applied bid for 3 to 4 weeks or **oxiconazole (Oxistat)** applied qd will correct the condition. If the lesion is moist and weeping, wet compresses of **Burow's solution** applied several times daily will hasten resolution.

If pruritus or inflammation is pronounced, mild steroids **(1% hydrocortisone)** or a combination antifungal/antibiotic/steroid such as **hydrocortisone-iodoquinol (Vytone)** may be applied bid for up to 2 weeks.

Systemic Agents

Itraconazole (Sporanox) 100 mg PO bid for 7 days may be necessary in severe or recalcitrant cases.

Indications for Referral

- Condition that does not respond to treatment

For Tinea Cruris ("Jock Itch") Patient Teaching information and materials, turn to p. 465.

TINEA CRURIS

- Is a fungal infection that can be prevented by keeping the skin dry and cool, changing out of damp clothing promptly, wearing cotton underwear and loose-fitting clothing, and using absorbent powder

- Has an affinity for skin-folds, making weight reduction an important component of treatment to decrease intertriginous areas

Tinea Manuum (Ringworm of the Hand)

Overview

Pathophysiology
Usually caused by *Trichophyton rubrum*.

Epidemiology
Tinea manuum is the least common of the superficial fungal infections. It is very rare in children and more common in persons of Asian descent.

Assessment

Clinical Presentation
Tinea manuum presents as an asymptomatic, dry, scaling hyperkeratotic lesion on an erythematous base. The palmar surface is more likely to be involved than the back of the hand (see Figure 3-9, *D*). It frequently occurs in association with tinea pedis but usually only one hand is involved ("one hand, two feet"). One or more nails on the same hand may be infected. Accentuation of the flexural creases is characteristic.

   Dermatophytid (Id reaction) should be considered if groups of minute, sterile papules or vesicles appear on the fingers or palms. Such a reaction may indicate an allergic response secondary to a dermatophyte infection.

Diagnostics
- Clinical presentation and history
- KOH examination

Differential Diagnosis
- Allergic contact or irritant dermatitis (lesions are usually distributed in areas where contact with the offending agent occurs) (see Figure 3-3, *A*)
- Atopic dermatitis (distribution of lesions primarily in popliteal and antecubital areas)
- Dyshidrosis (differentiated on basis of results of KOH testing)
- Psoriasis vulgaris (symmetric, erythematous lesions with gray-white scale) (see Figure 3-31, *A*)
- Poststreptococcal or poststaphylococcal exfoliation (history of previous sore throat or systemic disease)

TINEA MANUUM

- Can be minimized by keeping the hands supple and dry

- Will respond best to topical medication when it is applied to damp skin, since the skin on the hands is naturally quite thick and maximum penetration is required

Treatment

Nonpharmacologic

Keeping the hands dry and supple as much as possible is essential. If the condition occurs in conjunction with tinea pedis, the condition of the hands should resolve as the condition of the feet improves.

Pharmacologic

Topical agents

Antifungal creams and lotions such as **clotrimazole (Lotrimin, Mycelex), ketoconazole (Nizoral), or econazole (Spectazole)** may be applied bid.

If the disorder is an id reaction, steroids of medium to high potency such as **mometasone furoate (Elocon) 0.1%, fluocinonide (Lidex) 0.05%, diflorasone diacetate (Psorcon) cream 0.05%, or clobetasol propionate (Temovate) 0.05%** applied bid for not more than 2 weeks may be helpful.

Systemic Agents

Usually systemic agents are unnecessary, but they may be used if topical treatment is ineffective. **Griseofulvin ultramicrosize (Gris-PEG)** 250 mg PO qd to bid for up to 3 months is the treatment of choice. **Terbinafine (Lamasil)** 250 mg PO qd for 3 weeks is a viable alternative.

Indications for Referral

• Chronic infections unresponsive to therapy

Tinea Pedis (Athlete's Foot)

Overview

Pathophysiology

Trichophyton rubrum, Trichophyton mentagrophytes, and *Epidermophyton floccosum* are the most common pathogens. Trauma, increased bacterial flora, plus exposure to the fungus will produce clinical infection. The condition may be exacerbated by occlusive footwear, poor hygiene, and/or sweating. Recurrences are often due to coexistent onychomycosis rather than transmission from or to another individual.

Epidemiology

Tinea pedis is the most common of all fungal diseases, affecting as much as 70% of the population at some time. It rarely occurs before puberty and is most frequent in tropical climates and during the summertime. Males are affected two to four times more often than females. Relapse is common.

Assessment

Clinical Presentation

Commonly the condition occurs on **both feet and one hand** simultaneously when caused by *Trichophyton rubrum*. Infections usually appear as hyperkeratotic scaling lesions that present in a **moccasin-like distribution** along the sides of the feet and on the sole (see Figure 3-9, *E*).

Another form of tinea pedis presents as inflamed or scaly macules, typical of *T. mentagrophytes*. Macerated, pink, scaly, painfully **fissured skin is present between the toes** (see Figure 3-9, *F*). Lesions may be malodorous. **Pruritus** is the most common symptom, reported by almost 90% of patients. Simultaneous onychomycosis is frequent. *Candida* spp. and bacteria may produce a condition that is clinically indistinguishable from a dermatophyte infection or that may occur simultaneously.

Diagnostics

- Diagnosis is usually made on the basis of clinical presentation and history.
- KOH examination may be useful to distinguish the disorder from contact dermatitis and candidiasis.

Differential Diagnosis

- Irritant or contact dermatitis (lesions are usually distributed in the areas of contact with the offending agent; results of KOH testing will differentiate) (see Figure 3-3, *A*)
- Candidiasis, especially with erosions in the web spaces (results of KOH testing will differentiate)
- Psoriasis vulgaris (symmetric, erythematous lesions with gray-white scale) (see Figure 3-31, *A*)

Treatment

Nonpharmacologic

Prevention is key, especially in light of the high relapse rate. Feet should be kept as dry as possible by wearing **ventilated shoes or**

TINEA PEDIS

- Is somewhat contagious, being spread by contact with infected persons or items
- Can be minimized by not walking barefoot in public places or sharing shoes and socks
- Can be controlled through prevention: wearing cotton socks and changing them frequently, keeping feet dry, wearing well-ventilated shoes when possible

sandals with light cotton socks. Socks should be changed as necessary throughout the day as they become damp. Use of liberal amounts of over-the-counter (OTC) **antifungal powder** in the shoes and socks is helpful. Baby powder and talc should be avoided, since some contain elements that nourish fungi.

Pharmacologic

Topical Agents

Antifungal powders, creams, and/or lotions **(Zeasorb-AF powder, clotrimazole [Lotrimin, Mycelex], miconazole [Monistat-Derm], ketoconazole [Nizoral], econazole [Spectazole], or ciclopirox olamine [Loprox])** applied bid for 2 to 3 months will treat most cases.

Terbinafine (Lamasil) or **oxiconazole (Oxistat)** applied qd for 1 to 2 weeks is also effective.

Cool compresses of **Burow's solution,** applied four to five times daily, will be helpful in drying blisters or macerated, weeping lesions. To aid in the removal of dry, hyperkeratotic, scaling lesions, the application of **40% salicylic acid plasters** for 24 hours will desquamate the stratum corneum and remove the resident fungi.

Inflamed lesions may be calmed with the application of corticosteroids. Dry, scaling hyperkeratotic lesions along the sides of the feet or on the sole will require high-potency ointments **(betamethasone dipropionate [Diprolene] 0.05%, clobetasol propionate [Temovate] 0.05%, halobetasol propionate [Ultravate] 0.05%, or diflorasone diacetate [Psorcon] 0.05%).**

Inflamed skin that is soft, macerated, or in the toe webs will respond to a midpotency steroid such as **mometasone furoate (Elocon) 0.1% cream, fluticasone propionate (Cutivate) 0.05% cream, or hydrocortisone valerate (Westcort) 0.2% cream.**

With cracked or fissured skin, a bacterial infection may easily become established. Topical antibiotics, especially **gentamycin ointment,** should be used when a bacterial infection is suspected.

Systemic Agents

Oral antifungals such as **itraconazole (Sporanox)** 100 mg PO bid for 3 to 4 weeks may be necessary in severe cases, or for the treatment of coexisting onychomycosis.

For extensive secondary bacterial infections, **erythromycin** or **cephalexin** 250 mg PO q6h for 10 to 14 days may be required.

✴ Indications for Referral

- Extensive or recalcitrant infection not responding to treatment.
- Concomitant use of warfarin.
- Abnormal liver function test results.

For Tinea Pedis (Athlete's Foot) Patient Teaching information and materials, turn to p. 467.

Ichthyosis Vulgaris

Overview

Pathophysiology
Inherited as an autosomal dominant trait, associated with a familial history of atopic skin in approximately 50% of cases. The epidermal transit time is normal, indicating that the disorder is due to retention of scales resulting from increased adhesiveness of the stratum corneum (retention keratosis).

Epidemiology
Onset is usually in very early to middle childhood but is not present at birth. There is a marked seasonal variation with clearing associated with humidity.

Assessment

Clinical Presentation
Initially dry, white rectangular scales and follicular keratoses (keratosis pilaris) may be noted (see Figure 3-17). There are varying degrees of scaling, especially over the trunk and extensor extremities, as well as the scalp. Accentuation of normal palmar and sole creases is characteristic. Flexural areas and the nape of the neck are commonly spared. Pruritus and rough skin are frequent complaints. Many patients' conditions improves significantly with age, although it is a lifelong disorder.

Diagnostics
Diagnosis is based on history and clinical presentation. Skin biopsy will confirm the diagnosis. A thorough medical evaluation should be performed on patients with adult-onset disease.

Differential Diagnosis

Xerosis (thin, small scales on slightly erythematous base) (see Figure 3-39)

Treatment

Nonpharmacologic

Moisturization of the skin is the key to therapy. **Vaseline, Lubriderm, Eucerin, or Cetaphil cream,** applied several times throughout the day especially after a bath or shower, will help alleviate symptoms.

Pharmacologic

Topical Agents

Application of a lactic acid cream **(Lac-Hydrin 12%)** or a cream containing urea **(U-Lactin)** once or twice daily will hasten resolution. Use should be restricted to those patients whose skin is intact, since the acid component may cause burning or stinging in cracked skin.

For particularly recalcitrant cases **tretinoin (Retin-A)** cream 0.05% to 0.1.% may be applied every evening, but should be discontinued if irritation results.

Systemic Agents

Isotretinoin (Accutane) 1 to 2 mg/kg/day orally in divided doses is very effective but does carry the risk of substantial side effects (as described in the section on acne vulgaris). The risks and benefits of long-term therapy with this agent must be given careful consideration before implementing treatment.

ICHTHYOSIS VULGARIS

- Is a chronic condition that can be controlled but not cured
- Can be minimized by thorough and routine moisturization immediately after showering or bathing
- Is reduced by physical exfoliation and/or application of products containing alpha-hydroxyacids

Indications for Referral

- Adult-onset (acquired) ichthyosis to rule out associated disorders, including lymphoma, sarcoidosis, hypothyroidism, and systemic lupus erythematosus.
- Therapy not responding to topical moisturization, in which oral isotretinoin is a consideration.

Lichen Planus

Overview

Pathophysiology

Lichen planus is an idiopathic disease, thought to be caused by an underlying bacterial, viral, or yeast infection. Occasionally it is associated with exposure to drugs (thiazides are the most common), heavy metals, or photographic chemicals. An autoimmune cause is possible, and psychogenic factors may play a role in the onset and course of disease. Lesions tend to resolve spontaneously in 1 to 4 years, although scalp lesions may cause permanent alopecia, nails may be permanently destroyed, skin may be permanently hyperpigmented, and ulcerative changes in the mouth may lead to squamous cell carcinoma. Twenty percent of patients have a recurrence of lichen planus.

Epidemiology

The usual age of onset is between 30 and 70 years. About 10% of patients have a positive family history.

Assessment

Clinical Presentation

Lichen planus can be best described by the five *P's:* **pruritic, planar (flat-topped), polyangular, purple papules.** Shiny, violaceous, flat-topped papules with an irregular border, 1 to 4 mm in diameter, with **fine white lines and scales** (Wickham's striae, best demonstrated by placing a drop of oil on the lesion) are the hallmark of the disorder (see Figure 3-22). Lesions have a predilection for **flexor surfaces** (wrists, forearms, and ankles), **oral mucosa, genitalia, nails, and scalp.** Occasionally the papules coalesce into plaques. Nails become thin and atrophic with longitudinal striation. **Pruritus** is variable but may be intensely severe. Oral lesions cause eating to be painful and difficult. Scratching or injuring the skin may stimulate development of new lesions (Koebner's phenomenon).

Diagnostics

- A thorough drug history is essential.
- KOH examination of scrapings from the oral mucosa will identify oral candidiasis.
- A rapid plasma reagin (RPR) or Venereal Disease Research Laboratories (VDRL) serologic test will identify secondary syphilis

- Skin biopsy confirms the diagnosis.
- An increased incidence of chronic active hepatitis and abnormal liver function test results may occur.
- Abnormal glucose tolerance test results occur in more than 50% of cases.

Differential Diagnosis

- Drug-induced lichen planus (history of thiazide, quinidine, and benzodiazepines)
- Oral candidiasis (positive KOH finding; white cheesy membrane is easily scraped away)
- Flat warts (skin-toned, not shiny)
- Secondary syphilis (involves palms and soles; white membrane on buccal mucosa or genitals is absent; VDRL or RPR is positive; lesions are usually more generalized)
- Papulosquamous drug eruption (distribution is more generalized)
- Lichen simplex chronicus (lesions are usually solitary and larger than 1 cm in diameter) (see Figure 3-23)

Treatment

Nonpharmacologic

Elimination of drugs, chemicals, or other causative factors is essential. The disorder is very difficult to treat; mild disease can be treated topically, whereas more severe cases require systemic intervention. Wearing wool clothing (or other prickly garments) should be avoided to help prevent or relieve itching.

Pharmacologic

Topical Agents

High-potency topical corticosteroids **(clobetasol propionate [Temovate], betamethasone dipropionate [Diprolene], diflorasone diacetate [Psorcon])** applied bid will help relieve pruritus and encourage resolution of lesions. If high-potency corticosteroids contact the eyes, cataracts and glaucoma may develop. Application in the periorbital regions should therefore be avoided.

Triamcinolone acetonide dental paste (Kenalog in Orabase) applied bid to oral lesions helps relieve inflammation and discomfort. For more recalcitrant lesions, **tretinoin (Retin-A)** 0.05% cream applied for 10 minutes bid may be helpful. PUVA therapy (see Psoriasis) is gaining in popularity among practitioners, although it is still somewhat controversial.

LICHEN PLANUS

• Usually resolves spontaneously within 1 to 4 years

• Can be minimized by preventing causative agents such as wool clothing, thiazide medications, and photographic chemicals from coming into contact with the skin

• Responds to steroids, but because of the chronicity of the disorder, steroids must be used judiciously and only as directed

Intralesional Agents

Injections of **triamcinolone (Kenalog)** 5 mg/ml into hypertrophic lesions or into the nail matrix area (below the posterior nail fold) of affected nails may be beneficial. Limit the injected amount to no more than 0.1 ml per nail, to prevent nail dystrophy. Injections can be repeated on a monthly basis.

Systemic Agents

Prednisone 20 mg PO qAM for 1 week and tapered to 10 mg PO qAM the second week is appropriate for diffuse, highly symptomatic disease. After 2 weeks therapy should be switched to topical treatment. If underlying bacterial, fungal, or viral infections exist, appropriate treatment of those disorders can also be very effective in improving lichen planus. An antihistamine such as **hydroxyzine (Atarax)** 10 to 50 mg PO qid will help control pruritus.

   Isotretinoin (Accutane) has also demonstrated striking results.

Indications for Referral

- Referral to a dermatologist for unusually severe disease and consideration of long-term corticosteroid therapy or systemic retinoid **(Accutane)** therapy is appropriate.

Pityriasis Rosea

Overview

Pathophysiology

The cause is unknown, although 20% of patients report some form of an acute (usually viral) infection shortly before the eruption occurs. A single outbreak usually confers permanent immunity.

Epidemiology

Pityriasis rosea is the 10th most common dermatologic illness. Seventy-five percent of cases occur in persons between the ages of 10 and 35, with a peak incidence between ages 20 and 24. There is a possible female predominance. Most cases occur in the winter months, and there is a significant association with a personal or family history of asthma and/or atopic dermatitis.

Assessment

Clinical Presentation

A single oval, well-dermarcated salmon-colored patch **(herald patch)** with a fine collarette scale develops first (see Figure 3-28). One to two weeks later, smaller lesions of similar configuration develop on the trunk and proximal extremities. The lesions persist for 2 weeks, then fade over the next 2 weeks. The eruption typically follows skin lines in a **Christmas tree** pattern in non(sun-exposed areas. Lesions do not recur in 98% of cases. There are rarely any constitutional symptoms other than moderate pruritus.

Diagnostics

- Diagnosis is based on clinical presentation and history. Biopsy is not diagnostic.
- A serologic test for syphilis (RPR, VDRL) may be indicated if history is appropriate.

Differential Diagnosis

- Secondary syphilis (lesions occur on trunk, extremities, palms, and soles; moist papules may occur on oral mucosa and genitalia)
- Seborrheic dermatitis (distribution occurs on scalp, face, and central chest) (see Figure 3-35)
- Psoriasis vulgaris (symmetric, erythematous lesions with gray-white scale) (see Figure 3-31, *A*)
- Tinea corporis (positive KOH result; lesions are ring-shaped with central clearing) (see Figure 3-9, *B*)
- Tinea versicolor (positive KOH result; no herald patch or Christmas tree distribution) (see Figure 3-38)
- Papulosquamous drug eruption (oval to round erythematous macules, a few millimeters in diameter, with overlying scale, in a generalized distribution)

> **PITYRIASIS ROSEA**
>
> - Is not contagious
> - Will resolve spontaneously in time
> - Becomes more pruritic after periods of exercise or after a hot bath

Treatment

Nonpharmacologic

No nonpharmacologic therapy is known.

Pharmacologic

Topical Agents

Antipruritic lotions **(Sarna, Zonalon [Doxepin])** are soothing and helpful for pruritic symptoms. Ultraviolet-A and ultraviolet-B light treatments will also hasten disease resolution and limit pruritus.

Systemic Agents

Antihistamines **(diphenhydramine [Benadryl]** 25 mg PO qid, **hydroxyzine [Atarax]** 25 mg PO qid) may be helpful to relieve pruritus and enhance sleep. **Loratadine [Claritin]** 10 mg PO qd, or **citirizine [Zyrtec]** 10 mg PO qd help to relieve pruritus and are not sedating.

Indications for Referral

- Suspicion of other underlying disorder.
- Failure of condition to resolve

For Pityriasis Rosea Patient Teaching information and materials, turn to p. 455.

Pityrosporum Folliculitis

Overview

Pathophysiology

An infection of the hair follicles caused by the same organism that causes tinea versicolor *(Pityrosporum orbiculare)*.

Epidemiology

Most commonly occurs in young women. Patients with severely oily skin or diabetes mellitus and those who have recently completed a course of either corticosteroids or broad-spectrum antibiotics are at greater risk. Occasionally it occurs in association with either tinea versicolor or seborrheic dermatitis.

Assessment

Clinical Presentation

Moderately itchy, dome-shaped papules and pustules on the upper back, upper chest, and adjacent areas of arms and neck.

Diagnostics

- Diagnosis is confirmed when a KOH examination demonstrates budding yeast cells and hyphae.

Differential Diagnosis

- Acne (lesions are not all follicular in distribution; open and closed comedones are intermixed with pustules) (see Figure 3-1, *B*)
- Folliculitis caused by other organisms (e.g., *Staphylococcus aureus*; *Pseudomonas* spp.; presentations are very similar) (see Figure 3-11)

Treatment

Nonpharmacologic

Avoid contact with persons known to be infected.

Pharmacologic

Topical Agents

Selenium sulfide lotion (Selsun) applied to the entire upper trunk from the neck to the waist to the wrists for 10 minutes qd for 1 to 2 weeks. The scalp should also be shampooed to remove the subclinical reservoir of infection. Prolonged treatment may produce a contact dermatitis.

Topical antifungal agents **(econazole [Spectazole], miconazole [Monistat-Derm] and clotrimazole [Lotrimin, Mycelex])** applied bid, as well as **ketoconazole (Nizoral) and terbinafine (Lamisil)** applied qd, all for 1 to 2 weeks, may be helpful for unresponsive patients or for those sensitive to selenium sulfide. Usually, however, they are no more effective and are more expensive.

Systemic Agents

For resistant patients or those with extensive disease, oral **ketoconazole (Nizoral)** 400 mg one time only may be required. Alternately, 200 mg PO qd for 1 week may be prescribed. A 400 mg PO dose monthly may be helpful for prophylaxis. The patient should not have any hepatic irregularities and should not be taking other hepatotoxic drugs.

PITYROSPORUM FOLLICULITIS

- Is an infection of the hair follicles caused by a yeast
- Responds equally well to selenium sulfide lotion (Selsun) and the more expensive prescription products

 ## Indications for Referral

- Resistant cases in a patient with elevated liver function test results or who is taking other hepatotoxic drugs.

Psoriasis Vulgaris

Overview

Pathophysiology

The psoriatic epithelial cell takes 1.5 to 2 days (compared to 26 to 28 days for normal skin) to migrate from the basal layer to the skin surface to be normally exfoliated. The psoriatic cell cycle is 37 hours, whereas 300 hours is average for normal cells. Furthermore, almost 100% of the epidermal psoriatic cells are in a proliferative phase, compared to only 60% of normal cells. The result of these deviations is that normal maturation cannot take place.

Trauma (physical or psychologic) or any inflammation of the skin can be a precipitating event and induce skin lesions in 10 to 14 days. Environmental humidity, temperature, and sunburn can also trigger a flare.

Epidemiology

Psoriasis vulgaris is an apparently inherited trait, with an estimated heritability of 65%. The average age of onset is 27, but it can present at any age. It occurs most often in whites, five times less often in Asians, and least often in blacks. There is no sex difference in incidence. Ninety percent of patients notice a flare during winter months. In children flares frequently follow respiratory streptococcal infections by 7 to 10 days. In adults iodine, digoxin, clonidine, propranolol, lithium, and antimalarial drugs have been noted to exacerbate the condition.

Assessment

Clinical Presentation

Well-demarcated **erythematous papules and plaques with silver-white scales** (see Figure 3-31, *A*). A **symmetric distribution** is common. Lesions vary from coin-sized to extensive, maplike coalescing plaques that occur most commonly on the extremities (especially **knees and elbows**), **scalp, back, genitalia, intergluteal folds, and nails.** Lesions are sharply marginated. They are uncommon on the face but can occur anywhere. Pruritus is variable but occurs in approximately 20% of patients. Fifty percent of cases have associated scalp involvement.

Nails appear pitted with variable onycholysis (nail separation from the nail bed), with discoloration of the nail plate. A symmetric distribution of affected nails is common. A yellow-brown subungual discoloration (**"oil spot"**) is characteristic. Nail changes occur in 50% of adults and 70% of infants with psoriasis. Pinpoint bleeding occurs with removal of scales secondary to dilated dermal capillaries (Auspitz sign). A zone of nonerythematous hypopigmented skin often surrounds individual lesions, particularly after ultraviolet light therapy.

Marked with **exacerbations and remissions,** psoriasis often **flares during winter months** and improves with summer sun. Occasionally it resolves spontaneously.

Clinical variants include the following:

- **Guttate** psoriasis: "droplike" lesions that generally appear on the trunk after an upper respiratory streptococcal infection in children or a viral infection in adults (see Figure 3-31, *B*)
- **Localized pustular** psoriasis: discrete, sterile pustules and scaly plaques.
- **Generalized pustular** psoriasis (von Zumbusch's psoriasis): erythema with sheets of pustules over much of the body, usually accompanied by fever, polyarthralgias, chills, malaise, and leukocytosis. It commonly occurs after a course of systemic steroids (see Figure 3-31, *C*).
- **Erythrodermic (exfoliative)** psoriasis: almost total body exfoliation and erythroderma with localized or generalized edema. Generally occurs in chronic adult psoriatics after sunburn, systemic viral, or bacterial infection. Avoid use of tar, anthralin, and light.
- **Psoriatic arthritis:** distinguished from rheumatoid arthritis by the absence of rheumatoid factor and subcutaneous nodules. An asymmetric arthritis, first appears in the distal interphalangeal joints of the hands and feet in 50% of cases. Most often it follows the extent of skin manifestations with coinciding flares and remissions.
- **Psoriasis of the nails:** Pitting of the nails is the most common sign. In some cases the disorder may mimic onycholysis with the nail plate turning yellow or lifting from the nail bed (see Figure 9-7).
- **Scalp** psoriasis: Erythematous, scaling plaques occur on the scalp or near the hairline. The condition is easily confused with seborrheic dermatitis (see Figure 3-31, *D*)

Diagnostics
- Diagnosis is based on clinical impression, including distribution of lesions, and a thorough history with specific attention to family history of psoriasis, current medications, previous illness, and mental or physical stress.
- Skin biopsy may be helpful in difficult cases.
- KOH of scales to differentiate from fungal infection (especially in intertriginous folds)

- Fungal culture of nail clippings to differentiate from onychomycosis

Differential Diagnosis

- Tinea corporis (lesions have central clearing) (see Figure 3-9, *B*)
- Pityriasis rosea (herald patch occurs first; eruption follows skin lines in a Christmas tree pattern) (see Figure 3-28)
- Nummular eczema (lesions are more erythematous; scale less thick) (see Figure 2-1)
- Mycosis fungoides (lesions progress to violaceous, indurated plaques and nodules; begins on thighs, buttocks, and trunk)
- Pityriasis rubra pilaris (generalized erythematous lesions with areas of normal skin; some xerotic changes; palms and soles are usually erythematous)
- Seborrheic dermatitis (lesions usually occur on face, scalp, and central chest) (see Figure 3-35)

Treatment

Nonpharmacologic

Support groups are helpful to the patient and family.

Pharmacologic

Topical Agents

Emollient creams or ointments (over-the-counter products) are helpful in preventing cracking and fissuring of lesions, especially those on palms and soles. **Corticosteroids** may be needed during periods of flare and for exfoliative and erythrodermic lesions. They usually produce rapid but temporary remission with a flare common on discontinuation of therapy and must be tapered slowly to prevent rebound.

Higher-potency preparations **(groups I to IV)** used qd to qid may be necessary for persistent lesions on the extensor surfaces. The penetration will be increased with occlusion or if applied immediately after bathing. The potency should be decreased as soon as improvement is noted. A low-potency steroid **(groups V to VII)** should be used qd to bid to treat lesions on the face, intertriginous areas, breasts, and genitalia. Pulse dosing (2 weeks of treatment, 1 week of emollients only) for both mild and potent steroids may be beneficial.

For lesions on the scalp numerous shampoos are available, including selenium sulfide **(Exsel, Selsun)**, tar **(Denorex, DHS Tar, Ionil-T, Neutrogena T/gel)**, antimicrobial antiseborrheic **(DHS Zinc; FS Shampoo**, which requires a prescription; **Head and Shoulders** [equally effective and less expensive])**, and sulfur and

PSORIASIS

- Is a chronic condition that cannot be cured
- Will cycle through periods of remissions and flares
- Can be minimized with the use of topical steroids, which should be applied to moist skin exactly as directed
- Can be caused to flare by precipitating factors such as trauma to or inflammation of the skin, stress, increased humidity, sunburn, and high temperatures

salicylic acid **(Ionil Plus, Sebulex).** A scalp treatment, **clobetasol propionate 0.05% (Cormax)** lotion applied bid not exceeding 50 ml in a 1-week period, may be helpful during flares. **Derma-smoothe-FS** is particularly effective for removing thick lesions.

Trihydroxyanthracene (Anthralin) 0.1% to 3.0% ointment may be applied to affected areas other than intertriginous or facial. Care must be taken to prevent contact with the normal surrounding skin. At higher concentrations application for 10 to 20 minutes qd or bid is adequate. The ointment must be washed off with mineral oil, followed by soap and water. If overnight application is desired, a weaker concentration must be used. Patients should be warned about possible irritation and permanent staining of clothing. There is an additive effect if combined with ultraviolet A or ultraviolet B (UVA or UVB) light exposure. Remissions are usually longer than those obtained with topical steroids.

Salicylic acid preparations, in a 1% to 5% concentration, may be combined with any of these preparations to enhance penetration through thick lesions. They also function as keratolytic agents.

Phototherapy may be necessary for treatment of severe or generalized psoriasis, particularly if other treatment modalities fail. It may be administered in UVA or UVB wavelengths.

UVA light therapy, 320 to 400 nm, is most effective in conjunction with oral 8-methoxypsoralen **(Psoralen),** commonly known as **PUVA.** Treatment is two or three times weekly and is costly, in terms both of time and money. There are possible long-term premature aging and carcinogenic effects on the skin with prolonged therapy. Remissions after total clearing last 6 to 12 months, especially when weekly maintenance therapy is given.

UVB light therapy at 313 nm may be useful alone. Weekly maintenance therapy of 90% of the patient's final clearing treatment dose contributes to the duration of disease control.

Goeckerman therapy is a combination of tar preparations and ultraviolet B (UVB) light therapy. A 1% to 2% solution of crude coal tar cream or ointment or a tar-based lotion is applied at night from the neck down, avoiding the pubic area. The next morning after a tar bath the patient applies an emollient and is given a suberythrogenic UVB dose. An alternate outpatient regimen consists of applying a coal tar lotion **(T-derm)** 20 minutes to 2 hours before sunbathing to a suberythrodermic dose. It is best used in patients who note some improvement with sun exposure. An average 9-month remission is common.

Intralesional Agents
Triamcinolone acetonide (Kenalog) 10 mg/ml may be helpful for patients who have only a few, scattered plaques. The face and intertriginous areas should be avoided to prevent local atrophy.

Systemic Agents

Methotrexate 5 to 25 mg PO or IM weekly is indicated for generalized pustular psoriasis, generalized exfoliative psoriasis, severe psoriatic arthritis, severe uncontrolled psoriasis, and socially incapacitating psoriasis. The dosage is tapered individually for each patient to obtain the maximal effect with the lowest possible dose. It may be combined with other modalities in particularly resistant cases. Pretreatment evaluation includes a complete blood count, renal function tests, and liver biopsy. Weekly to monthly blood chemical evaluations should be obtained throughout treatment. Liver biopsies should be obtained every 1 to 2 years or as indicated by abnormal chemical findings.

Retinoid therapy, specifically **etretinate (Tegison),** is best reserved for erythrodermic pustular recalcitrant psoriasis. The initial dose is 1 mg/kg/day and is decreased to a maintenance dose of 0.5 to 0.75 mg/kg/day. Treatment is usually prolonged for 6 to 12 months to prevent relapse. It is most useful when combined with other treatment modalities, especially PUVA. It is best to begin etretinate 1 week before PUVA and continue until complete clearance occurs. Combination therapy usually reduces total PUVA treatment time by 1 to 2 weeks. Side effects mimic those of isotretoin **(Accutane).**

Indications for Referral

- Severe, recalcitrant, or unstable disease
- Liver biopsy before methotrexate administration
- Before phototherapy, if unfamiliar with light dosages or combination therapies
- Consultation encouraged unless familiar with systemic agents methotrexate and etretinate

Seborrheic Dermatitis

Overview

Pathophysiology

Exact cause is unknown but several theories exist:

1. Prolonged retention of sebum on the skin may alter the epidermal function or act as an irritant.

2. Androgenic hormones may exacerbate the disease course.

3. The condition may be precipitated by medications such as antidepressants, tranquilizers, and cimetidine.

4. Seborrheic dermatitis may be precipitated by stress, fatigue, inadequate nutrition, or infection.

5. The yeast *Pityrosporum ovale* may be the causative factor.

Epidemiology

Seborrheic dermatitis occurs during the first few months of life ("cradle cap") and then is rare until after puberty. Thirty percent of nursing home residents are afflicted. It is more common in males and during winter months. It is a common manifestation of acquired immunodeficiency syndrome (AIDS).

Assessment

Clinical Presentation

Seborrheic dermatitis is a chronic, recurrent disorder with exacerbations and remissions. Commonly originates in hairy skin and involves the **scalp, central face, eyebrows, eyelids, nasolabial folds, external ear, midsternal and interscapular regions, umbilicus, and intertriginous areas.** Lesions are dull to yellowish-red in color, sharply marginated, and covered with **greasy scales** (see Figure 3-35). They are variably pruritic. Infantile forms are not pruritic and clear spontaneously within 8 to 12 months. It is the most common cause of otitis externa. Temporary hair loss may also occur.

Diagnostics

- Diagnosis is made primarily by clinical evaluation.
- KOH is used to rule out fungal infection.
- Patch test rules out allergic contact dermatitis.
- Skin biopsy may be necessary to differentiate from psoriasis.

Differential Diagnosis

- Psoriasis vulgaris (symmetric, erythematous lesions with gray-white scale) (see Figure 3-31, *A*)
- Tinea faciale (well-demarcated round patch of erythematous skin with peripheral scale)
- Lupus erythematosus (erythematous, slightly scaly symmetric lesion usually on the face, in a "butterfly" distribution)
- Actinic keratosis (erythematous macules or papules with dry, rough scale; more discrete, less plaquelike) (see Figure 3-2)

Treatment

Nonpharmacologic

Eliminating aggravating factors may help reduce the frequency of exacerbations. Infants with cradle cap may be treated by applying warm mineral oil to the scalp and then washing the oil off in several hours with liquid detergent **(Dawn)** to remove the scale.

Pharmacologic

Topical Agents
Mild corticosteroids such as 1% hydrocortisone **(Hytone 1.0%)** or desonide **(Desowen 0.05%)** may be used twice daily on the face and intertriginous areas or on the scalp of infants. As the condition clears, dosing should taper over a 2-week period. During periods of remission topical steroids should be avoided, since prolonged use may lead to atrophic changes in the skin.

Ketoconazole **(Nizoral),** clotrimazole **(Lotrimin),** or econazole (Spectazole) may be applied bid either alone or in combination with hydrocortisone and may be used for extended periods without fear of atrophy. Washing the face with an antiseborrheic shampoo may be a helpful adjunct in controlling the scale. In cases of seborrheic blepharitis patients should be encouraged to wash the eyelids and lashes qd with an antiseborrheic shampoo.

Frequent shampooing (at least three to four times weekly) with an antiseborrheic shampoo, left on for 10 minutes, will help control scale on the scalp of infants, as well as adults. Rotation among various shampoos may be more effective than continuous use of the same one. Any one of several may be effective, and the efficacy may vary from patient to patient. Selenium sulfide **(Selsun Blue),** salicyclic acid **(Sebulex, Ionil),** tar **(T/Gel, Sebutone),** and zinc pyrithione **(Head and Shoulders, DHS-Zinc)** are the most effective. Combination shampoos of tar and salicyclic acid **(T-Sal)** are also available.

Midpotency corticosteroids such as mometasone 0.1% **(Elocon),** halcinonide 0.025% **(Halog),** alclometasone dipropionate 0.05% **(Aclovate),** betamethasone valerate 0.1% **(Valisone),** or hydrocortisone 0.2% **(Westcort)** may be applied to the body twice daily. Long-term use (over 2 to 3 weeks of continuous treatment) should be discouraged and therapy reserved for exacerbations only. For especially recalcitrant cases of scalp seborrheic dermatitis, **clobetasol propionate topical solution 0.05% (Cormax)** may be helpful.

Systemic Agents
Systemic agents are not indicated in therapy.

Indications for Referral

- Failure to respond to therapy.

For Seborrheic Dermatitis Patient Teaching information and materials, turn to p. 463.

SEBORRHEIC DERMATITIS

- Is a chronic but controllable condition
- Is not contagious
- Can be minimized by eliminating precipitating factors such as retained oil on the skin, certain male hormones, certain medications, stress, fatigue, and infection

Tinea Versicolor (Pityriasis Versicolor)

Overview

Pathophysiology

Tinea versicolor is a superficial fungal infection that occurs with the transition of a normal component of the skin flora, *Pityrosporum orbiculare*, into a pathogen that affects the outer layers of the stratum corneum, *Malassezia furfur*. Overgrowth of this pathogen may result in either hyperpigmentation or hypopigmentation. Hyperpigmentation results from an inflammatory reaction to the fungus. Hypopigmentation occurs because the fungi physically filter out ultraviolet A and/or B rays, resulting in nonpigmented patches on tanned skin. Furthermore the pathogen produces azelaic acid, which decreases the production of melanin.

The disease may be spread by contact to a susceptible person. Pregnancy, serious underlying disease, malnutrition, and elevated plasma cortisol level are predisposing factors. Most important exogenous factors are high temperatures and relative high humidity. In cases of recurrent infection the scalp should be evaluated as a possible reservoir for *P. orbiculare*. Repigmentation after treatment may take months.

Epidemiology

Tinea versicolor is a universal disease, affecting up to 40% of the population in temperate climates. It occurs most commonly in young adults, with a peak incidence in the early twenties. It is rare in childhood or old age. There is an increased incidence of familial disease and an equal sex distribution.

Assessment

Clinical Presentation

The disorder begins as small **asymptomatic** white-pink to brown **macules** with an overlying fine scale (see Figure 3-38). The macules gradually enlarge and may coalesce. On tanned skin they may appear lighter; on light skin they may appear darker. **Back, chest, and upper arms** are the most frequently affected areas.

Diagnostics

- KOH examination reveals the characteristic **"spaghetti and meatballs."**
- Wood's lamp examination may show orange-gold fluorescence of the involved areas.
- Fungal culture is difficult and not recommended.

Differential Diagnosis
- Vitiligo (lesions are chalk-white and nonscaling) (Figure 6-15)
- Pityriasis rosea (lesions are more papular; begins with a single "herald patch") (see Figure 3-28)
- Pityriasis alba (lesions are confined to the face, upper arms, neck, or shoulders) (see Figure 3-27)
- Secondary syphilis (lesions on trunk and extremities, palms, and soles; moist papules may occur on oral mucosa and genitalia)

Treatment

Nonpharmacologic
Avoid contact with persons known to be infected.

Pharmacologic

Topical Agents
Selenium sulfide lotion (Selsun) applied to the entire upper trunk from the neck to the waist to the wrists for 10 minutes qd for 1 to 2 weeks. The scalp should also be shampooed to remove the subclinical reservoir of infection. Prolonged treatment may produce a contact dermatitis.

Topical antifungal agents **(econazole [Spectazole], miconazole [Monistat-Derm], and clotrimazole [Lotrimin, Mycelex]** applied bid, as well as **ketoconazole [Nizoral], oxiconazole (Oxistat)** and **terbinafine [Lamisil]** applied qd, all for 1 to 2 weeks, may be helpful for unresponsive patients or for those sensitive to selenium sulfide. Usually, however, they are no more effective and are more expensive.

Systemic Agents
For resistant conditions or patients with extensive disease, **oral ketoconazole (Nizoral)** 400 mg one time only may be required. Alternately, 200 mg PO qd for 1 week may be prescribed. A 400 mg PO dose monthly may be helpful for prophylaxis. The patient should not have any hepatic irregularities and should not be taking other hepatotoxic drugs.

Indications for Referral

- Resistant cases in a patient with elevated liver function test results or taking other hepatotoxic drugs.

TINEA VERSICOLOR

- May be spread by person-to-person contact, although the exact degree of contagion is unknown
- May leave abnormally pigmented lesions that take months to return to a normal color

Erythematous Disorders

Figure 4-1 ACNE

A, *Teenage male with both open and closed comedones.* **B,** *Teenage male with nodular cystic acne, inflammatory lesions, and open and closed comedones.*

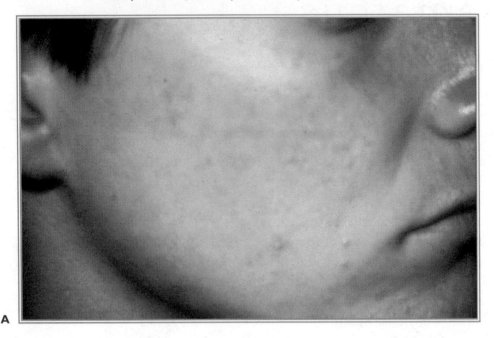

A

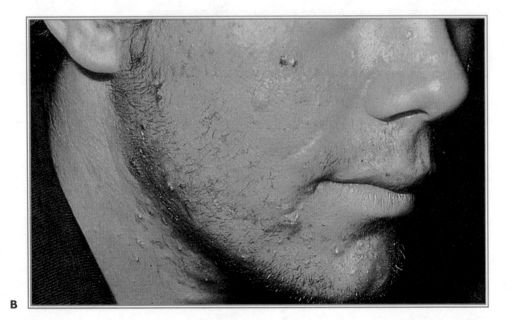

B

Figure 4-2 ACTINIC KERATOSIS

Slightly erythematous, rough, scaling papules and plaques on sun-damaged skin.

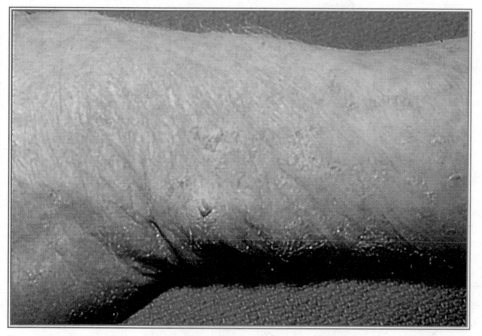

(From Goldstein BG, Goldstein AO: *Practical dermatology,* ed 2, St Louis, 1997, Mosby.)

Figure 4-3 ACUTE NUMMULAR ECZEMA

Multiple coinlike, hyperkeratotic erythematous lesions on the medial aspect of the thigh, with surrounding erythematous papules.

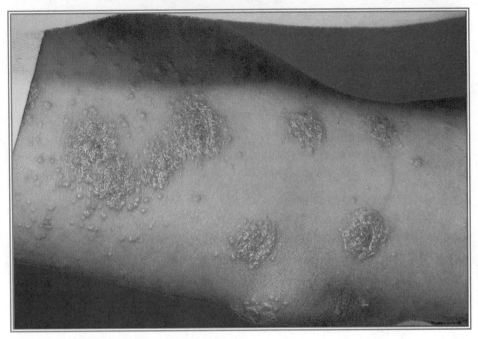

(Courtesy of Stacy R. Smith, MD.)

Figure 4-4 **ALLERGIC CONTACT DERMATITIS**

A, *Well-demarcated, erythematous macule caused by contact with the undersurface of a nickel-plated watch.* **B,** *Rhus variety: Linear vesicular lesions on the thigh and knees are characteristic of poison ivy exposure.*

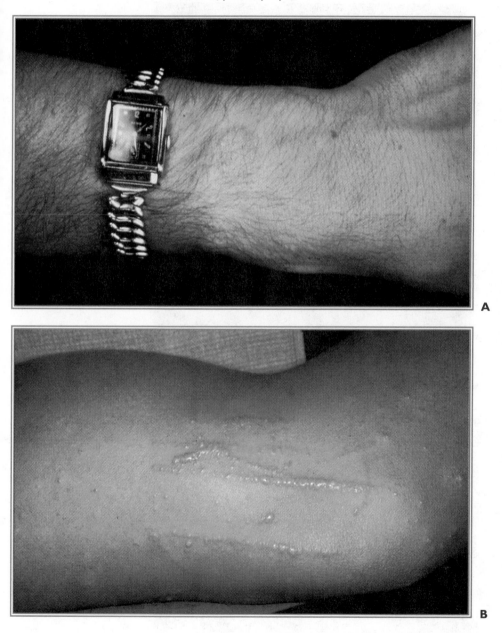

A

B

Figure 4-5 ATOPIC DERMATITIS

Blotchy, erythematous lesions on the face with accentuation in the central facial area.

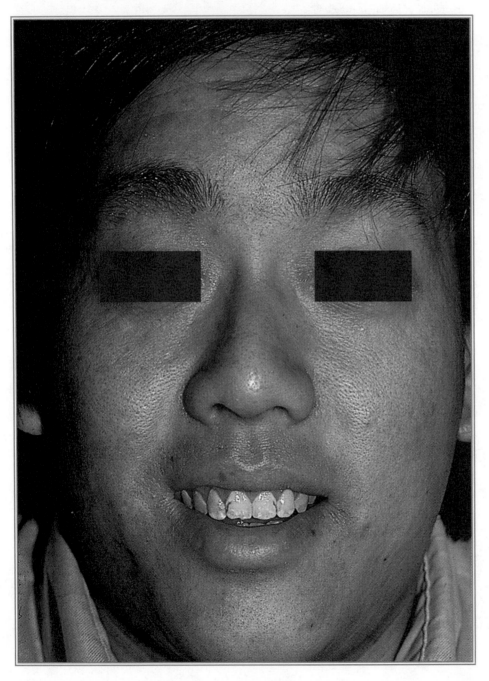

Figure 4-6 **BOWEN'S DISEASE**

Erythematous, keratotic, poorly marginated lesion on the arm of a 57-year-old male.

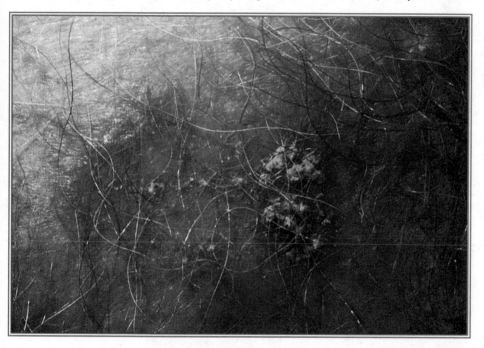

Figure 4-7 ACUTE CANDIDA INTERTRIGO

Note peripheral fringe of scale and satellite lesions.

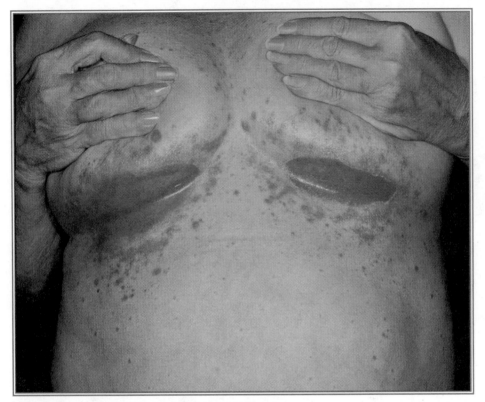

(From Habif TP: *Clinical dermatology,* ed 3, St Louis, 1996, Mosby.)

Figure 4-8   CELLULITIS

Poorly marginated erythematous plaque on the forearm.

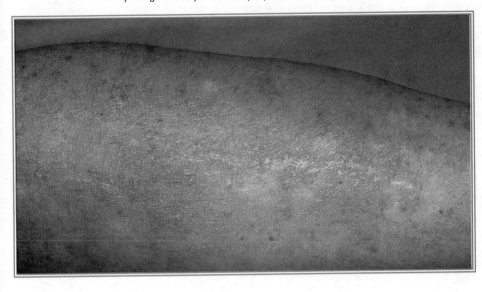

Figure 4-9   CHICKENPOX

Small vesicles on an erythematous macular base, in a generalized distribution on the back. Lesions vary in size from (early) papular lesions to (later) macular lesions.

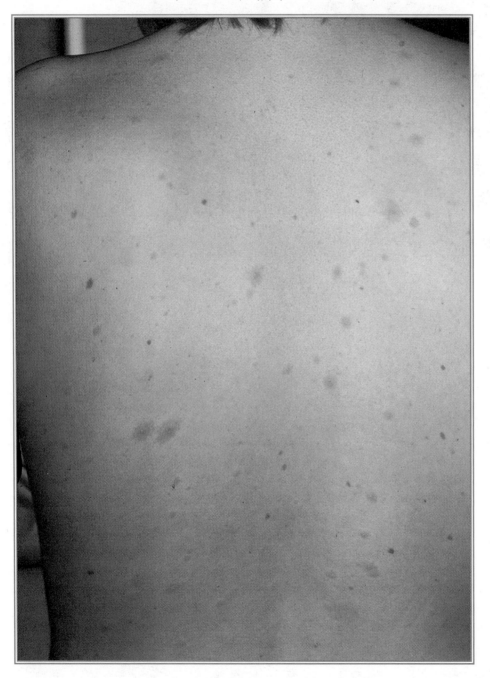

Figure 4-10

A, *Tinea capitis: Thick scale and crust on the apical aspect of a child's head.*
B, *Tinea corporis: Annular lesion with a sharply marginated erythematous border. Note central clearing with appearance of normal skin.*

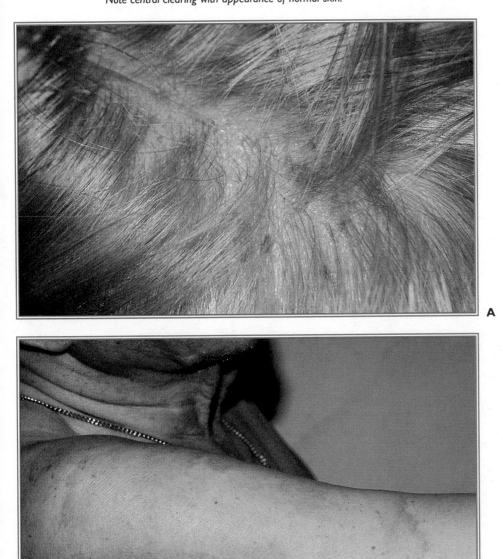

A

B

(**C through F**, From Habif TP: *Clinical dermatology*, ed 3, St. Louis, 1996, Mosby.)

continued

Figure 4-10

C, *Tinea cruris: A half-moon-shaped erythematous plaque with a slightly scaling border. Note sparing of the scrotum.* **D,** *Tinea manus: Tinea of the palm. Note thickened, dry, scaly skin.*

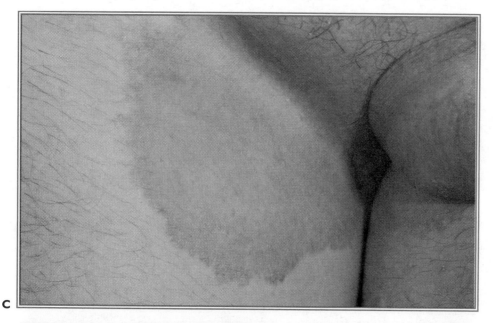

C

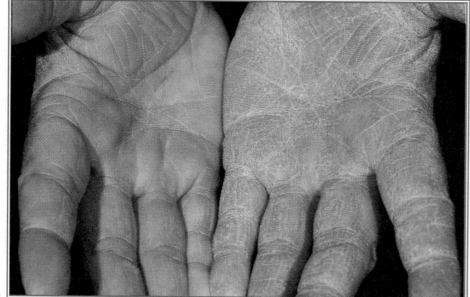

D

Figure 4-10

E, *Tinea pedis: Inflammation of the sole and lateral edges of the foot give it a moccasin-like appearance.* **F,** *Tinea pedis: The infection has macerated the skin in the toe web. Inflammation extends to the dorsum of the foot.*

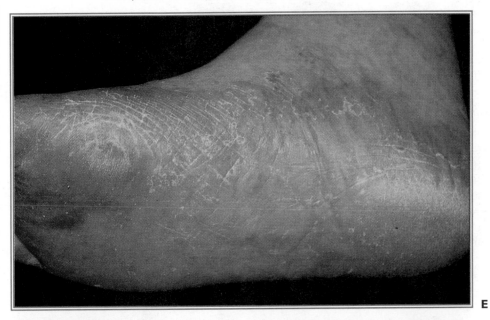

E

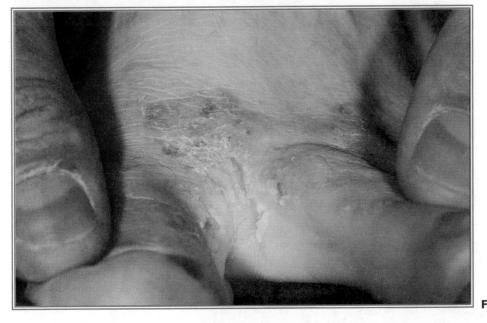

F

Figure 4-11   DYSHIDROTIC ECZEMA

Erythematous palms with only small areas of normal skin. Many areas are hyperkeratotic.

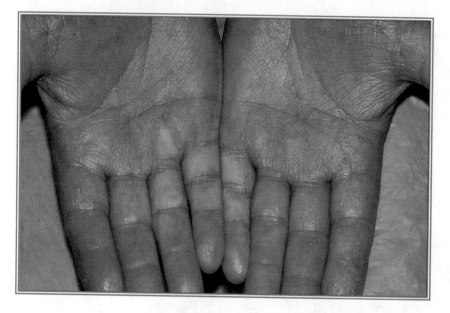

Figure 4-12   ERYSIPELAS

Sharply marginated, brightly erythematous plaque on the distal leg.

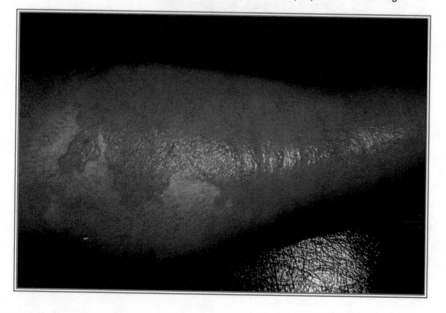

Figure 4-13 **ERYTHEMA INFECTIOSUM**

Facial erythema ("slapped cheek"), sparing the nasolabial fold and circumoral region.

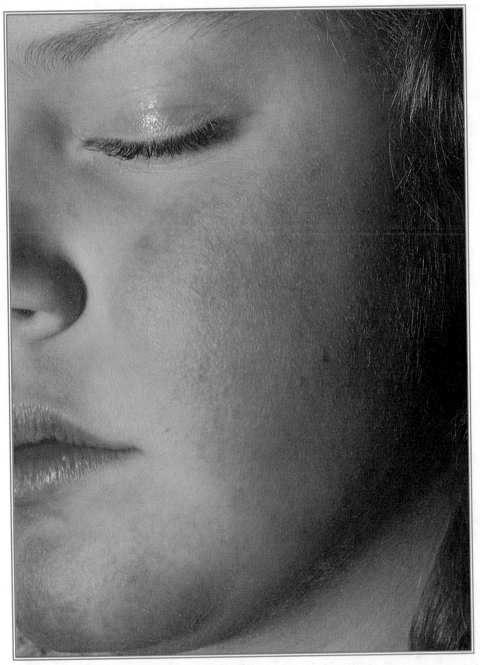

(From Habif TP: *Clinical dermatology*, ed 3, St Louis, 1996, Mosby.)

Figure 4-14 ERYTHEMA MULTIFORME

Erythematous, macular, targetlike lesions on the palms.

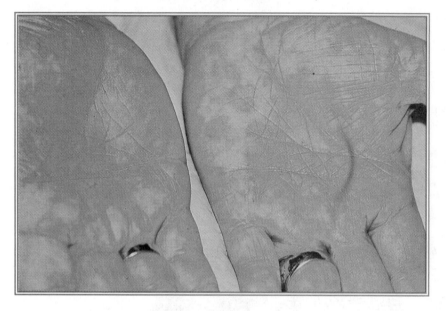

Figure 4-15 FOLLICULITIS

Extensive number of inflammatory closed comedones centered around hair follicles on the cheek of a male electrical worker exposed to fluorocarbons.

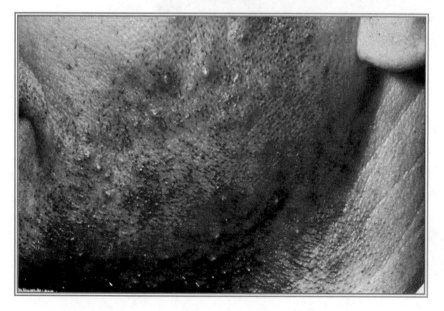

Figure 4-16 **FURUNCLE**

Pustular deep nodule on the posterior aspect of the right neck.

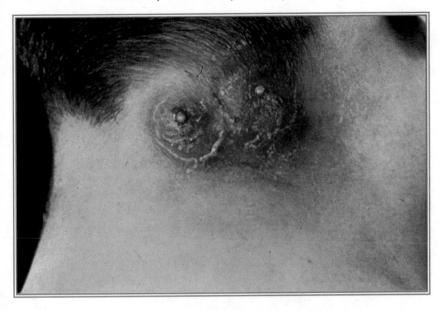

Figure 4-17 **CARBUNCLE**

Multiple pustular nodules on the posterior aspect of the neck. Many of the nodules have a confluent nature and exude pus.

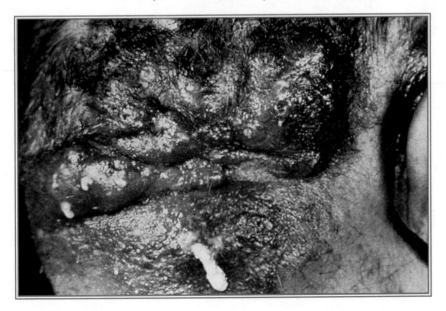

Figure 4-18   RUBELLA

Faint pink maculopapules, paler than the lesions characteristic of measles.

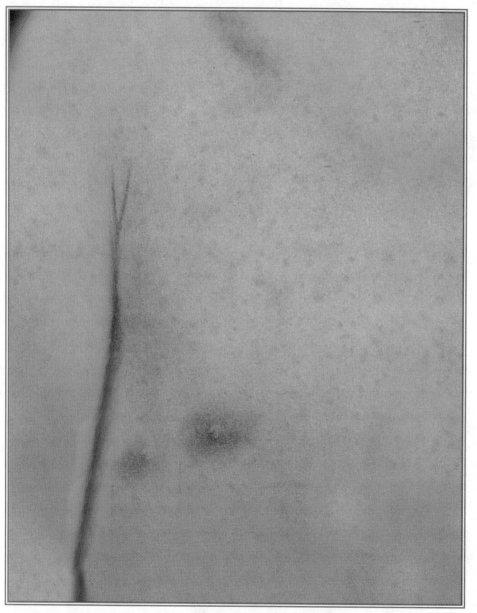

(From Habif TP: *Clinical dermatology*, ed 3, St Louis, 1996, Mosby.)

Figure 4-19   **HERPES SIMPLEX**

A, *Oral: Slightly crusted vesicular lesion on the upper lip.* **B,** *Genital: A small group of vesicles on an erythematous base.*

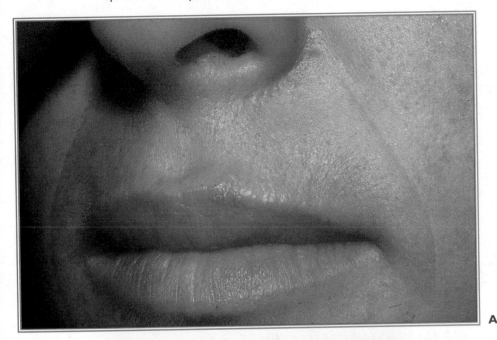

A

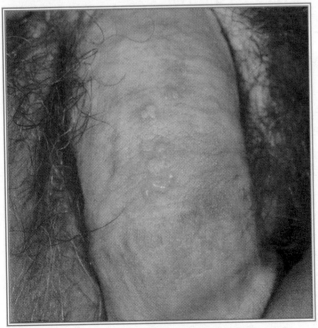

B

(**B,** From Habif TP: *Clinical dermatology,* ed 3, St Louis, 1996, Mosby.)

Figure 4-20 HERPES ZOSTER

Vesicular lesion on an erythematous base in a dermatomal pattern, extending from the right midback across the anterior and lateral aspect of the nipple line.

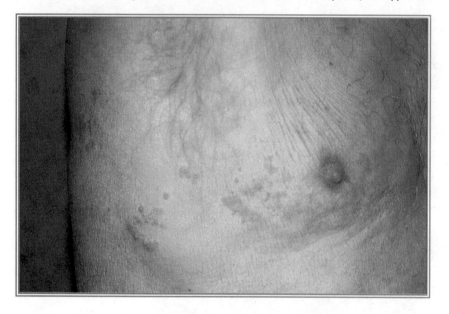

Figure 4-21 HIDRADENITIS SUPPURATIVA

Inflammatory dermatitis of the axilla with multiple sinus tracts, some of which are draining pustular fluid. Note presence of scarring.

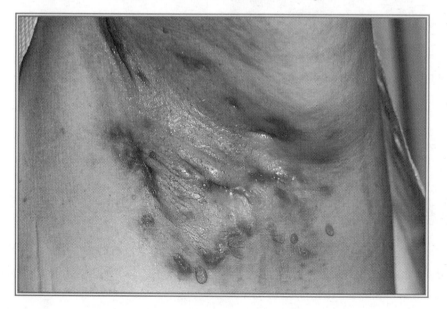

Figure 4-22   **ICHTHYOSIS VULGARIS**

Polygonal, scalelike lesions of brown hyperkeratotic skin of the lower extremities.

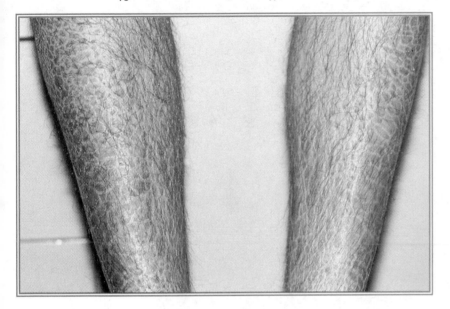

Figure 4-23   **IMPETIGO**

Erythematous lesions with honey-colored crust on the posterior thighs and buttocks region.

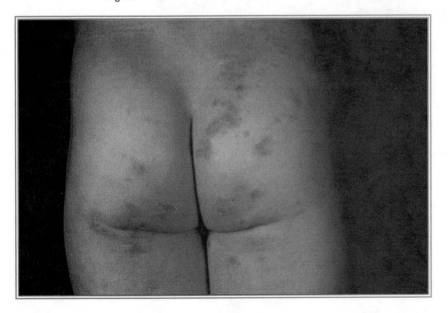

Figure 4-24 **INSECT BITES**

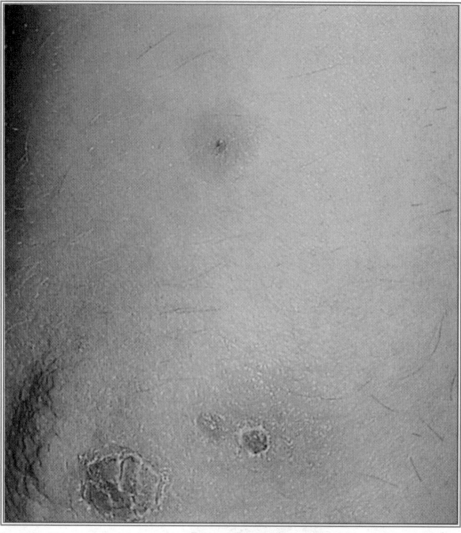

(From Cox N, Lawrence C: *Diagnostic problems in dermatology,* St Louis, 1998, Mosby.)

Figure 4-25 **KERATOSIS PILARIS**

Lateral aspect of the arm in a teenage girl, showing erythematous hyperkeratotic papules overlying hair follicles.

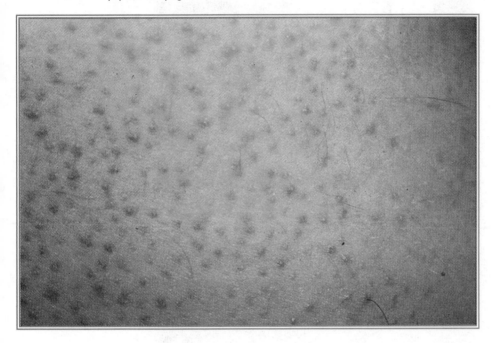

Figure 4-26 RUBEOLA

Erythematous macules on the lateral aspect of an adult male.

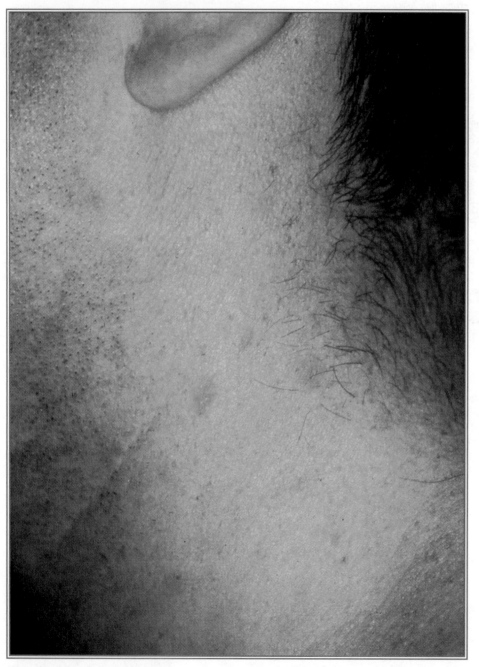

(Courtesy of Stacy R. Smith, MD.)

Figure 4-27 **PERIORAL DERMATITIS**

Inflammatory closed comedones and generalized inflammation in a perioral distribution.

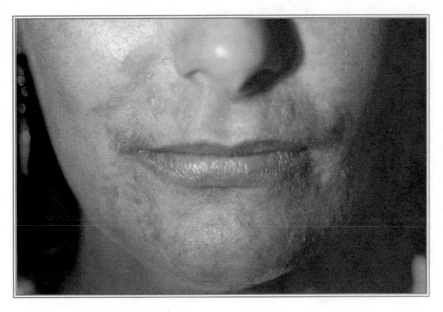

Figure 4-28 **PHOTOALLERGIC REACTION**

Erythematous to violaceous dermatitis on the dorsal aspect of the hand of a photographer who uses multiple chemicals to develop film.

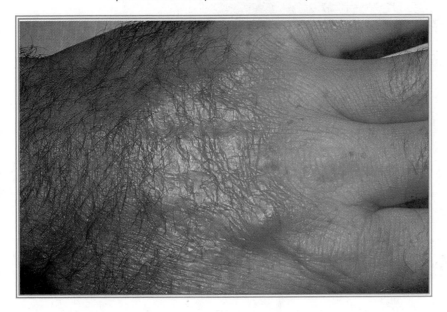

Figure 4-29   POLYMORPHOUS LIGHT ERUPTION

Diffuse, erythematous eruption, noted predominantly over sun-exposed areas.

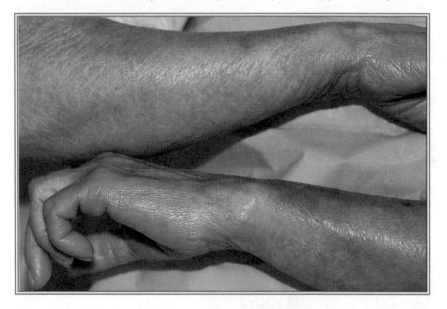

Figure 4-30   PSEUDOFOLLICULITIS

Inflammatory lesions with some pustules in the mandibular angle. Note curled hairs, some of which are embedding back into the skin.

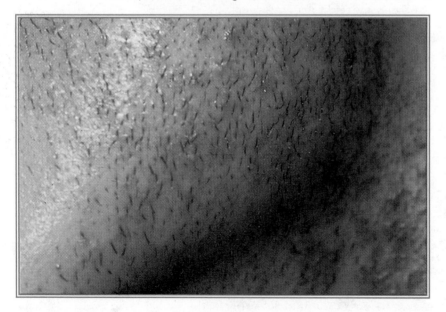

Figure 4-31 **PSORIASIS**

A, *Psoriasis vulgaris:* Thick, lichenlike plaques with some erythematous excoriation on the foot. Note hyperkeratotic nails. **B,** *Guttate psoriasis:* Generalized erythematous papular eruption on the trunk.

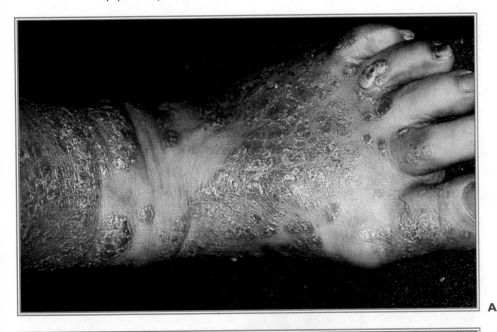

A

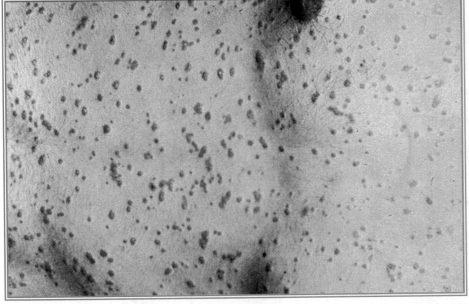

B

(**A,** Courtesy of Stacy R. Smith, MD.)

continued

Figure 4-31   PSORIASIS

C, *Pustular psoriasis: An erythematous plaque with multiple pustules.* **D,** *Scalp psoriasis: Erythematous plaquelike lesion on the anterior aspect of the scalp extending to the forehead, with overlying hyperkeratosis and lichenlike scales.*

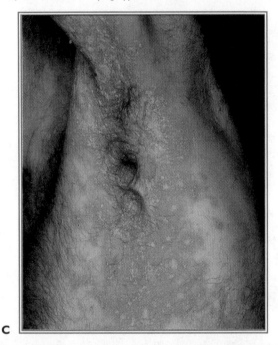

C

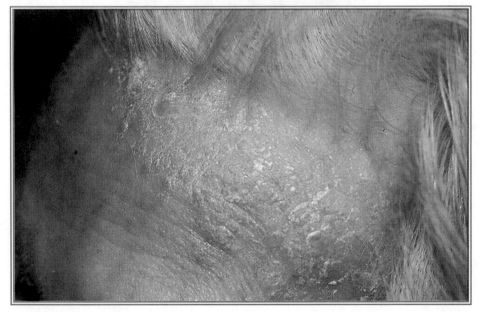

D

Figure 4-32 **PRURITIC URTICARIAL PAPULES AND PLAQUES OF PREGNANCY (PUPPP)**

Erythematous macular eruption with multiple urticarial and papular lesions on the central aspect of the abdomen in a pregnant woman.

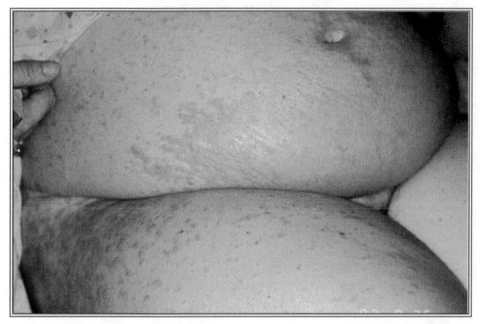

(Courtesy of Stacy R. Smith, MD.)

Figure 4-33   ROSACEA

Generalized inflammation with multiple closed comedones, predominantly located on the central aspect of the face and nose.

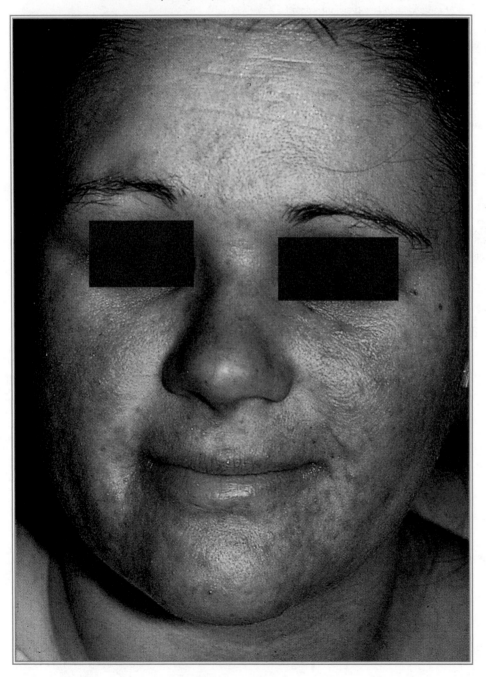

Figure 4-34 ROSEOLA INFANTUM

Erythematous macular lesions of the cheeks and generalized over the trunk of an infant.

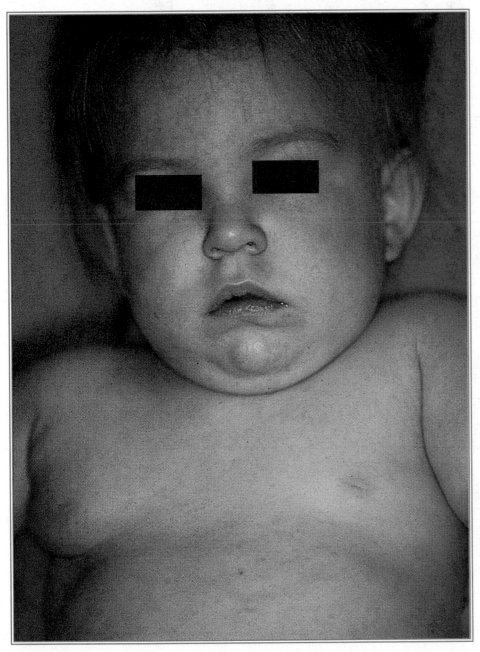

(Courtesy of Stacy R. Smith, MD.)

Figure 4-35 SEBORRHEIC DERMATITIS

Erythematous patches with some evidence of scale in the usual facial distribution.

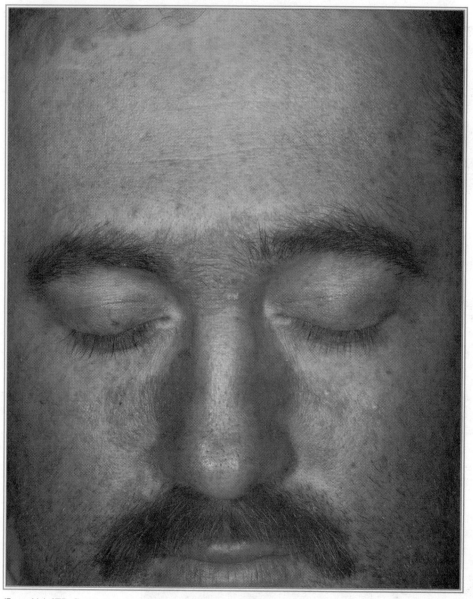

(From Habif TP: *Clinical dermatology,* ed 3, St Louis, 1996, Mosby.)

Figure 4-36 **SUNBURN**

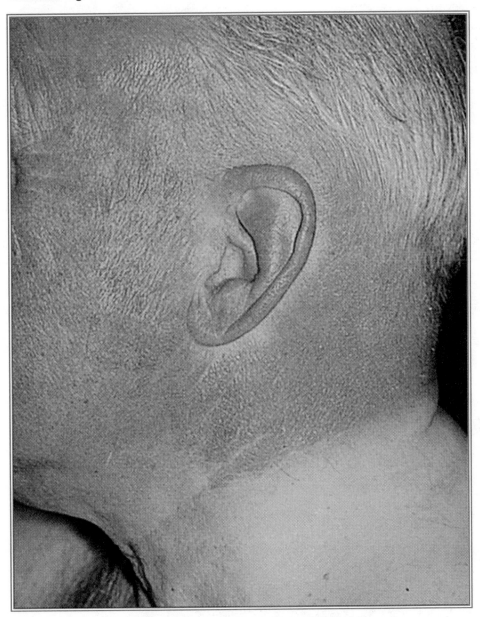

(From Cox N, Lawrence C: *Diagnostic problems in dermatology,* St Louis, 1998, Mosby.)

Figure 4-37

A, *Urticaria: Typical urticarial lesions, showing edematous macules over slightly erythematous skin.* **B,** *Dermatographism: Erythematous urticarial lesions that appeared within 1 to 2 minutes after drawing on the patient's back with a blunt object.*

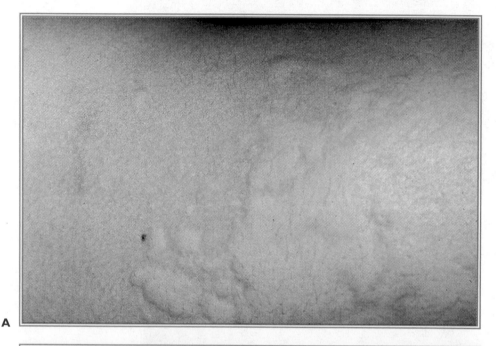

A

B

Figure 4-38 VIRAL EXANTHEM

A maculopapular eruption without follicular orientation.

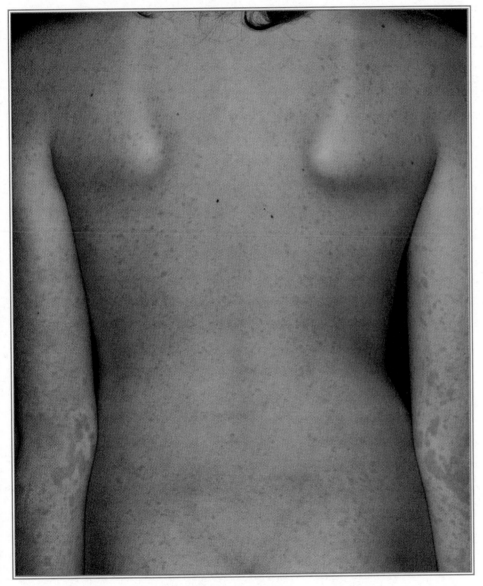

(From Habif TP: *Clinical dermatology,* ed 3, St Louis, 1996, Mosby.)

Figure 4-39   XEROSIS

Parchmentlike skin with overlying scales on a background of erythema.

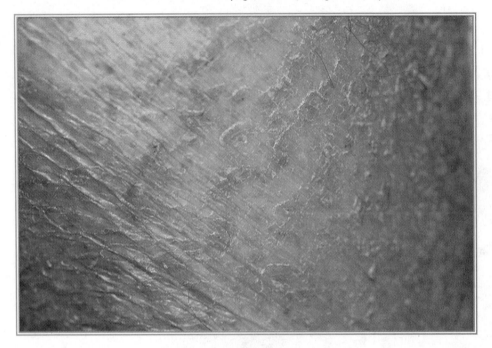

Table 4-1

Differential Diagnosis of Erythematous Disorders

DISORDER	TEXT	KEYS TO DIAGNOSIS
Acne vulgaris	Ch. 1, p. 29 (Figure 4-1)	Comedones, papules, pustules, and cysts are present on face, neck, shoulders, chest, back; peak age 14 to 15 for females, age 16 to 17 for males.
Actinic keratosis	Ch. 5, p. 235 (Figure 4-2)	Skin-colored to slightly erythematous macules with dry, rough scale.
Acute nummular eczema	Ch. 7, p. 332 (Figure 4-3)	Pruritic, coin-shaped plaques or papulovesicles on an erythematous base, which may become exudative and crusted.
Allergic contact dermatitis	Ch. 7, p. 333 (Figure 4-4)	Intensely inflammatory, pruritic papulovesicular eruption in distribution of contact with allergen.
Atopic dermatitis	Ch. 7, p. 336 (Figure 4-5)	Severe pruritus; dermatographism. Palmar markings and infraorbital folds increase. Red cheeks in infancy; sides of neck and flexural surfaces most commonly affected after age 12.
Bowen's disease	Ch. 5, p. 240 (Figure 4-6)	Erythematous, flat to slightly raised scaly plaque with erythematous and irregular surface.
Candidiasis	Ch. 1, p. 33 (Figure 4-7)	Satellite pustules; sharp, scaling border; erythematous, macerated patches; favors warm, moist environment; may be pruritic or tender.
Cellulitis	Ch. 4, p. 182 (Figure 4-8)	Erythematous, edematous, tense, painful tissue surrounding lesion. Lymphatic streaking may be prominent. Usually occurs on an extremity or the face. Diffuse border.
Chickenpox (varicella)	Ch. 2, p. 64 (Figure 4-9)	Maculopapular rash that begins on chest and back, then forms small, superficial vesicles on an erythematous base ("dewdrop on a rose petal"); intensely pruritic.
Dermatophyte infections	Ch. 3, p. 116 (Figure 4-10)	Presentation depends on area of involvement: patchy loss of hair; erythematous ring-shaped patches with central clearing and advancing scaling border; fissured, macerated skin between toes. Pruritus is common.
Dyshidrotic eczema (pompholyx)	Ch. 7, p. 339 (Figure 4-11)	Pruritus with bilateral, symmetric vesicles on eczematous soles and palms. Sides of fingers may resemble tapioca; hands are erythematous and damp.
Erysipelas	Ch. 4, p. 182 (Figure 4-12)	Erythematous, edematous, tense, painful tissue surrounding lesion. Lymphatic streaking is more obvious than in cellulitis. Border is sharply marginated.
Erythema infectiosum	Ch. 4, p. 183 (Figure 4-13)	Erythematous, bright red macules and papules occur suddenly on the cheeks. Lacy rash on trunk, buttocks and upper arms. Generally known as "slapped cheek appearance."

continued

Table 4-1 *continued*

DISORDER	TEXT	KEYS TO DIAGNOSIS
Erythema multiforme	Ch. 4, p. 185 (Figure 4-14)	Macules, papules, vesicles, and bullae all may be present ("multiform"). Hallmark is the iris or target lesion, usually on extensor surfaces, palms, and soles. Some may appear urticarial.
Folliculitis	Ch. 1, p. 36 (Figure 4-15)	Follicular, erythematous papules and pustules on any hair-bearing surface; *Pseudomonas* folliculitis occurs 1 to 3 days after use of a hot tub.
Furuncles and carbuncles	Ch. 1, p. 38 (Figures 4-16 and 4-17)	*Furuncles:* 1 to 5 cm tender nodules with surrounding erythema. May become fluctuant *Carbuncles:* 3 to 10 cm tender erythematous nodules that drain pus from multiple follicular orifices.
German measles (rubella)	Ch. 4, p. 187 (Figure 4-18)	Dusky red, blotchy macular eruption on face or neck that develops into small, discrete pink macules and papules over trunk and extremities.
Herpes simplex	Ch. 2, p. 66 (Figure 4-19)	Grouped vesicles with clear to cloudy fluid on an erythematous and edematous base. Eruption may be preceded by a prodrome of burning and tingling.
Herpes zoster	Ch. 2, p. 70 (Figure 4-20)	Grouped vesicles on an erythematous, tender base along a sensory nerve (dermatome). Lesions usually unilateral and painful. Thoracic, trigeminal, and cervical distributions are most common.
Hidradenitis suppurativa	Ch. 1, p. 41 (Figure 4-21)	Double comedone; foul-smelling discharge. Subcutaneous sinus tracts; adenopathy; axillae, groin, perineum.
Icythyosis vulgaris	Ch. 3, p. 126 (Figure 4-22)	Dry, white rectangular scales on an erythematous base, especially over extensor extremities. Accentuation of palmar and sole creases. Pruritus and rough skin are common.
Impetigo	Ch. 2, p. 73 (Figure 4-23)	Vesicles on an erythematous base that rupture to form honey-colored crusts, usually around mouth. Regional adenopathy and pruritus are common.
Insect bites	(Figure 4-24)	Erythematous papule with central punctum. Usually pruritic.
Keratosis pilaris	Ch. 1, p. 43 (Figure 4-25)	Small, discrete follicular papules on posterior pilaris, upper arms, and anterior thighs. May be erythematous.
Measles (rubeola)	Ch. 4, p. 189 (Figure 4-26)	Prodrome of cough, coryza, conjunctivitis, and high fever with cervical lymphadenopathy. Erythematous, pruritic macules become papular on face, neck, trunk, and extremities.
Perioral Dermatitis	Ch. 1, p. 44 (Figure 4-27)	Pruritic, burning, discrete erythematous or flesh-colored papules and pustules around mouth and in nasolabial folds.
Photoallergic Reaction	Ch. 4, p. 190 (Figure 4-28)	Erythematous papular rash in sun-exposed reaction areas. No sharp borders; pruritus; occurs 24 hours or more after sun exposure.

Table 4-1 *continued*

DISORDER	TEXT	KEYS TO DIAGNOSIS
Polymorphous light eruption	Ch. 4, p. 192 (Figure 4-29)	Pruritic, erythematous papules scattered over sun-exposed areas. Occurs within a few hours of sun exposure and lasts for 2 or 3 days.
Pseudofolliculitis	Ch. 1, p. 46 (Figure 4-30)	Erythematous papules and pustules on shaved areas, especially beards of men with coarse, curly hair. May be asymptomatic or painful and pruritic.
Psoriasis	Ch. 3, p. 134 (Figure 4-31)	Erythematous papules, and plaques with silver-white scales. Symmetric distribution is common. Frequently on knees, elbows, scalp, back, genitalia, intergluteal folds, and nails.
Pruritic urticarial papules and plaques pregnancy (PUPPP)	Ch. 7, p. 345 (Figure 4-32)	Tiny, erythematous pruritic plaques and papules. Occurs late third trimester in primigravidas. Usually begins on abdomen and spreads to buttocks, arms, and hands.
Rosacea	Ch. 1, p. 48 (Figure 4-33)	Facial papules and pustules but no comedones; flushing, telangiectasias, rhinophyma; triggered by hot foods, emotional stress.
Roseola infantum	Ch. 4, p. 194 (Figure 4-34)	Usually occurs before 2 years of age. High fever, which subsides as pink macular rash develops.
Seborrheic dermatitis	Ch. 3, p. 138 (Figure 4-35)	Sharply marginated yellowish-red patches with sharp borders and greasy scales. Scalp, central face, eyebrows, eyelids, nasolabial folds, and external ear are most commonly affected. May be pruritic.
Sunburn	Ch. 4, p. 195 (Figure 4-36)	Erythema develops with sun exposure. Sharp boundaries of sun-exposed areas. Blisters occur with severe forms.
Urticaria	Ch. 4, p. 198 (Figure 4-37)	Intense pruritus; primary lesion is the wheal; migration of lesions; angioedema; dermatographism.
Viral exanthem	(Figure 4-38)	Dry, slightly scaly skin with variable erythema and superficial fissuring. Pruritus is common. Most prominent on extremities.
Xerosis (dry skin)	Ch. 7, p. 349 (Figure 4-39)	Dry, slightly scaly skin with variable erythema and superficial fissuring. Pruritus is common; most prominent on extremities.

Cellulitis and Erysipelas

Overview

Pathophysiology

Cellulitis and erysipelas both occur as a complication of a wound, ulcer, bite, fissure, or other break in skin integrity. **Cellulitis** is caused by the invasion of *Staphylococcus* or *Streptococcus* spp. (in adults), *Hemophilus influenzae* (in children less than 2 years), or gram-negative bacteria. **Erysipelas** is a form of cellulitis, which results from the invasion of group A beta-hemolytic *streptococcus*. In both cases the invading organism penetrates the dermis and subcutaneous tissues, resulting in a deep infection. Without treatment the morbidity rate approaches 80% in infants and 75% in the frail or elderly.

Epidemiology

Persons with malnutrition, alcoholism, recent infections, or edema of any origin are at increased risk. Erysipelas is most common in infants, young children, and older adults. Patients who have recovered from one episode of cellulitis are predisposed to recurrences, possibly as a result of lymphatic damage caused during the initial episode.

Assessment

Clinical Presentation

Skin surrounding the offending lesion is usually erythematous, edematous, tense, and painful. Lymphatic involvement ("streaking") may be prominent. Fever, chills, headache, malaise, and vomiting are common sequelae. If left untreated, the condition may progress to lymphadenopathy and septicemia. While **cellulitis** presents without a well-marginated border, **erysipelas** displays a sharply marginated periphery and streaking is more obvious. The usual site of predilection is an extremity or face. In infants, the abdominal wall is usually affected.

Diagnostics

Obtaining a **culture of material** from the wound is appropriate, especially if there is drainage. Without obvious drainage, biopsy is the easier method of obtaining a sample. A **blood culture** should be performed if septicemia is suspected. A complete blood count **(CBC)** may show an elevated white blood cell count **(WBC)** with shift to the left, and a mildly elevated sedimentation rate. **Allergic patch testing** may be indicated to rule out contact dermatitis.

Differential Diagnosis
- Hives (lesions are more generalized)
- Allergic contact dermatitis (lesions are usually distributed in areas where contact with the offending agent occurs.)

Treatment

Nonpharmacologic
Bed rest with elevation of an affected extremity may help relieve pain. Hot packs hasten resolution of cellulitis.

Pharmacologic

Topical Agents
Pain can be lessened with cool **Burow's solution** compresses.

Systemic Agents
Dicloxacillin (Dynapen) 250 mg PO qid or **penicillin with clavulanate potassium (Augmentin)** 500 mg PO bid should be used.

If group A *streptococcus* has been identified as the offending organism, **penicillin V** 250 mg PO qid is prescribed.

Either clindamycin (Cleocin) 300 mg PO q6h for 10 to14 days or **azithromycin (Zithromax)** 500 mg PO the first day, followed by 250 mg PO qd for 4 days, is recommended for patients allergic to penicillin.

Pain management is always a consideration, and **acetaminophen with codeine** (1 to 2 tablets q4-6h prn) is appropriate.

CELLULITIS
- Discomfort can be lessened by elevating the affected extremity and using cool compresses; bed rest may be recommended
- Is usually due to a bacterial infection; therefore, antibiotics should be taken as prescribed
- If left untreated, or if not responding to treatment, may have severe consequences

Indications for Referral

- *H. influenzae* cellulitis (prompt treatment is essential).
- Septicemia.
- Hospitalization with intravenous antibiotic or other supportive therapy.

Erythema Infectiosum

Overview

Pathophysiology
A mildly contagious viral disease, erythema infectiosum ("slapped cheek," fifth disease) is caused by the B19 parvovirus.

Epidemiology

The disorder occurs most often in children between 2 and 10 years of age, although it may also occur in adults. There is a female-to-male predominance of 2:1. It usually occurs in the spring and summer in epidemics every 5 to 6 years. Exposure during pregnancy causes an increase in the rate of miscarriages, although no increase in birth defects.

Assessment

Clinical Presentation

Prodromal symptoms are usually mild or absent. There is no lymphadenopathy, although older individuals may complain of joint pain.

Erythematous, bright red macules and papules occur suddenly on the cheeks. They coalesce but spare the nasolabial folds and perioral area. Fading occurs in 3 to 4 days.

A lacy rash on the trunk, buttocks, and extremities (especially upper arms) appears 24 hours or so after the slapped cheek presentation and persists for 6 to 10 days. Headache and gastrointestinal symptoms may be present. A characteristic feature is that the condition may recur briefly a few times.

Adults (especially women) who acquire the disease may experience pruritus and migratory arthritis, which may last for several months.

Diagnostics
- No specific diagnostic test is available.
- Eosinophilia may occur transiently for a few weeks.

Differential Diagnosis
- Other viral exanthem (lesions are usually more generalized) (see Figure 4-38).

Treatment

Only supportive therapy is given. The disease resolves spontaneously.

ERYTHEMA INFECTIOSUM

- Is a mildly contagious viral infection
- Requires supportive therapy only to relieve headache and gastrointestinal (GI) symptoms
- Resolves spontaneously

Indications for Referral

- None.

Erythema Multiforme: Minor

Overview

Pathophysiology

Erythema multiforme (EM) is believed to be a hypersensitivity disorder triggered by a specific immune response to a precipitating factor. It may present in either a mild or a severe form. The disorder is idiopathic and self-limiting in 20% to 50% of cases. Precipitating factors include the following:

- Herpes simplex infections, both type I and type II (usually occurs 4 to 10 days after the herpes outbreak)
- Drugs, including penicillin, sulfonamides, birth control pills, salicylates, barbiturates, and dilantin
- Pregnancy, usually the third trimester
- Internal infections, including *Streptococcus*, deep fungal, and viral
- Immunizations to poliomyelitis, tuberculosis, or smallpox

Epidemiology

Erythema multiforme is most common in young, healthy adults ages 20 to 40 but may present at any age. Severe bullous forms are most common in children and adolescents. It occurs most frequently in winter and early spring. About one third of cases are recurrent.

Assessment

Clinical Presentation

Mild prodromal symptoms of malaise and sore throat may occur up to 1 week before the development of skin lesions. As the name suggests, the lesions are of many forms (multiform), including macules, papules, vesicles, and bullae. Although the hallmark is the **iris or target lesion,** a lesion with a reddish or reddish-blue center, pale ring, and surrounding darker ring, many of the lesions are arcs and semicircles. Lesions can occur anywhere on the skin and mucus membranes but are usually found on extensor surfaces, palms, and soles. Mucosal involvement usually occurs simultaneously with skin involvement as edematous, erythematous lesions that progress within hours to erosions. Postinflammatory hyperpigmentation is common. The condition usually resolves within 2 to 3 weeks.

A variant of EM minor is EM major **(Stevens-Johnson syndrome).** This disorder involves the mucus membranes and severe blistering. It begins with a sudden high fever, malaise, cough, sore throat, myalgias, and arthralgias, which may last up to 2 to 3 weeks. Vesicles and ulcerations occur on the oral mucus membranes, lips, nasal passages, eyes, and genitalia.

Diagnostics

- Thorough history taking is essential to identify any precipitating factors.
- CBC with differential may show an elevated eosinophil count if the cause is a drug reaction.
- A skin biopsy may be helpful but is not always diagnostic.

Differential Diagnosis

- Urticaria (lesions are more generalized, extremely pruritic; wheals and angioedema are common
- Nummular eczema (lesions usually on arms, legs, and neck)
- Aphthous stomatitis or canker sores (lesions are usually a few millimeters in diameter and solitary)
- Drug eruptions (difficult to differentiate, but lesions are not "targetoid")
- Viral exanthems (lesions are usually smaller [a few millimeters in diameter] and not "targetoid")
- Vasculitis (lesions are smaller [a few millimeters in diameter]; palpable purpura is a characteristic sign; subcutaneous nodules, ulcerations, and ecchymoses are common)

Treatment

Nonpharmacologic

Cool or lukewarm compresses for erosive or bullous lesions are soothing.

Pharmacologic

Topical Agents

Topical agents should be used cautiously if numerous lesions are present (extensive disruption of the skin's barrier function could increase systemic absorption). **Hydrogen peroxide mouthwash** is helpful for cleansing and débriding. **Viscous lidocaine (Xylocaine)** may be used for the anesthetic effects on oral lesions.

In younger children **diphenhydramine (Benadryl)** as an oral rinse has less risk of aspiration and is more easily tolerated. Group IV topical steroids such as **mometasone furoate 0.1% (Elocon) or triamcinolone acetonide 0.1% (Kenalog)** may be applied bid to pruritic lesions.

ERYTHEMA MULTIFORME

- Is an inflammatory disorder for which no cause can be found in about 50% of cases
- Is recurrent in about one third of cases; it is therefore important to reduce or eliminate precipitating factors such as herpes simplex virus (HSV) type 1 or type 2 infections, mycoplasma infections, immunizations, and certain medications
- May cause lesions on the oral mucosa; if so, a soft or liquid diet may be more easily tolerated
- Pruritus can be relieved with oral antihistamines
- Blisters can be soothed with cool Burow's solution compresses

Systemic Agents

An empirical course of **valacyclovir (Valtrex)** 500 mg PO tid for 10 days or **famciclovir (Famvir)** 250 mg PO bid for 10 days is recommended even if a history of herpes simplex virus is not obtained.

Oral corticosteroids (**prednisone** 1 to 2 mg/kg/day orally in three divided doses) are standard treatment unless an underlying infection is present. A course of 1 to 2 weeks is usually sufficient.

Antihistamines such as **hydroxyzine (Atarax)** 25 mg PO q4h are useful for pruritic symptoms.

Tetracycline or erythromycin 250 mg PO qd is appropriate if mycoplasmal infection is present.

If lesions become secondarily infected, **dicloxacillin (Dynapen)** 250 mg PO qid for 10 to 14 days; for the penicillin-allergic patient, **clindamycin (Cleocin)** 300 mg PO q6h also for 10 to 14 days is appropriate.

Indications for Referral

- Stevens-Johnson syndrome.
- Ocular involvement (refer to ophthalmologist).

German Measles (Rubella)

Overview

Pathophysiology

Transmission of the virus results from droplet spread from the nasopharynx of infectious individuals. The virus is spread up to 1 week before and 2 weeks after the clinical onset of the disease. Birth defects occur in 25% of cases in which the pregnant mother was infected with rubella during the first trimester. The disease confers long-term immunity; however, reinfection of previously immune individuals does occur.

Epidemiology

German measles occurs throughout the world and is endemic in large cities. Epidemics occur at irregular intervals (6 to 9 years), usually during the winter and spring. It mainly affects older children and young adults.

Assessment

Clinical Presentation

After a 2- to 3-week incubation period mild prodromal symptoms of headache, malaise, and low-grade fever occur. Pain on lateral gaze, as well as occipital and postauricular lymphadenopathy, characteristically occurs 3 to 5 days before the cutaneous eruption. Small erythematous macules on the palate may also precede the appearance of the rash.

The rash develops on the face or neck as a dusky red, blotchy macular eruption that rapidly extends to the trunk and extremities. It may be absent in up to 50% of exposed children but is present in virtually all adults and is characteristically pruritic. The lesions are discrete, small, pinkish round or oval macules and papules. They fade in 1 to 2 days.

Diagnostics

- Diagnosis is based on clinical presentation and history.
- Lab tests results may reveal transient thrombocytopenia and leukopenia.

Differential Diagnosis

- Enteroviral and adenoviral illness (generalized maculopapular eruption of acute onset)
- Rubeola (lesions begin on the face but are larger and coalesce)
- Drug eruption (no enlargement of occipital nodes occurs)
- Roseola infantum (lesions occur on the face and are larger; lesions are rare on the trunk)
- Infectious mononucleosis (maculopapular eruption usually occurs after a course of ampicillin or amoxicillin)

Treatment

Nonpharmacologic

Bed rest is recommended.

Pharmacologic

Topical Agents

None is necessary.

Systemic Agents

Symptomatic relief with **acetaminophen (Tylenol)** or nonsteroidal antiinflammatory agents such as **ibuprofen (Motrin, Advil, Aleve)** may be helpful.

GERMAN MEASLES

- Is contagious through droplet spread 1 week before and 2 weeks after skin lesions are visible
- Causes birth defects in 25% of cases when it occurs during the first trimester
- Symptoms can be reduced with acetaminophen, ibuprofen, and bed rest

---

✳ | **Indications for Referral**

> • Referral is not indicated unless complications develop.

Measles (Rubeola)

Overview

Pathophysiology

Infection of measles occurs through transmission of droplets from the nasopharynx and upper respiratory tract of infectious people. After a 10- to 14-day incubation period a viremia occurs; it disappears as the rash emerges.

Epidemiology

There is a worldwide distribution with a high prevalence in persons 10 years of age or older. Maternal antibody gives passive immunity to the newborn for 6 to 7 months. One episode produces lifelong immunity.

Assessment

Clinical Presentation

The prodromal symptoms are characterized by the "three C's": cough, coryza, and conjunctivitis. The fever is high for 1 to 2 days, returns to normal, and then becomes elevated again. Additionally the anterior cervical lymph nodes become enlarged and tender. The prodrome lasts 3 to 4 days, followed by the appearance of tiny white spots with an erythematous base on the buccal mucosa (Koplik's spots). The eruption of erythematous, pruritic macules begins 24 to 36 hours later. The macules become papular, then enlarge and coalesce, resulting in a blotchy appearance. The rash begins on the face and extends down to the neck, trunk, and extremities. It reaches its peak in 3 to 5 days before fading over the next few days.

Diagnostics

• The diagnosis is based on the clinical presentation and history.

Differential Diagnosis

• Roseola infantum (lesions occur on the face and are larger; lesions are rare on the trunk)

MEASLES

• Is a highly contagious viral disease spread by droplets from the nasopharynx of infected individuals

• Can be spread from a few days before the prodrome until 4 days after the rash is evident

• Symptoms can be reduced with acetaminophen, ibuprofen, and bed rest

- Rubella (prodrome consists of fatigue, headache, and mild fever; Koplik's spots do not occur)
- Infectious mononucleosis (maculopapular eruption usually occurs after a course of ampicillin or amoxicillin)

Treatment

Nonpharmacologic
Bed rest is recommended.

Pharmacologic

Topical Agents
Antipruritic lotions such as **Sarna** or **Calamine** are beneficial; **Aveeno bath treatments** for itchy skin may also be soothing.

Topical diphenhydramine (Benadryl) should be avoided because allergic reactions are not uncommon and large doses may cause pediatric toxicity, especially if combined with oral doses.

Systemic Agents
Acetaminophen (Tylenol) and antihistamines such as **diphenhydramine (Benadryl)** or **hydroxyzine (Atarax)** 25 mg PO tid and qhs will help relieve symptoms.

Indications for Referral

- Development of a secondary bacterial infection or encephalitis.

Photoallergic Reaction

Overview

Pathophysiology
Photoallergic reactions result from a combination of factors, any of which alone causes no problem. Rather, it is the combined effects that lead to a photoallergic disorder. The reaction requires a photosensitizing substance (topical or oral) plus ultraviolet light. Common oral photosensitizers include tetracyclines, thiazide diuretics, sulfonamides, psoralens, and promethazines. Topical photosensitizers include perfumes, mangos, limes, wild celery, coal tar derivatives, and para-aminobenzoic acid (PABA) sunscreen.

Epidemiology

No age, sex, or skin type prevalence. It is less common than phototoxic reactions (sunburn).

Assessment

Clinical Presentation

The predominant sign is an **erythematous macular to papular eruption,** concentrated in **sun-exposed areas.** There are **no sharp borders.** Lesions may also occur in non–sun-exposed areas. The eruption usually occurs 24 hours or more after exposure to light. The chief complaint is **pruritus.**

Diagnostics

- Diagnosis can usually be made on the basis of clinical presentation and history alone.
- Photopatch testing (applying suspected contact sensitizer to the skin and exposing to sunlight) may be helpful.
- Antinuclear antibody (ANA) serologic studies (to differentiate from lupus erythematosus).

Differential Diagnosis

- Allergic contact dermatitis (lesions are usually distributed in areas where contact with the offending agent occurs)
- Lupus erythematosus (positive ANA test result; lesion on face forms a "butterfly" pattern)
- Polymorphous light eruption (lesions also occur on sun-protected areas and may be macular, papular, or vesicular)

Treatment

Nonpharmacologic

Resolution occurs spontaneously if either sunlight or the photosensitizing agent is avoided.

Pharmacologic

Topical Agents

Sunscreens may be helpful but are usually not completely effective. For lesions on the face low- to mid-potency steroids may be used bid for short periods: **hydrocortisone (Hytone) 2.5%, desonide (Desowen) 0.05%, triamcinolone acetonide (Kenalog) 0.1%,** or **alclometasone dipropionate (Aclovate) 0.05%.**

For *nonfacial* lesions, middle- to high-potency steroids may be of help: **triamcinolone acetonide (Aristocort) 0.5%** or **mometasone furoate (Elocon) 0.1%,** both used bid

---

PHOTOALLERGIC REACTION

- Results from a combination of factors, all of which must be present for the disorder to occur
- May cause a pruritus that can be relieved with oral antihistamines and cool compresses
- Will resolve spontaneously if either of the photosensitizing agents is removed
- Can be prevented or minimized with conscientious sun protection (sunscreens, protective clothing, etc.)

Systemic Agents

For severely pruritic lesions unrelieved by topical steroids, **prednisone** 20 mg PO qd for 3 to 7 days may be helpful. For insomnia resulting from pruritus, **hydroxyzine (Atarax)** 25 to 50 mg PO qhs is recommended.

Indications for Referral

- Failure of the lesions to resolve within a few days.

Polymorphous Light Eruption

Overview

Pathophysiology

The exact causative mechanism is unknown, but most probably is a cutaneous reaction that can develop in anyone under adequate irradiation and certain environmental conditions.

Epidemiology

Polymorphous light eruption (PLE) is second only to sunburn in prevalence of a photosensitive eruption. It is most common in American Indians, Northern European races, and North American Anglo-Saxons, but is rare in Australians and people in the tropics. The age of onset ranges from 2 to 74 years with the majority between 11 and 30 years. Females are more often affected than males. Attacks usually occur in the spring (especially during the first few days of vacationing at the beach or in high altitudes) and early summer. Remission or improvement in late summer is attributed to thickening of the stratum corneum through tanning. There is a 15% familial history.

Assessment

Clinical Presentation

A few hours to days after sun exposure (typically 18 hours) a crop of pruritic, erythematous papules erupt, widely scattered, over any sun-exposed area. Lesions may coalesce into plaques and spread to nonexposed areas. Occasionally the lesions are vesicular. The submental, midupper lip, and eyelids are usually spared. Pruritus usually precedes the eruption and may (rarely) be severe. Lesions spontaneously clear in 1 to 2 weeks with avoidance of sun exposure. Sunburn is not a prominent feature.

Diagnostics
- ANA serologic results rule out lupus erythematosus.
- Skin biopsy may be necessary to make a definitive diagnosis

Differential Diagnosis
- Lupus erythematosus (positive ANA test result; lesions are limited to areas exposed to sunlight, especially upper cheeks, scalp, neck, and arms)
- Erythema multiforme (lesions are targetoid and more generalized)
- Photo contact dermatitis (lesions are limited to sun-exposed areas with sparing on sun-protected areas)
- Solar urticaria (lesions are more urticarial, larger, and more common on the trunk)

Treatment

Spontaneous resolution occurs in 30% to 50% of cases.

Nonpharmacologic
Avoidance of sunlight is paramount. When avoidance is impossible, the use of sunscreens and protective clothing is essential.

Pharmacologic

Topical Agents
Diflorasone diacetate (Psorcon) 0.05% ointment (or another class I corticosteroid) applied bid will help reduce pruritus and erythema. **Mometasone furoate (Elocon 0.1%)** cream or lotion (or another class IV corticosteroid) is suitable for less intense reactions.

Desensitization phototherapy (controlled and repeated exposure to ultraviolet B [UVB] radiation) is also effective. Patients wear protective clothing over the involved areas and receive five treatments per week for 3 weeks with gradually increasing exposure times. For resistant or recalcitrant cases, ultraviolet A therapy with 8-methoxypsoralen (PUVA) therapy may be effective (see Psoriasis).

Systemic Agents
Prednisone 0.5 to 1.0 mg/kg/day PO qAM for 5 days may be appropriate for severe inflammations. **Hydroxyzine (Atarax)** 25 to 50 mg q6h will help relieve the itching but will not reduce erythema. Antimalarials (**hydroxychloroquine** 100 mg PO bid)

POLYMORPHOUS LIGHT ERUPTION

- Resolves spontaneously in 30% to 50% of cases when either sunlight or the photosensitizing agent is avoided
- Pruritus can be reduced with oral antihistamines
- Will not occur unless all precipitating factors are present; thus can be prevented or minimized with conscientious sun protection (sunscreens, protective clothing, etc.)

should be considered for patients who do not respond to more conventional therapy.

Indications for Referral

- Desensitization phototherapy.
- Psoralen UVA (PUVA).

Roseola Infantum (Exanthem Subitum)

Overview

Pathophysiology
The disorder roseola infantum probably represents a syndrome caused by several different viruses, one of which may be herpesvirus 6.

Epidemiology
Roseola occurs in infants aged 6 months to 4 years. Ninety percent of cases occur in the first 2 years of life. Roseola is the most common cause of febrile convulsions in this age group.

Assessment

Clinical Presentation
The disorder begins as an abrupt fever that may reach as high as 106° F. Periorbital edema is common. The child is otherwise asymptomatic except for perhaps slight anorexia or nausea. The fever precedes skin manifestations by 3 to 4 days and subsides as the rash begins. Numerous pink macules erupt and fade after 24 hours. Cervical and occipital lymph nodes are usually enlarged.

Diagnostics
- Laboratory tests are not yet available for confirmation.

Differential Diagnosis
- Rubeola (lesions begin on the face but are larger and coalesce)
- Rubella (small pink maculopapules; begins on face and spreads to trunk)
- Scarlet fever (associated with finely thickened, scaly skin, especially on the arms)

ROSEOLA INFANTUM

- May result in dehydration if vomiting occurs; fluid replacement is therefore essential
- Fever may be lessened with cool compresses, acetaminophen, and/or ibuprofen
- Bed rest is recommended

- Infectious mononucleosis (maculopapular eruption usually occurs after a course of ampicillin or amoxicillin)
- Allergic drug eruptions (usually presents with overlying scale; prior history of drug ingestion)

Treatment

Nonpharmacologic
Bed rest and fluid management are recommended, especially when the condition is associated with nausea and vomiting. Cool compresses help control fever.

Pharmacologic

Topical Agents
None are recommended.

Systemic Agents
Acetaminophen (Tylenol) or nonsteroidal antiinflammatory agents such as **ibuprofen (Motrin)** control fever and provide comfort.

Indications for Referral

- Febrile convulsions.

Sunburn (Phototoxic Reaction)

Overview

General Information
In general about two thirds of the total amount of ultraviolet light (UVL) reaches the earth between the hours of 10:00 AM and 2:00 PM and varies with the season, weather, and air pollution. The ultraviolet A wave dosage (UVA) in winter is only 23% of the summertime dose. Complete cloud cover decreases UV exposure by about 50%. Thin cloud cover on a bright day allows 60% to 80% of UVA penetration. Reflection of sunlight from sand is about 23%; from water, anywhere from 0% to 100% depending on the angle of sunlight; and from snow, about 70% to 90%. About 50% of UVL penetrates through water. Fluorescent sun lamps in sun-

tanning booths emit 26 times more deoxyribonucleic acid (DNA)-damaging UVL than an equivalent amount of sunlight.

Pathophysiology

Erythema is produced by dilatation of venules, terminal arterioles, and capillaries as either a direct effect on the vascular wall or an indirect effect from photochemically induced mediators. The epidermis reflects and scatters about 10% of ultraviolet B (UVB) light. About 20% of UVB penetrates the stratum corneum into the dermis. UVA has a relatively greater histologic effect on the dermis than on the epidermis. UVB rays are the most efficient carcinogenic rays. UVA markedly accentuates UVB damage.

Variation in the minimal erythema dose (MED) on a seasonal basis is probably related to an increase in horny layer thickness and induced melanogenesis. Multiple exposures to UVL markedly decrease the threshold for subsequent UV-induced inflammation and pigmentation.

Immediate tanning occurs with 8 to 10 minutes of midday sun exposure, reaches a peak within 60 minutes, and rapidly fades after 1 hour. After exposure of 2 hours the skin may remain pigmented for 1 to 2 days, after which newly synthesized melanin, produced by a proliferation and hypertrophy of melanocytes, causes a delayed tanning reaction.

Epidemiology

Sunburn is most prevalent in fair-skinned individuals. Pregnancy increases the susceptibility and extent of sunburning by decreasing the MED by 50%. Common nomenclature for distinguishing skin types and anticipating sunburn potential is as follows:

Type I: Always burns, never tans
Type II: Burns easily, tans minimally
Type III: Burns moderately, tans gradually
Type IV: Burns minimally, tans well
Type V: Rarely burns, tans profusely
Type VI: Never burns, deeply pigmented

Assessment

Clinical Presentation

Mild forms present as erythema, which develops over a latent period of 3 to 4 hours and persists from a few hours to a few days. Increased doses of sunlight decrease the latency and increase the persistence of erythema. Symptoms usually peak in 16 to 24 hours.

There are sharp boundaries distinguishing the sun-exposed from the non-sun-exposed skin. Severe forms present with edema, blistering, and desquamation. In the absence of superinfection scarring does not occur.

Differential Diagnosis

- Phototoxic drug eruptions (tetracycline, thiazide diuretics, phenothiazines, sulfonamides, and psoralens can increase sensitivity to sunlight)
- Polymorphous light eruption (lesions may be macular, papular, urticarial, or vesicular and are more generalized with areas of normal skin)

Treatment

Nonpharmacologic

Prevention is the best treatment. Patients should be encouraged and reminded to use **sunscreen,** wear **protective clothing,** and **minimize exposure** to the sun during midday (10:00 AM to 2:00 PM). The amount of protection derived from clothing is related to the tightness of the weave, not the color or thickness of material.

Cool compresses provide soothing relief to the irritation and pain of a sunburn.

Diagnostics

- Diagnosis is made by clinical presentation and history.

Pharmacologic

Topical Agents

Hydrocortisone 1% lotion, applied bid will help decrease erythema and pain or itching.

Systemic Agents

Aspirin 325 to 500 mg PO q4h, **indomethicin (Indocin)** 25 mg PO bid to tid, or **ibuprofen (Advil, Motrin, Aleve)** 400 mg PO q4-6h helps to reduce discomfort.

Prednisone given in rapidly tapering doses of 60 mg, 40 mg, and 20 mg PO qAM over 3 days may help reduce inflammation and erythema.

Antihistamines such as **hydroxyzine (Atarax)** 25 to 50 mg PO qhs and **Loratadine (Claritin)** 10 mg PO qAM may reduce sunburn development.

SUNBURN

- Prevention is key
- Can be minimized through the use of sunscreen applied every 2 hours when outdoors (more frequently if swimming or perspiring heavily), wearing sun-protective clothing, and avoidance of the sun between 10 AM and 2 PM
- Can occur on a cloudy day
- Discomfort can be minimized with cool compresses and acetaminophen

---

✳ | Indications for Referral

- Sunburn will resolve with or without treatment. If a suspected case of sunburn does not resolve over 1 week, consultation with a dermatologist may be indicated to evaluate other potential diagnoses.

Urticaria (Hives)

Overview

Pathophysiology

Multiple stimuli may produce urticaria by immunologic or nonimmunologic mechanisms. The most common causes include **drugs** (aspirin, penicillin, sulfonamides, codeine, morphine), **ingestants** (food additives and colorings, shellfish, tomatoes, milk, chocolate, eggs, nuts, pork, and strawberries), and **insect bites** (especially bee, hornet, wasp, and mites). A less frequently identified cause is **occult infection** (parasitic infestations; viral hepatitis; dermatophyte or yeast infections; sinus; dental; or urinaty tract infections). **Heat, fever, alcohol, exercise, and emotional stress** are all aggravating rather than causative factors. No cause is identifiable in 30% to 50% of chronic cases and in up to 80% of acute reactions.

Probably the most common mechanism is a type I hypersensitivity reaction in which an antigen-immunoglobulin E (IgE) interaction leads to a release of histamine. The result is an increase in capillary permeability and subsequent edema of the dermis.

Epidemiology

Twenty percent or more of the population is affected by urticaria at some time in life. Urticaria may be associated with a personal or family history of atopic disorders. Acute urticaria has no sex predominance but may be more common in young patients. Chronic urticaria is more common in females ages 20 to 50.

Assessment

Clinical Presentation

Pruritus is usually intense and is the chief complaint. Lesions typically have a pale edematous center with a sharply marginated erythematous halo in an annular or serpiginous pattern. The primary lesion is the **wheal**, a swelling due to intradermal edema. Individual lesions are transient, lasting only a few hours, with new lesions appearing and disappearing over days. The result appears to be a **migration of lesions. Angioedema** (swelling of any area, but specifically of the mouth, eyelids, hands, and tongue) may occur. **Laryngeal edema** is rare but may be fatal as part of the anaphylaxis syndrome. **Dermagraphism** (a sign of urticaria in which wheals are produced by pressure on the skin) may or may not be present.

Clinical variants include the following:

- **Acute urticaria:** persisting for less than 2 months.
- **Chronic urticaria:** persisting for more than 2 months.
- **Cold urticaria:** Lesions can be readily induced by a cold challenge (ice cube test).
- Mucus membranes are not usually involved and patients are often able to tolerate cold foods and liquids.
- **Cholinergic urticaria** (generalized heat urticaria or physical urticaria): Precipitated by an increase in body temperature (hot showers, exercise, emotional upset, or fever), small macular and papular lesions appear, preceded by pruritus and erythema. The palms, soles, and axillae are spared.

Diagnostics

- A detailed **history and physical examination** are essential to identify the cause of the urticaria.
- A **CBC, eosinophil count, erythrocyte sedimentation rate, liver function tests, urinalysis, and hepatitis screen** may be useful in identifying causative factors.
- **Cultures** may be indicated if infection is suspected. Stool should be cultured for **ova and parasites in chronic urticaria**
- **Skin biopsy** is necessary if individual lesions persist for more than 48 hours.
- **Antinuclear antibody (ANA)** testing may be indicated if collagen vascular disease is suspected.
- **An elimination diet** (avoiding legumes, for example) may be helpful if foods are suspected as a causative factor.

Differential Diagnosis

- Insect bite reactions (usually have a central punctum that is persistent for days, not hours; eruption is more localized to areas of bites)
- Erythema multiforme (lesions are more targetoid)

Treatment

In the great majority of cases spontaneous improvement occurs even in the absence of treatment. In many cases the history reveals a probable explanation.

URTICARIA

- Usually resolves spontaneously
- May be appropriate to note on a medical bracelet
- To soothe pruritus use cool compresses and antihistamines
- May be minimized by preventing an increase in body temperature (resulting from hot showers, exercise, emotional upset, or fever) and by avoiding bath brushes and rough clothing

Nonpharmacologic

Remove causative or exacerbating factors. Detailed food diaries can be useful in determining the causative agent. Medical alert bracelets should be given to patients who have anaphylactic reactions to allergens. Attacks of cholinergic urticaria can be abated by application of cold water or ice to the skin after sweating occurs. Avoidance of irritating factors such as hot showers, bath brushes, drying soaps and rough clothing can help prevent the exacerbation of pruritus.

Pharmacologic

Topical Agents

Antipruritic lotions such as **calamine, menthol camphor (Sarna), or doxepine hydrochloride (Zonalon)** qid are recommended. **Benadryl-**containing lotions should be avoided because a contact dermatitis may result.

Systemic Agents

Doxepine (Sinequan) 10 mg PO tid is useful in cold and chronic urticaria and is less sedating than **Benedryl** or **Atarax.**

For symptomatic dermatographism a combination of **hydroxyzine (Atarax)** 10 mg PO qid and **cimetidine (Tagamet)** 400 mg PO qid may be the most efficacious regimen.

For intractable cases a combination of **hydroxyzine (Atarax)** 50 mg PO q6h and **propantheline (Pro-Banthine)** 15 mg PO q6h may be tried but should be used with caution since it may have an excessive anticholinergic effect.

Epinephrine 0.1 ml/10 kg SQ, with a maximum dose of 0.3 ml in children and 0.5 ml in adults, is effective in acute attacks and may be repeated every 20 to 30 minutes for up to three doses.

Sus-Phrine (a longer-acting epinephrine) may be prescribed as an alternative. The adult dose is 0.1 to 0.3 ml SQ depending on patient response. For children 30 kg or less, the maximum single dose is 0.15 ml. Subsequent doses for both children and adults should be administered only when necessary and not more often than q6h.

A short course of **prednisone,** 40 mg PO qAM for 4 days, may be tried in cases of severe, recalcitrant acute urticaria. This short course is helpful in symptom reduction, and side effects are prevented.

Indications for Referral

- Anaphylactic or other life-threatening reactions.
- Presence of collagen vascular disease.

Chapter 5

Cysts, Nodules, Papules, and Skin Cancer

Figure 5-1 ACNE

A, Teenage male with both open and closed comedones. *B,* Teenage male with nodular cystic acne, inflammatory lesions, and open and closed comedones.

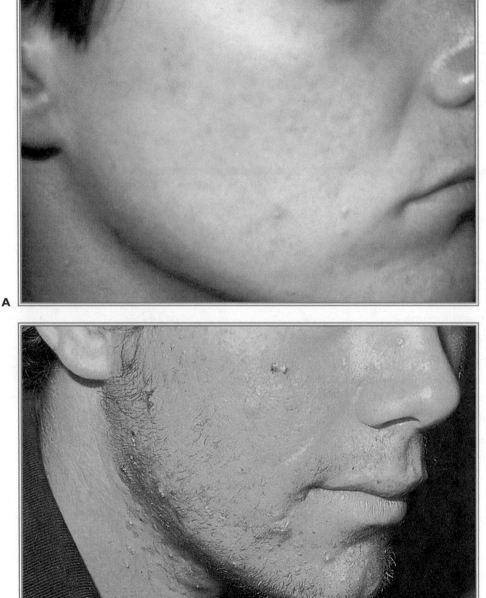

A

B

Figure 5-2 **ACROCHORDON**

Papular, pedunculated lesions on the lateral aspect of the neck.

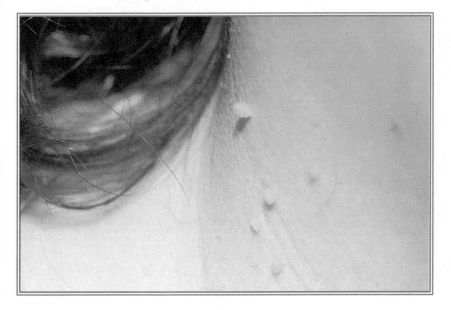

Figure 5-3 **ACTINIC KERATOSIS**

Slightly erythematous, rough, scaling papules and plaques on sun-damaged skin.

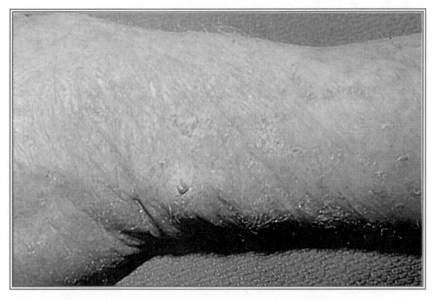

(From Goldstein BG, Goldstein AO: *Practical dermatology,* ed 2, St Louis, 1997, Mosby.)

Figure 5-4   **BASAL CELL CARCINOMA**

Pearly papule with slight erythema.

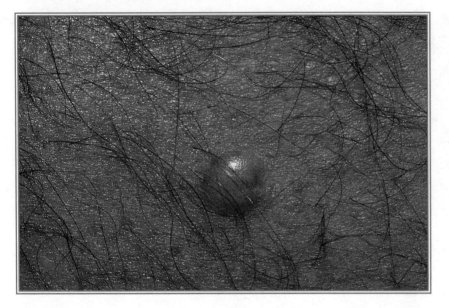

Figure 5-5   **BLUE NEVUS**

Uniformly pigmented blue-black macule on the neck.

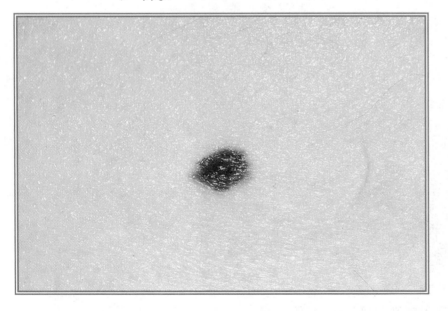

Figure 5-6 **BOWEN'S DISEASE**

Erythematous, keratotic, poorly marginated lesion on the arm of a 57-year-old male.

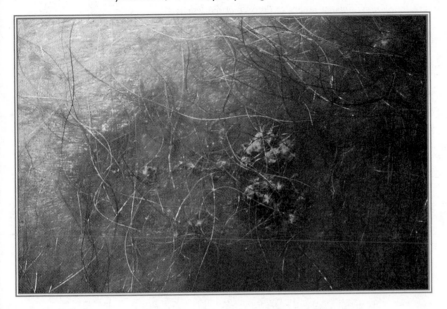

Figure 5-7 **ACUTE CANDIDA INTERTRIGO**

Note peripheral fringe of scale and satellite lesions.

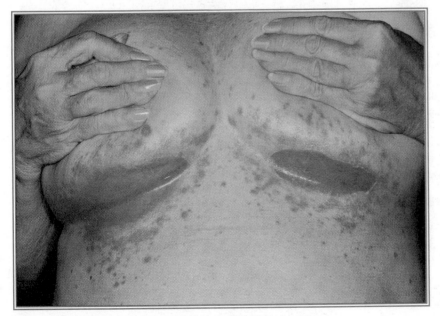

(From Habif TP: *Clinical dermatology,* ed 3, St Louis, 1996, Mosby.)

Figure 5-8   CHICKENPOX

Small vesicles on an erythematous macular base, in a generalized distribution on the back. Lesions vary in size from (early) papular lesions to (later) macular lesions.

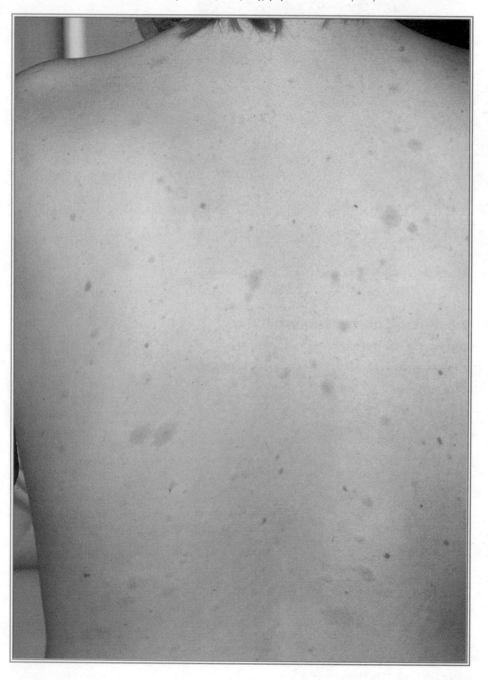

Figure 5-9 NEVUS

A, *Becker's nevus: Light-brown macule with overlying hair.* **B,** *Compound nevus: Well-circumscribed tan-brown papule on the cheek.*

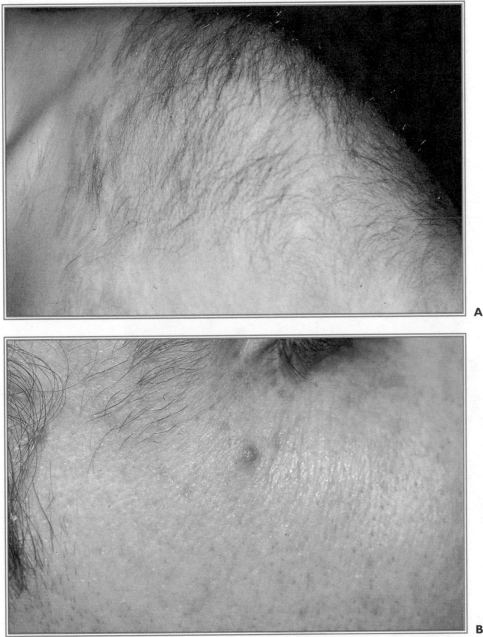

A

B

continued

Figure 5-9 NEVUS

C, Halo nevus: Pigmented, slightly irregular nevus with surrounding stark hyperpigmentation. **D,** Intradermal nevus: Well-marginated, deeply pigmented papule in the nasolabial groove.

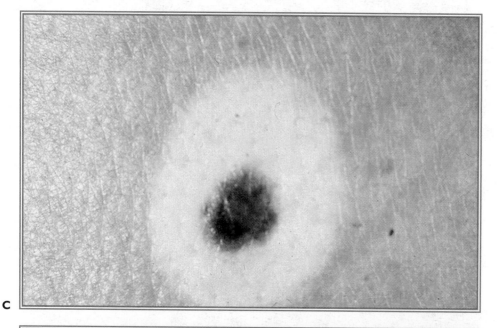

C

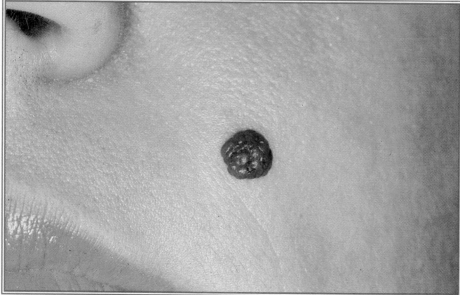

D

Figure 5-9   NEVUS

E, Nevus spilus. Light tan, macular lesion with multiple small black/brown macules within.

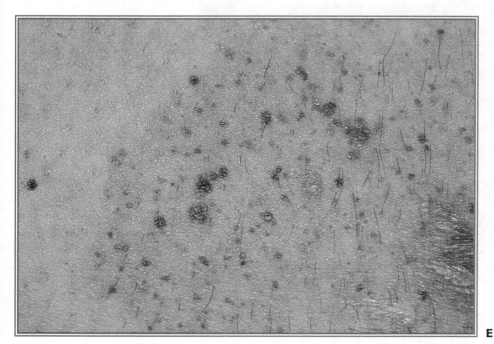

E

Figure 5-10   **CONGENITAL NEVUS**

Dark brown, hairy nevi on a young child, present since birth.

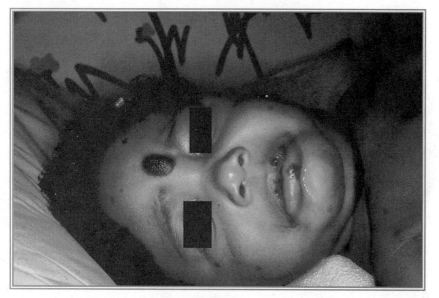

(Courtesy of Stacy R. Smith, MD.)

Figure 5-11   **DERMATOFIBROMA**

Light brown, dome-shaped nodule on the lateral aspect of the leg.

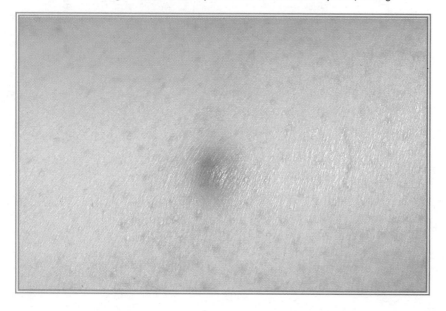

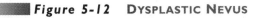 *Figure 5-12* **DYSPLASTIC NEVUS**

Multiple nevi larger than 1 cm and irregularly pigmented.

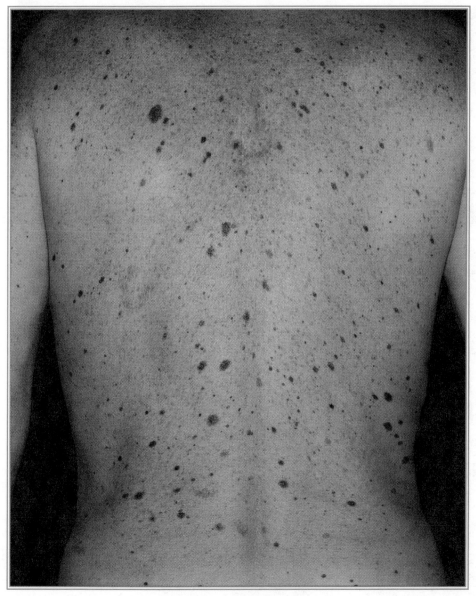

(From Habif TP: *Clinical dermatology*, ed 3, St Louis, 1996, Mosby.)

Figure 5-13 EPIDERMAL CYST

The posterior auricular fold is a common location of many epidermal cysts.

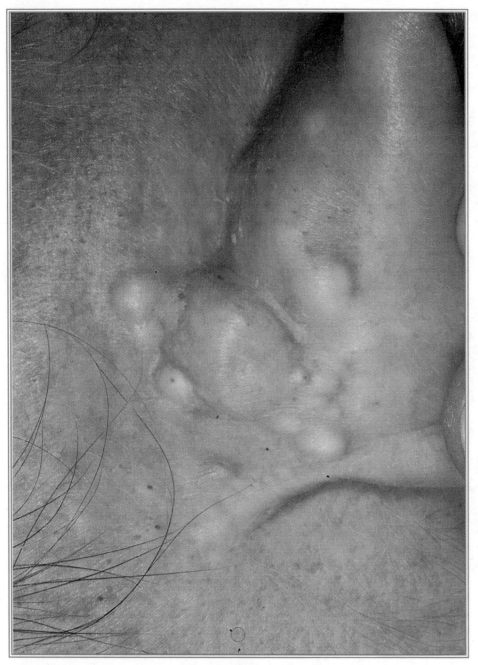

(From Habif TF: *Clinical dermatology* ed 3, St Louis, 1996, Mosby.)

Figure 5-14 ERYTHEMA INFECTIOSUM

Facial erythema ("slapped cheek"), sparing the nasolabial fold and circumoral region.

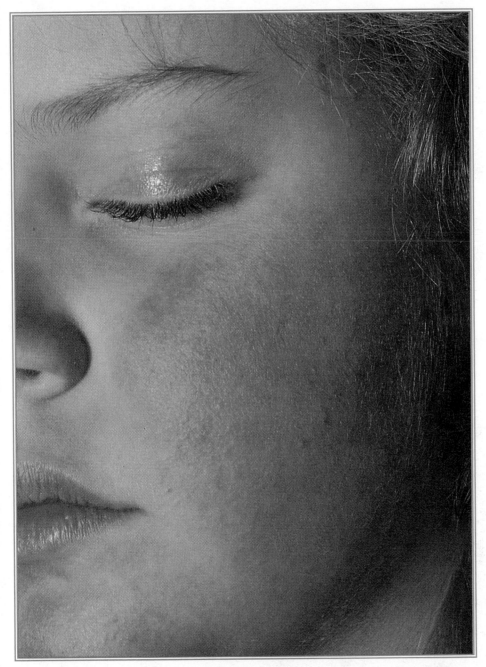

(From Habif TF: *Clinical dermatology*, ed 3, St Louis, 1996, Mosby.)

Figure 5-15   ERYTHEMA MULTIFORME

Erythematous macular targetlike lesions on the palms.

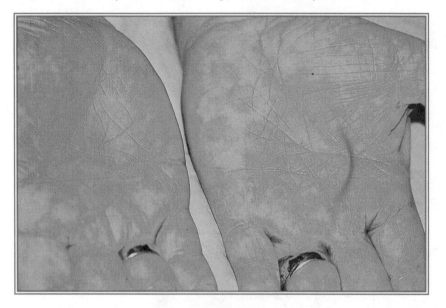

Figure 5-16   FOLLICULITIS

Extensive inflammatory closed comedones centered around hair follicles on the cheek of a male electrical worker exposed to fluorocarbons.

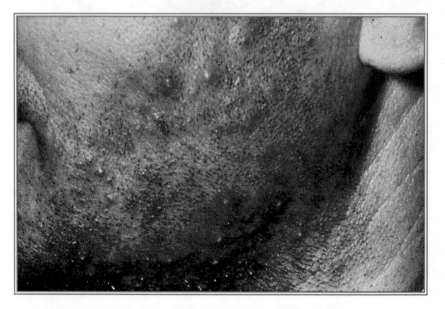

Figure 5-17 **FURUNCLE**

Pustular deep nodule located on the posterior aspect of the right side of the neck.

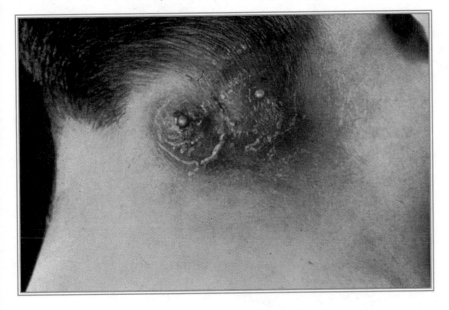

Figure 5-18 **CARBUNCLE**

Multiple pustular nodules located on the posterior aspect of the neck. Many of the nodules have a confluent nature and exude pus.

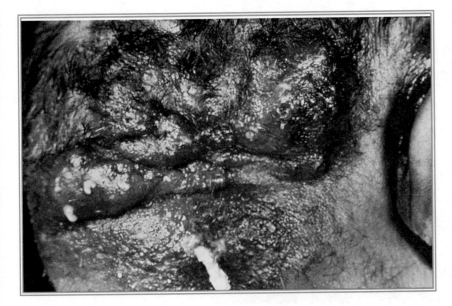

Figure 5-19 HIDRADENITIS SUPPURATIVA

Inflammatory dermatitis of the axilla with multiple sinus tracts, some of which are draining pustular fluid. Note presence of scarring.

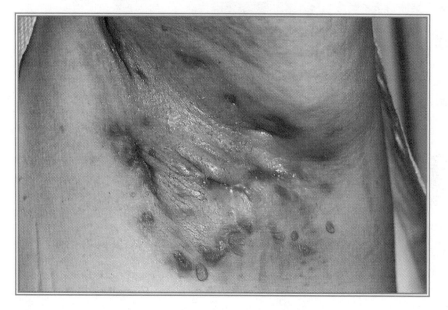

Figure 5-20 IMPETIGO

Erythematous lesions with honey-colored crust on the posterior thighs and buttocks region.

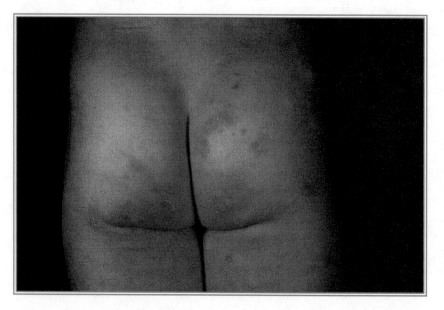

Figure 5-21 **INSECT BITES**

Insect bites with characteristic purpuric spots in center of papule. A central punctum is typical.

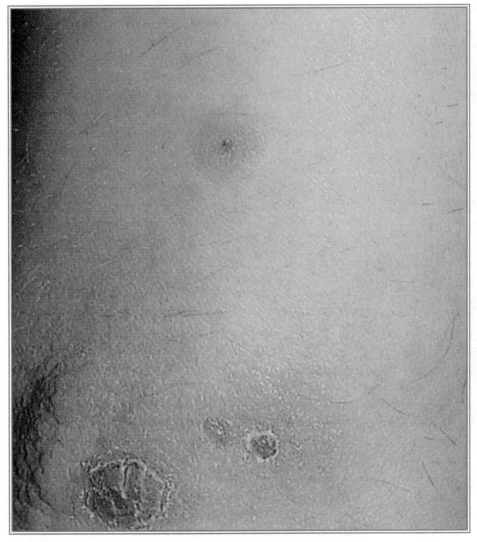

(From Cox N, Lawrence C: *Diagnostic problems in dermatology,* St Louis, 1998, Mosby.)

Figure 5-22   KELOID

Exuberant growth of hyperpigmented tissue along and well beyond the surgical aspect of the scar.

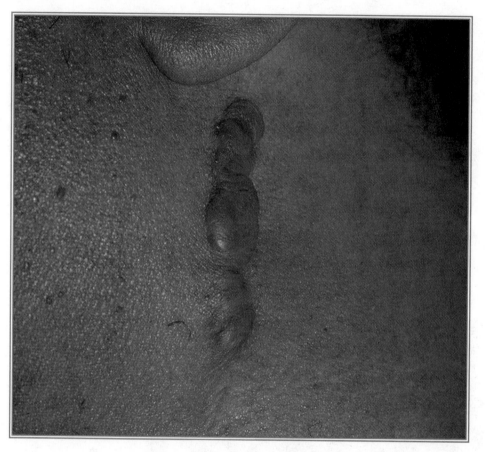

Figure 5-23 **KERATOACANTHOMA**

Rapidly enlarging nodule with a central crateriform crust.

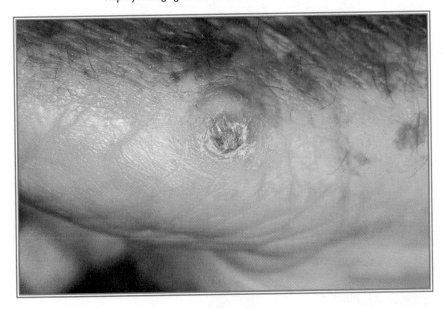

Figure 5-24 **KERATOSIS PILARIS**

Lateral aspect of the arm in a teenage girl, showing erythematous hyperkeratotic papules overlying hair follicles.

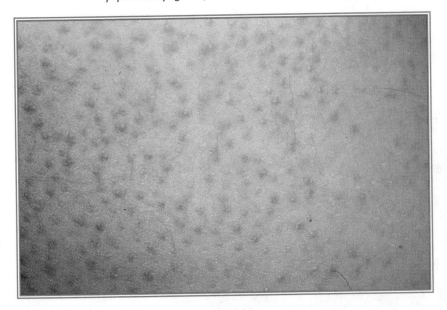

Figure 5-25 LICHEN PLANUS

Erythematous to violaceous, flat-topped polygonal papules on the dorsal and lateral aspect of the foot.

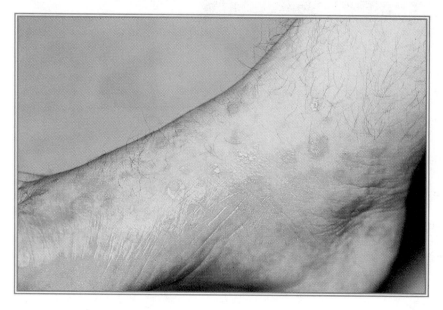

Figure 5-26 LIPOMA

This yellow semiencapsulated nodule of fatty tissue was extruded with external pressure immediately after excision of a subcutaneous nodule.

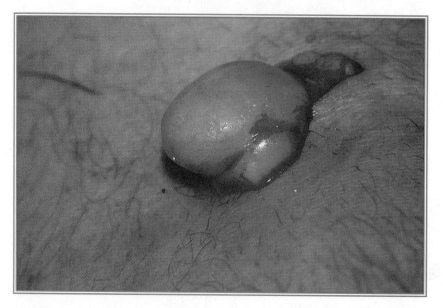

Figure 5-27 **MALIGNANT MELANOMA**

A, Variably pigmented asymmetric nevus on the midback. Note normal-appearing nevus to the right, and a slightly dysplastic nevus inferiorly. *B,* Superficial spreading melanoma: Annular pigmented lesion with irregular border and a variegated color.

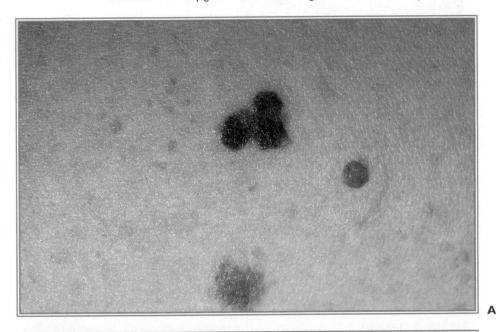

A

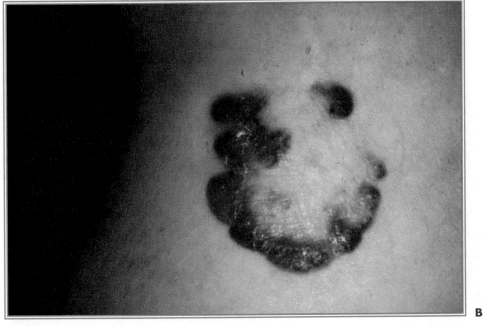

B

Figure 5-28 MOLLUSCUM CONTAGIOSUM

Pearly, dome-shaped papule in the pubic region of a teenager.

Figure 5-29 NEVUS SEBACEUS

Pearly, slightly pink papule on the scalp.

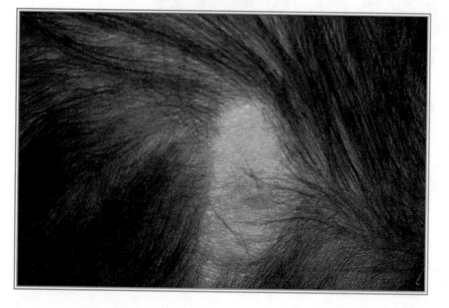

Figure 5-30 **PERIORAL DERMATITIS**

Inflammatory closed comedones and generalized inflammation in a perioral distribution.

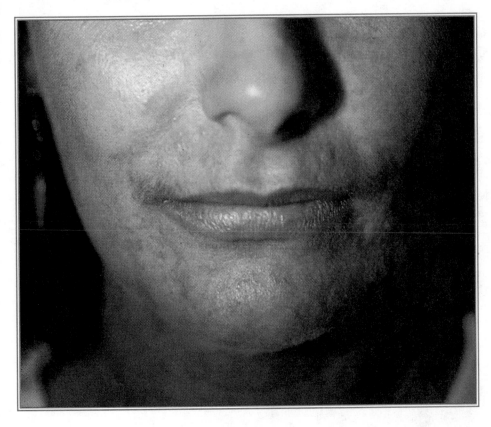

Figure 5-31 PSEUDOFOLLICULITIS

Inflammatory lesions with some pustules in the mandibular angle. Note curled hairs, some of which are embedding back into the skin.

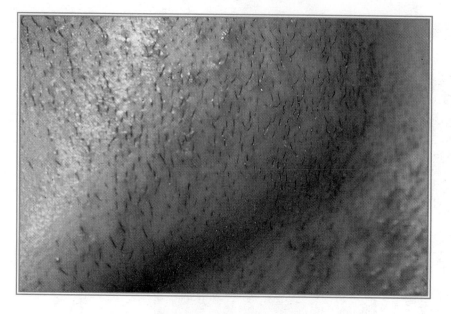

Figure 5-32 PYOGENIC GRANULOMA

Rapidly growing necrotic papule on the posterior aspect of the neck.

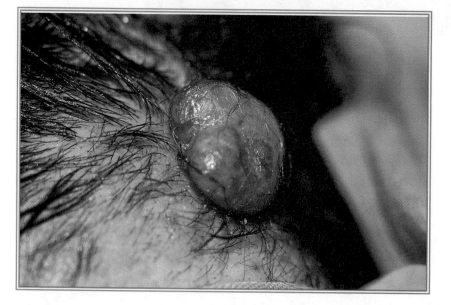

Figure 5-33 ROSACEA

Generalized inflammation with multiple closed comedones, predominantly on the central aspect of the face and nose.

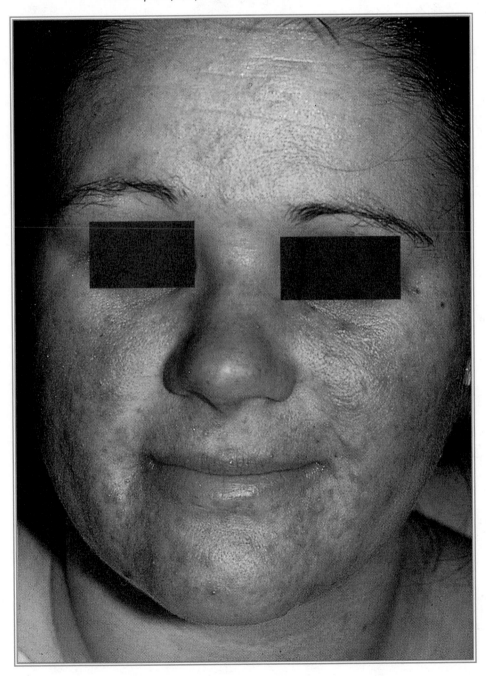

Figure 5-34 SCABIES

Black linear tract with surrounding erythema.

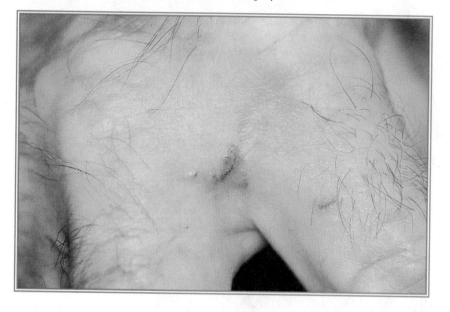

Figure 5-35 SEBACEOUS HYPERPLASIA

Multiple yellow and erythematous papules on the forehead.

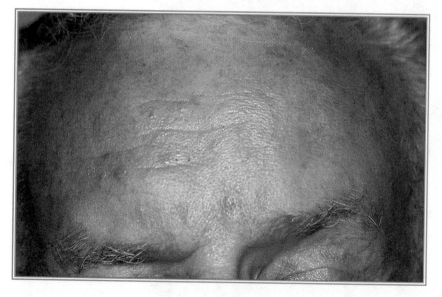

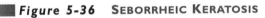

Figure 5-36 **SEBORRHEIC KERATOSIS**

Extensive greasy, "stuck-on" hyperkeratotic lesions of the face.

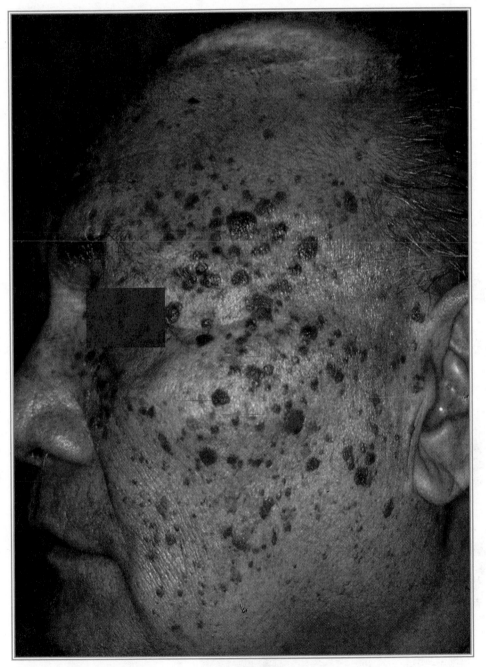

(Courtesy of Stacy R. Smith, MD.)

Figure 5-37   SPITZ NEVUS

A poorly demarcated papule on the cheek of a 7-year-old girl. Note the range of colors.

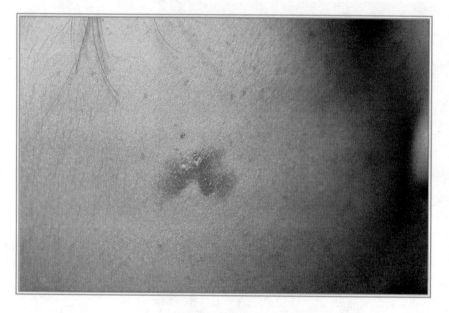

Figure 5-38   SQUAMOUS CELL CARCINOMA

A firm, elevated mass with central crust, occurring on sun-damaged skin of the lower lip.

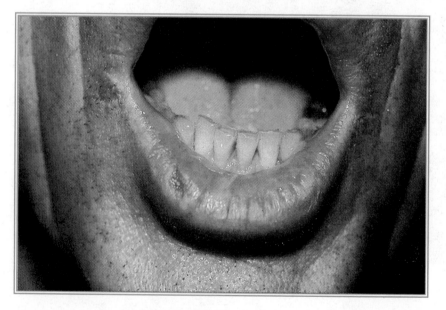

Figure 5-39 WARTS

A, *Common warts: Multiple hyperkeratotic growths with characteristic black dots.*
B, *Filiform warts: An extruding papular growth with fingerlike projections on the right cheek.*

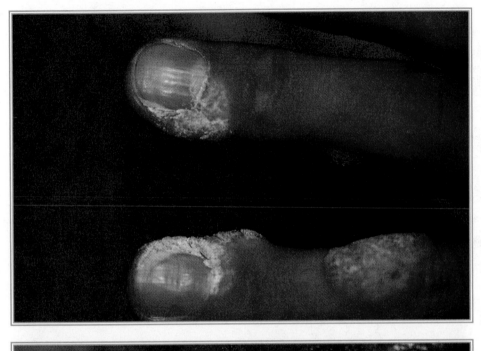

A

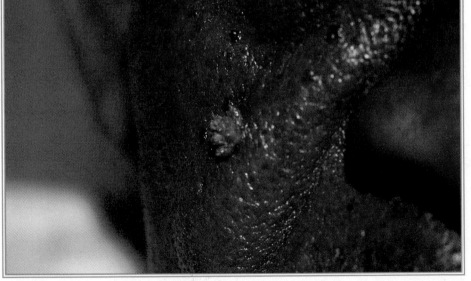

B

continued

Figure 5-39 WARTS

C, Genital warts: Broad-based wart on the shaft of a penis. Note verrucous surface texture. *D,* Plantar warts: Firm, keratotic macule with multiple black dots on the plantar aspect of the great toe.

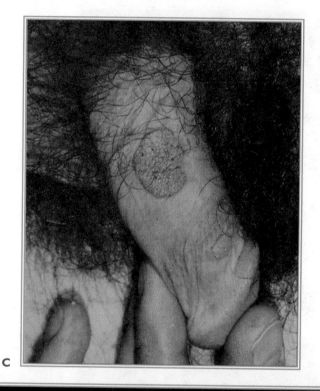

C

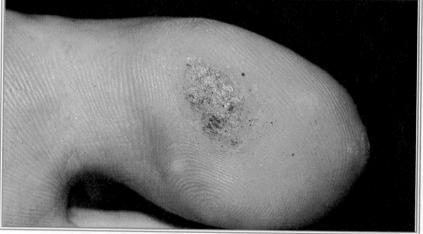

D

(**C,** From Habif TF: *Clinical dermatology,* ed 3, St Louis, 1996, Mosby.

Table 5-1

Differential Diagnosis of Cysts, Nodules, Papules, and Skin Cancer

DISORDER	TEXT	KEYS TO DIAGNOSIS
Acne vulgaris	Ch. 1, p. 29 (Figure 5-1)	Comedones, papules, pustules, cysts are present on face, neck, shoulders, chest, back; peak age 14 to 15 for females, age 16 to 17 for males
Acrochordon	Ch. 5, p. 234 (Figure 5-2)	Soft, skin-colored to brown pedunculated growth; usually on neck, axillae, groin, eyelids, and trunk
Actinic keratosis	Ch. 5, p. 235 (Figure 5-3)	Skin-colored to slightly erythematous macules with dry, rough scale
Basal cell carcinoma	Ch. 5, p. 237 (Figure 5-4)	Pearly or waxy papule that may have a central depression or ulceration, often with fine telangiectasias
Blue nevus	Ch. 5, p. 239 (Figure 5-5)	Asymptomatic, slightly elevated, round papule with a blue tint; usually occurs on dorsum of hands, feet, face, or buttocks
Bowen's disease	Ch. 5, p. 240 (Figure 5-6)	Erythematous, flat to slightly raised scaly plaque with erythematous and irregular surface
Candidiasis	Ch. 1, p. 33 (Figure 5-7)	Satellite pustules; sharp, scaling border; erythematous, macerated patches; favors warm, moist environment; may be pruritic or tender
Chickenpox (varicella)	Ch. 2, p. 64 (Figure 5-8)	Maculopapular rash that begins on chest and back, then forms small, superficial vesicles on an erythematous base ("dewdrop on a rose petal"); intensely pruritic
Common acquired nevus (mole)	Ch. 6, p. 286 (Figure 5-9)	Most common as a flat or slightly raised tan-brown lesion less than 6 mm in diameter; sharp margins; may have hair or light halo; may be flesh-toned with dark flecks of color
Congenital nevus	Ch. 6, p. 289 (Figure 5-10)	Asymptomatic, dark brown raised lesion with irregular surface and sharp border; usually has hair; present at birth
Dermatofibroma	Ch. 5, p. 241 (Figure 5-11)	Round, firm tan to light brown cutaneous nodule; may "dimple" when pinched; often occurs at site of previous trauma
Dysplastic nevus	Ch. 6, p. 290 (Figure 5-12)	Asymptomatic, red or brown maculopapular lesion with indistinct, irregular border; occurs most often on trunk and extremities; first appears in midchildhood and develops abnormal characteristics in adolescence or adulthood
Epidermal cyst	Ch. 5, p. 243 (Figure 5-13)	Subcutaneous, fluctuant swelling; central opening may exude pasty, odoriferous material; usually on scalp, face, neck, or trunk
Erythema infectiosum	Ch. 4, p. 183 (Figure 5-14)	Erythematous, bright red macules and papules that appear suddenly on the cheeks; lacy rash on trunk, buttocks, and upper arms; generally known as "slapped cheek appearance"
Erythema multiforme	Ch. 4, p. 185 (Figure 5-15)	Macules, papules, vesicles, and bullae all may be present ("multiform"); hallmark is the iris or target lesion, usually on extensor surfaces, palms, and soles; some may appear urticarial

continued

Table 5-1 *continued*

Disorder	Text	Keys to Diagnosis
Folliculitis	Ch. 1, p. 36 (Figure 5-16)	*Follicular,* erythematous papules and pustules on any hair-bearing surface; *Pseudomonas* folliculitis occurs 1 to 3 days after use of a hot tub
Furuncles and carbuncles	Ch. 1, p. 38 (Figure 5-17 and 5-18)	*Furuncles:* 1 to 5 cm tender nodules with surrounding erythema; may become fluctuant. *Carbuncles:* 3 to 10 cm tender erythematous nodules that drain pus from multiple follicular orifices
Hidradenitis suppurativa	Ch. 1, p. 41 (Figure 5-19)	Double comedone, foul-smelling discharge; subcutaneous sinus tracts; adenopathy; axillae, groin, perineum
Impetigo	Ch. 2, p. 73 (Figure 5-20)	Vesicles on an erythematous base that rupture to form honey-colored crusts, usually around mouth; regional adenopathy and pruritus common
Insect bites	(Figure 5-21)	Erythematous papule with central punctum; usually pruritic
Keloids and hypertrophic scars	Ch. 5, p. 244 (Figure 5-22)	Firm, rubbery, erythematous or tan plaques with telangiectasias; occur over areas of previous trauma
Keratoacanthoma	Ch. 5, p. 247 (Figure 5-23)	Red, dome-shaped nodule with central crater; has raised, rolled borders, frequently covered with crust
Keratosis pilaris	Ch. 1, p. 43 (Figure 5-24)	Small, discrete follicular papules on posterior upper arms and anterior thighs; may be erythematous
Lichen planus	Ch. 3, p. 128 (Figure 5-25)	Pruritic, flat, irregular purple papules with fine white lines and scales; commonly on flexor surfaces, nails, and scalp
Lipoma	Ch. 5, p. 249 (Figure 5-26)	Soft subcutaneous, freely mobile nodule; asymptomatic; commonly occurs on neck, shoulders, and back
Malignant melanoma	Ch. 5, p. 250 (Figure 5-27)	Lesions have asymmetric, irregular border; color variegation; diameter usually greater than 6 mm
Molluscum contagiosum	Ch. 5, p. 253 (Figure 5-28)	Multiple asymptomatic, flesh-colored, firm, domed umbilicated papules
Nevus sebaceus	Ch. 5, p. 255 (Figure 5-29)	Sharply circumscribed, solitary raised lesion with irregular surface, covered with multiple yellow to dark brown papules; asymptomatic
Perioral dermatitis	Ch. 1, p. 44 (Figure 5-30)	Pruritic, burning, discrete erythematous or flesh-colored papules and pustules around mouth and in nasolabial folds
Pseudofolliculitis	Ch. 1, p. 46 (Figure 5-31)	Erythematous papules and pustules on shaved areas, especially beards of men with coarse, curly hair; may be asymptomatic or painful and pruritic
Pyogenic granuloma	Ch. 12, p. 434 (Figure 5-32)	Solitary, rapidly growing dark red papule with moist or scaly surface; usually on fingers, face, shoulders, or feet; common in children, during pregnancy, or after trauma
Rosacea	Ch. 1, p. 48 (Figure 5-33)	Facial papules and pustules but no comedones; flushing, telangiectasias, rhinophyma; triggered by hot foods, emotional stress

Table 5-1 *continued*

DISORDER	TEXT	KEYS TO DIAGNOSIS
Scabies	Ch. 7, p. 346 (Figure 5-34)	Crusted papules or burrows on genitals, wrists, finger webs, belt line; intensely pruritic
Sebaceous hyperplasia	Ch. 5, p. 256 (Figure 5-35)	Soft, yellowish cauliflower-like papule on forehead or cheek; usually umbilicated and asymptomatic
Seborrheic keratosis	Ch. 5, p. 257 (Figure 5-36)	Warty, greasy, sharply marginated pigmented lesion; appears "stuck-on"
Spitz nevus	Ch. 5, p. 259 (Figure 5-37)	Asymptomatic, rapidly growing firm round nodule with pink or deep red color; bleeds readily when traumatized; usually occurs in childhood
Squamous cell carcinoma	Ch. 5, p. 260 (Figure 5-38)	Firm, skin-colored or reddish-brown nodule on sun-damaged skin; ulceration, scaling, and crusting frequently present
Verrucae	Ch. 5, p. 262 (Figure 5-39)	Skin-colored lesions with rough surface; normal skin lines obscured; multiple black dots sometimes visible within lesion

Acrochordon (Skin Tag, Papilloma)

Overview

Pathophysiology

The exact cause is unknown; it may be the result of a senile degeneration of the skin.

Epidemiology

Acrochordons are extremely common in the middle-aged and elderly. They may be associated with obesity, pregnancy, menopause, or a family history of acrochordons. The incidence is frequently higher in diabetics.

Assessment

Clinical Presentation

Acrochordons are **soft, skin-color to brown pedunculated growths** (see Figure 5-2). They most commonly occur on the **neck, axillae, inframammary folds, groin, eyelids, and trunk.** The lesions are asymptomatic but may become irritated or inflamed if exposed to repeated trauma.

Diagnostics

Diagnosis is usually made by clinical appearance alone. A biopsy is generally not needed unless the lesion is pigmented or erythematous.

Differential Diagnosis

- Verruca (surface usually rougher, more papillomatous) (see Figure 5-39, *A*)
- Nevus (usually pigmented) (see Figure 5-9, *B*)
- Neurofibroma (usually larger with a more solid feel)

Treatment

Nonpharmacologic

Electrodesiccate until the lesion "bubbles up."

Perform simple scissor excision: grasp the acrochordon with forceps and lift it away from the skin surface; excise at the base.

Employ cryotherapy: treat lightly to prevent permanent hypopigmentation.

ACROCHORDON

- Is in most cases a cosmetic disorder only
- May indicate colonic polyps or colon cancer if multiple lesions occur rapidly over only a few months; the patient should be referred for colonoscopy or sigmoidoscopy

Pharmacologic

Topical Agents
No topical therapy is indicated.

Systemic Agents
None is indicated.

Indications for Referral

- Rapid occurrence over a few months may indicate associated colonic polyps.
- Appropriate patients (especially those above age 50 with a family history of colon cancer) should be referred for colonoscopy or sigmoidoscopy.

Actinic Keratosis

Overview

Pathophysiology
Sun-induced damage to epidermal cells, cumulative from birth, causes a proliferation of abnormal, premalignant, dystrophic cells that may eventually transform (20% within 5 years) into squamous cell carcinoma. Lesions may also occur on postirradiation sites.

Epidemiology
Since the cell changes are caused by cumulative damage by the sun, the lesions are most common in persons above age 50. There is an increased incidence in redheads, blonds, and those who freckle easily. The disorder occurs in 40% to 50% of Australians after age 40.

Assessment

Clinical Presentation
Lesions appear as **flat hyperkeratotic skin-colored macules with a dry, hard, rough scale on an erythematous base** (see Figure 5-3). They most commonly occur on sun-exposed areas (face, lower arms and legs, tops of ears, dorsa of hands) and are chronic with repeated episodes of scaling (after sun exposure) and quiescence (after sun avoidance). They may be described as **"better felt than seen,"** referring to the rough texture of the skin, even without visible signs.

Diagnostics

- Lesions are usually diagnosed by clinical presentation alone. To confirm the diagnosis, a skin biopsy is required.

Differential Diagnosis

- Seborrheic keratosis (greasy, scaly, pigmented lesion with stuck-on appearance) (see Figure 5-36)
- Squamous cell carcinoma in situ (more indurated and erythematous) (see Figure 5-38)
- Verruca vulgaris (hyperkeratotic without erythema) (see Figure 5-39, *A*)

Treatment

Nonpharmacologic

Avoidance of the sun through protective clothing, chemical sunscreens, or prevention of midday (10:00 AM to 2:00 PM) sun exposure is essential. Since patients are at increased risk for other cutaneous neoplasms, close follow-up evaluation is mandatory.

Pharmacologic

Topical Agents

Sunscreens (with a sun protection factor [SPF] of 15 or greater) are mandatory for the prevention of new lesions and possibly for the treatment of existing ones.

Cryosurgery, with the application of **liquid nitrogen** for 5 to 15 seconds (depending on the degree of hyperkeratosis), is common practice.

5-Fluorouracil (5-FU) cream or ointment is appropriate for multiple lesions scattered over an area. It is applied q.h.s. to the affected skin for 3 to 6 weeks, or until the inflammatory response is at the ulcerative and necrotic stage. Alternatively it may be applied weekly for 3 to 6 months to prevent inflammation. For single lesions that do not respond to treatment, a shave excision may be indicated.

Systemic Agents

None is indicated.

ACTINIC KERATOSIS

- Is caused by cumulative sun damage to the skin over many years
- Treatment must include avoidance of the sun between 10:00 AM and 2:00 PM, consistent and liberal use of sunscreen (SPF ≥15), routine full body skin examinations every 6 to 12 months, and wearing protective clothing
- Should be suspected in any lesion that is scaly and red and does not heal
- Evolves into squamous cell carcinoma in 20% of cases

Indications for Referral

- Refer to a dermatologist if squamous cell carcinoma should develop.

Basal Cell Carcinoma

Overview

Pathophysiology
The tumor arises from the epidermis. There are multiple causes, including chronic exposure to sunlight or ionizing radiation and genetic predisposition. The inability to tan may be the single most important risk factor. There is a low tendency for metastasis but it commonly expands locally.

Epidemiology
Basal cell carcinoma (BCC) is the most common malignant tumor affecting the white population. It is very rare in Latin and Asian peoples and extremely rare in blacks. Accounting for 75% of all skin cancers, it comprises 700,000 cases per year in the United States. The highest incidence occurs in fair-skinned people with red or blond hair. Over 75% of patients are above 40 years of age.

Assessment

Clinical Presentation
Basal cell carcinoma can take several forms: Initially with *nodule-ulcerative tumor* the lesion begins as a small **pearly or translucent waxy papule** that enlarges peripherally and develops a **central depression,** which often becomes ulcerated or scaly (see Figure 5-4). The border becomes translucent, elevated, and shiny with fine characteristic telangiectasias. Lesions are rarely pigmented and do not respond to steroid therapy.

   In *superficial BCC* the lesion appears initially as an **erythematous scaly macule or patch with an elevated threadlike border.** Multiple lesions are characteristically present, especially on the back and chest.

   With *sclerosing, morpheaform, or fibrosing BCC* the lesion begins as a slowly enlarging pore, which when fully developed appears as a **slightly indurated yellowish-white plaque with an indistinct border.** The plaque **blanches with pressure or with stretching** of the surrounding skin. It is seldom ulcerated. The most frequent location is the head or neck.

Diagnostics
• A skin biopsy is required for confirmation of the diagnosis.

Differential Diagnosis
• Sebaceous hyperplasia (waxy, pink cauliflower appearance) (see Figure 5-35)

- Seborrheic keratosis ("stuck-on" appearance) (see Figure 5-36)
- Squamous cell carcinoma (more erythematous, scaling, macular) (see Figure 5-38)
- Actinic keratosis (more macular appearance) (see Figure 5-3)
- Malignant melanoma (irregularly pigmented) (see Figure 5-27, *A*)
- Molluscum contagiosum (central depression present) (see Figure 5-28)
- Angiofibroma (tan, erythematous papule)

Treatment

Nonpharmacologic

All of the following treatment methods leave atrophic, hypopigmented scars:

Curettage and electrodesiccation are indicated for lesions less than 1 cm in diameter and in a nonfacial location. There is better than an 85% cure rate with this technique. The lesion must be destroyed beyond the limits of the visible tumor border. Cancerous tissue (which is soft) must be distinguished from normal tissue (which is dense).

Cryosurgery is best for superficial lesions, except those around the nose, ears, eyelids, forehead, and temples.

In *excision* the excised tissue must be examined microscopically to assure clear borders and complete removal of the lesion. If it is located on the head or neck, Mohs' surgery is indicated to obtain the best cosmetic result.

Pharmacologic

Topical Agents

Prevention is essential and consists of liberal use of sunscreens every day and frequent dermatologic checkups for those with a history of skin carcinomas.

Systemic Agents

None is indicated.

BASAL CELL CARCINOMA

- Is caused by cumulative sun damage to the skin over many years
- Treatment must include avoidance of the sun between 10:00 AM and 2:00 PM, as well as consistent and liberal use of a sunscreen of SPF >15 and wearing protective clothing
- Patients with a history of extensive sun exposure should have routine full body skin examinations every 6 to 12 months
- Is the most common malignant tumor in the white population

Indications for Referral

- Location of lesion in a cosmetically prominent location such as the face, eyelids, inner canthus, nose, or ears. (Refer to Mohs' surgery.)

Blue Nevus

Overview

Pathophysiology

A blue nevus occurs in the dermis and results from the proliferation of melanocytes, which produce a blue-black papule. These nevus cells are thought to be melanocytes that never complete the migration to the epidermis. The exact cause of this proliferation is unknown.

Epidemiology

Blue nevi are commonly present at birth or in early childhood and progress for 10 to 15 years. The female/male ratio is 2:1. There is an increased incidence among darker-skinned races.

Assessment

Clinical Presentation

A blue nevus is an asymptomatic, slightly elevated, round, small solitary lesion with a blue tint that usually occurs on the dorsum of the hands, feet, face, or buttocks (see Figure 5-5). The color is due to intensely pigmented melanocytes in the deep dermis. The margin of the lesion is regular but indistinct. These lesions remain benign throughout life.

Diagnostics

Clinical presentation is usually adequate to differentiate a blue nevus from a malignant melanoma. If any doubt exists, however, the patient should be referred to a dermatologist for surgical excision or biopsy.

Differential Diagnosis

- Malignant melanoma (variegated color, irregular border, changing characteristics) (see Figure 5-27, *A*)
- Dermal tattoo (history of trauma from pencil lead or other sharp object)

Treatment

Nonpharmacologic

Most blue nevi require no treatment unless they are cosmetically unacceptable. If they are, surgical excision is indicated.

BLUE NEVUS

- Results from the proliferation of melanocytes
- Is a benign lesion with no metastatic potential
- Should be removed if the patient finds it aesthetically unacceptable or it is becoming irritated

Pharmacologic

Topical Agents
None is indicated.

Systemic Agents
None is indicated.

Indications for Referral

- The patient should be referred to a dermatologist if there is any question that the diagnosis could be a malignant melanoma.

Bowen's Disease
(Squamous Cell Carcinoma in Situ)

Overview

Pathophysiology
Bowen's disease is synonymous with squamous cell carcinoma in situ (confined to the epidermis). The vast majority of lesions remain as carcinoma in situ throughout the patient's lifetime, but 10% progress to invasive squamous cell carcinomas.

Epidemiology
This disorder is very common in patients exposed to inorganic arsenic. There is an equal sex distribution, with an average age of onset between 50 and 60 years. Non-sun-exposed lesions may have a 20% to 25% incidence of internal malignancy, but this association is debatable at present.

Assessment

Clinical Presentation
Lesions present initially as **chronic erythematous flat, slightly scaly plaques, often with an eczematous appearance and an irregular surface** (see Figure 5-6). They enlarge very slowly and may occur on any body surface, predominantly on **unexposed areas of the trunk or mucus membranes.**

Diagnostics
- A biopsy is required to confirm the diagnosis, usually made on the basis of clinical presentation.

Differential Diagnosis
- Psoriasis vulgaris (symmetric, erythematous plaques with gray-white scale) (see Figure 3-30, *A*)
- Tinea corporis (annular lesions with central clearing) (see Figure 3-9, *B*)
- Basal cell carcinoma (less scaly, rolled borders; more pearllike) (see Figure 5-4)
- Lichen simplex chronicus (ankles and posterior neck are most common locations) (see Figure 3-23)
- Actinic keratosis (smaller, less indurated lesion, which occurs on sun-exposed areas) (see Figure 5-3)
- Nummular eczema (pruritic, coin-shaped lesions; most occur in winter) (see Figure 2-1)

Treatment

Nonpharmacologic
Conservative surgical removal is appropriate.

Pharmacologic

Topical Agents
None is indicated.

Systemic Agents
None is indicated.

Indications for Referral
- Refer to a dermatologist for excision of lesions located in cosmetically prominent locations.

Dermatofibroma

Overview

Pathophysiology
The exact cause is unknown; it is known that the lesion is a localized accumulation of fibroblasts that either develop spontaneously or arise from a reaction to localized trauma (usually an insect bite).

BOWEN'S DISEASE

- Is the first, very superficial stage of squamous cell carcinoma
- Ninety percent of squamous cell lesions remain in situ (Bowen's disease) throughout the patient's life, but 10% progress to become invasive thus illustrating the importance of frequent check-ups and/or excision of any suspicious lesion

They are benign lesions.

Epidemiology

A common lesion, more frequently occurring in females and seen mostly in middle age. Twenty percent of patients have more than one lesion.

Assessment

Clinical Presentation

The dermatofibroma presents as an asymptomatic **single, round, firm, tan to brown papule** (see Figure 5-11). The lesion often **"dimples" when gently pinched** between the thumb and forefinger. A surrounding ring of pigmentation is common. Dermatofibromas most often occur on the lower extremities, near the elbows, or on the lateral trunk. Often they occur at the **site of previous trauma,** such as an insect bite or splinter.

Diagnostics

- The diagnosis is usually based on the clinical presentation; a biopsy is optional.

Differential Diagnosis

- Lipoma (freely moveable, slightly compressible; usually 1 cm or larger) (see Figure 5-26)
- Basal cell carcinoma (more pearly appearance) (see Figure 5-4)

DERMATOFIBROMA

- Is a benign lesion with no metastatic potential
- Frequently arises at the site of previous trauma to the skin, such as an insect bite

Treatment

Dermatofibromas require treatment only for cosmetic reasons or for confirmation of the diagnosis. There is little tendency to spontaneous regression.

Nonpharmacologic

Cryosurgery every 3 to 4 weeks causes gradual involution.

Pharmacologic

Topical Agents
None is indicated.

Systemic Agents
None is indicated.

✳️ | Indications for Referral

• Refer to a dermatologist for excision of lesions in cosmetically prominent locations.

Epidermal Cyst
(Pilar Cyst, Keratin Cyst, Sebaceous Cyst)

Overview

Pathophysiology
The exact cause of an epidermal cyst is not certain; however, the wall of the cyst is probably formed from occluded pilosebaceous follicles. In some cases the lesion may be a result of a traumatizing event on the cutaneous surface, where a portion of epithelium is forced into the superficial dermis. The cyst contains keratin and is usually noninflammatory unless it ruptures, in which case a foreign body reaction occurs. Although the inflammation is usually sterile, it can also be infected.

Epidemiology
A common disorder with a slight male predominance.

Assessment

Clinical Presentation
An epidermal cyst presents as a subcutaneous fluctuant, easily movable **tense swelling** (see Figure 5-13). Commonly there is a **central opening**, which may exude a **pasty, cheesy, odoriferous material** composed of necrotic keratin. It most commonly occurs on the scalp, face, neck, or trunk. Cysts are usually asymptomatic unless inflamed or infected.

Diagnostics
• Diagnosis is usually made by clinical presentation or examination of expressed material. Biopsy results will confirm the diagnosis.

Differential Diagnosis
• Lipoma (softer, without central pore) (see Figure 5-26)
• Metastatic tumor (hard, bound-down lesion without central pore)
• Furuncle (pustular, fluctuant lesion; always inflamed) (see Figure 5-17)

EPIDERMAL CYST

• Is a benign lesion with no metastatic potential

• Should be removed to eliminate the potential of its becoming infected

Treatment

Nonpharmacologic

Incision and drainage
Lesions can be excised before rupturing or they can be allowed to heal (inflammation subsides) before they are excised. Cyst contents may be removed through a small puncture wound or a 3 to 4 mm punch biopsy hole, after topical intradermal anesthesia. If cyst contents are removed, the lesion should be allowed to heal for at least 1 week before the wall is excised.

Pharmacologic

Topical Agents
None is indicated.

Systemic Agents
Antibiotics are optional. **Dicloxacillin** 250 mg PO q6h for 7 to 10 days may be prudent. For those allergic to penicillin, **azithromycin (Zithromax)** 250 mg PO, two tablets on the first day of therapy, followed by one tablet daily for the next 4 days, may be employed.

Indications for Referral

- Referral to a dermatologist for excision may be appropriate if the lesion is located in a cosmetically prominent or logistically difficult area.

Keloids and Hypertrophic Scars

Overview

Pathophysiology
Keloids and hypertrophic scars are caused by an excessive development of connective tissue (collagen) that occurs in response to skin trauma. Androgens and estrogens may also play a role in the pathogenesis. Histamine release in lesions may be responsible for the physical discomfort and itchy sensation associated with them.

Epidemiology

The incidence of keloid development in the United States is 3 to 15 times higher in blacks and Asians than in white races. Approximately 1.5% of the entire U.S. population is affected. Keloids are not present at birth and are rare before puberty. There is an increased incidence in patients with severe acne and hidradenitis suppurativa. A positive family history is obtained in about 10% of non-Asian and non-black patients.

Assessment

Clinical Presentation

Keloids develop over areas of trauma in 3 to 5 weeks and begin as pink, firm, rubbery plaques with telangiectasias (see Figure 5-22). They are smooth, irregularly shaped, and hyperpigmented. Claw-like prolongations are characteristic and lesions may continue to enlarge, **extending outside the area of injury.** Frequently affected areas are the earlobes (after piercing), neck, abdomen, chest, and upper back. Lesions are more exuberant than hypertrophic scars and **may resist therapy** for years. They may be tender, painful, pruritic, or burning. There is about a 60% recurrence rate after surgery in patients with keloids elsewhere.

    Hypertrophic scars usually occur over the sternum, deltoid, mandible, or upper lip and are less exuberant than keloids. Additionally they tend to be **restricted to the area of injury.** They **involute spontaneously** and resolve without treatment within 6 to 18 months. Occasionally they are pruritic but more often are completely **asymptomatic.**

Diagnostics

- Diagnosis is made clinically and confirmed with skin biopsy if necessary.

Differential Diagnosis

- Dermatofibroma (round, firm nodule; dimples when pinched) (see Figure 5-11)
- Lymphoma (occurs without prior history of trauma to skin; tendency to central clearing)

Treatment

Nonpharmacologic

Prevention (avoidance of both accidental and intentional trauma to the skin) is essential in those prone to keloid. When skin disruption occurs, pressure dressings over the area 8 hours a day for 4 to

---

HYPERTROPHIC SCAR

- Results from skin trauma in genetically predisposed individuals
- Usually resolves spontaneously in 6 to 18 months
- Is restricted to the area of injury

KELOID

- Results from skin trauma in genetically predisposed individuals
- Physicians should be informed of potential before surgery
- May continue to grow and extend beyond edges of initial scar
- Does not resolve spontaneously

6 months may be beneficial. Topical **silicone gel sheeting may also minimize the extent of scarring and promote gradual resolution.**

Pharmacologic

Topical/Intralesional

Liquid nitrogen with a 10- to 15-second freeze, used immediately before the injection of intralesional steroids **(triamcinolone [Kenalog-10 or Kenalog-40])** every 3 to 4 weeks may increase collagenase production in addition to inhibiting collagen synthesis. Cryotherapy not only produces temporary anesthesia, but its mild edematous effect softens the tissue to allow easier injection of the corticosteroid.

Intralesional **5% 5-fluorouracil (5% 5 FU)** mixed 1:8 with **triamcinolone (Kenalog 10 mg/ml)** injected every week until lesions flatten is also effective. Medication should be injected only until lesions blanch.

Indications for Referral

- If the preceding treatment does not minimize the keloid to a painless or cosmetically acceptable level, surgical excision is indicated and should be performed by a dermatologist.
- Laser treatment by physicians familiar with various lasers and their use may also be helpful in minimizing keloids. Here the Ultrapulse CO_2 and Er:Yag lasers work best to vaporize the lesion. The healing wound is then covered with a silicone dressing. Weekly follow-up and injection of 5% 5 FU/triamcinolone until the lesion is healed and flat may be performed by the nurse practitioner.
- The 585 nm Pulse Dye Laser and PhotoDerm VL have been found effective when used at monthly intervals to promote involution and elimination of the telangiectatic, erythematous component of keloids and hypertrophic scars.
- Systemic methotrexate has been useful postoperatively in patients with lesions recalcitrant to treatment and may be combined with laser therapy.

Keratoacanthoma

Overview

Pathophysiology
The exact cause is unknown; the lesion may be of viral origin. There is an increased incidence in sites with exposure to tar, mineral oil, or trauma. There is no association with internal malignancy.

Epidemiology
Keratoacanthoma has a peak incidence between ages 50 and 60. The male/female ratio is almost 3:1. It is uncommon in Asian and dark-skinned people but has a higher incidence in those who smoke cigarettes. It is most common in immunosuppressed patients. Up to 30% of patients with keratoacanthoma may have an associated squamous cell carcinoma.

Assessment

Clinical Presentation
The lesion presents suddenly as a **red dome-shaped nodule with a central keratin plug** (see Figure 5-23). It has **raised, rolled borders,** often with **overlying telangiectasias,** and may be tender. A fully developed tumor retains its red dome-shaped appearance but has a central keratin-filled crater.

Keratoacanthoma grows spontaneously over 2 weeks to 3 months and may reach a final size of 5 to 15 mm, occasionally much larger. Lesions tend to involute spontaneously with scarring in up to 30% of those affected.

Lesions most commonly occur on the head, neck, dorsal hands, and forearms but may occur anywhere, including the oral mucosa. It is rare to find keratoacanthoma on the palms or soles.

Diagnostics
- Because of the clinical similarity of the lesion to squamous and basal cell carcinomas, all excised tissue should be submitted for pathology evaluation.

Differential Diagnosis
- Squamous cell carcinoma (slower growth without a central core) (see Figure 5-38)
- Basal cell carcinoma (much slower growth) (see Figure 5-4)

KERATOACANTHOMA

- Is a benign lesion that has no malignant potential
- Has similar characteristics to malignant lesions (basal cell carcinoma [BCC] and squamous cell carcinoma [SCC]); therefore biopsy may be prudent
- May resolve spontaneously over time

- Dermatofibroma (no central core) (see Figure 5-11)
- Verruca vulgaris (not crateriform) (see Figure 5-39, *A*)
- Molluscum contagiosum (smaller lesion with dome-shaped papule) (see Figure 5-28)
- Hyperkeratotic actinic keratosis (more irregular border)

Treatment

Nonpharmacologic

In asymptomatic lesions on noncosmetically prominent areas, close observation may be sufficient. Lesions should be accurately measured and documented for later comparison. Photographs may be helpful.

The use of *curettage and electrodesiccation* is curative in 90% of lesions.

Shave excision is best for lesions not larger than 15 mm in diameter. It is usually followed by topical therapy with **5-fluorouracil, 20% to 50% podophyllin** qod × 3, or cryotherapy

Pharmacologic

Topical Agents

5-Fluorouracil cream (Efudex) applied tid with occlusion during the growth phase may be effective. Lesions resolve in 1 to 6 weeks. To enhance penetration of the medication, the central crust should be removed and the lesion pretreated with 6% salicylic acid gel **(Keralyt)** or 20% urea cream **(Carmol 20).**

Systemic Agents

Acitretin (Soriatane) 25 to 50 mg q12h, taken with the main meal, may be especially useful for multiple lesions. Therapy should be terminated when lesions have resolved. A patient advisory regarding the possibility of birth defects caused by acitretin should be signed by all females of childbearing age.

Indications for Referral

- Refer to a dermatologist for excision of lesions in cosmetically prominent locations.
- Refer to a dermatologist for excision if biopsy results indicate squamous or basal cell carcinoma.

Lipoma

Overview

Pathophysiology

Lipomas represent a proliferation of histologically normal adipose tissue, of unknown origin.

Epidemiology

At least 3% of all benign tumors are lipomas. Thirty-five percent occur in the fourth and fifth decades, with females more often affected than males.

Assessment

Clinical Presentation

Soft, single or multiple, freely mobile, slightly compressible growths (see Figure 5-26) that are very slow growing appear. The size may vary from 1 cm to several centimeters in diameter. They are most commonly located on the **shoulders, legs, arms, buttocks, and back.** Most are asymptomatic.

Diagnostics

- The diagnosis is made clinically; excised tissue should be sent for pathology evaluation.

Differential Diagnosis

- Epidermal cyst (fluctuant lesion with central clearing; odoriferous contents; usually on the scalp, neck, face, or trunk) (see Figure 5-13)

Treatment

No treatment is necessary unless the lesion is bothersome to the patient or cosmetically unacceptable. In cases where it is desired, treatment is by surgical excision.

LIPOMA

- Is a benign accumulation of adipose tissue
- Does not require treatment unless it is cosmetically unacceptable to the patient

Indications for Referral

- Referral to a dermatologist for excision of large lesions or those in cosmetically prominent or logistically difficult locations is appropriate.

Malignant Melanoma

Overview

Pathophysiology

Malignant melanomas (MMs) develop from benign melanocytic cells (congenital nevi, dysplastic nevi); their exact causative factors remain unknown. Ultraviolet B radiation may play a role in this malignant transformation. Spread occurs by several methods including local extension and lymphatic drainage. The radial (horizontal) growth phase occurs as the cells spread through the epidermis. Cells that have begun to grow down into the dermis are characterized as being in the vertical growth phase.

There are four commonly recognized classifications of melanoma:

- *Superficial spreading melanoma (SSM):* Very common, accounting for approximately 70% of all melanomas. It usually begins in the fifth decade, especially in women. A prolonged radial (horizontal) growth phase of up to 10 years is characteristic with the lesions reaching 1 to 2 cm before the vertical growth phase begins. It is characterized by **variegated colors, irregular borders,** and an eventual diameter of 2 to 3 cm (see Figure 5-27). **Margins may be elevated.** The vertical growth phase is characterized by nodule formation, bleeding, or ulceration, with a subsequent increase in the probability of metastasis. Early presentation is of a slightly elevated, brown pigmented lesion. **Notching of the margin** of the lesion is common. Partial regression may cause central pigment loss.
- *Nodular melanoma (NM):* Constituting 15% of malignant melanomas, it presents most commonly between age 40 to 60 with a male/female incidence of 2:1. NM presents as a round or irregular, **slightly elevated papule of gray-blue color on a dark background** embedded beneath the surface. There is no apparent radial growth, but rather an immediate vertical growth, which begins with rapid appearance of a dark or occasionally nonpigmented nodule. These lesions **ulcerate and bleed** frequently. Metastasis occurs early with a subsequent poor prognosis.
- *Lentigo maligna melanoma (LMM):* A fairly uncommon melanoma, constituting 5% of malignant melanomas. It usually occurs on sun-exposed areas, especially the face. On individuals age 50 to 70, 10% occur on the hand or leg. The lesion tends to be a **flat (stainlike) macule a few centimeters in diameter** with areas of regression and loss of skin markings. The color

gradually darkens overall but may demonstrate flecks of **irregular pigmentation.**

- *Acral-lentiginous malignant melanoma (ALM):* A **flat, variably pigmented brown-black macule** commonly on the **tips of the fingers and toes or under the nail bed,** this lesion enlarges peripherally and develops blue and depigmented areas. It can present as a **black nail** or with loss of a nail. It is the most common form of melanoma among the black population and occurs predominantly in the sixth and seventh decades.

In general, females have a better prognosis than males. Palpable lymph node involvement bodes a worse prognosis than nonpalpable nodes, with a 10% to 19% 5-year survival rate. Site of the lesion is also important; distal extremity sites are less likely to become fatal. Primary lesions on the upper trunk have a poorer prognosis than those on the lower trunk. Lesions in the nasal cavity, pharynx, oral cavity, or larynx are almost always fatal.

Metastases can develop 10 to 15 years after removal of the primary tumor. Melanoma is one of the few tumors that consistently metastasize to the spleen and may cause unexplained splenomegaly. It also frequently metastasizes to the heart.

Biopsied **lesions are staged by the pathologist,** according to the amount of penetration discerned, as follows:

- Level 1: Confined to the epidermis (also referred to as *in situ*)
- Level 2: Invasion of papillary dermis
- Level 3: Invasion of interface of papillary and reticular dermis
- Level 4: Invasion of reticular dermis
- Level 5: Invasion of subcutaneous fat

The exact depth of the invasion (in millimeters) is given. Lesions less than 0.76 mm in depth are almost always 100% cured with simple excision of 0.5 to 1 cm borders.

Epidemiology

Malignant melanoma is most common in persons with fair skin, red hair, blue eyes, and freckles. The number of new cases reported annually is rising, perhaps as a result of the decreasing amount of protection provided by the atmosphere, as well as increased recreational sun exposure. The greatest number of cases occur in individuals 30 to 49 years old, among whom it is the second most prevalent cancer among men and the fourth among women. There is an increased incidence in the southern United States and countries closer to the equator, with Australia having the highest reported incidence.

Assessment

Clinical Presentation

The early development of a malignant lesion produces so few warning symptoms that it is often unobserved. Twenty-five percent of patients remember the lesion's being present for up to 3 years before diagnosis. The signs of malignancy are rapid change in size or color, development of inflammation, bleeding, and ulceration. Key clues to diagnosis are the **ABCD's of MM:**

A: **Asymmetry** of border
B: **Border** irregularity
C: **Color** variegation
D: **Diameter** greater than 6 mm

The most common sites are the head, neck, and trunk in males and the distal lower extremities in females. MM may also occur on the mucus membranes and in internal organs.

(Specific distinguishing characteristics of the four common types of melanoma are discussed under Pathophysiology.)

Diagnostics

- Many conditions can imitate MM, and the clinician must be extremely careful in differentiating benign from malignant. If any doubt exists, the lesion should be biopsied to establish a confirmatory diagnosis. However, because a shave biopsy does not preserve the anatomic relationships necessary to permit accurate staging and diagnosis, an **excisional biopsy** is preferable.

Differential Diagnosis

- Other benign melanocytic lesions (refer to sections on junctional nevus, compound nevus, Spitz nevus)
- Pigmented, inflamed, or hemorrhagic seborrheic keratosis (appears more stuck-on and greasy; may remain unchanged for years) (see Figure 5-3)
- Pigmented basal cell carcinoma (rolled border with telangiectasias; more pearllike) (see Figure 5-4)
- Dermatofibroma (tan to light brown nodule; dimples when pinched) (see Figure 5-11)

Treatment

Nonpharmacologic

Surgical excision is performed. The lesion must be completely excised to ensure the prevention of metastasis.

MALIGNANT MELANOMA

- Characteristics are summarized by the ABCDs of melanoma: Asymmetry of border, Border irregularity, Color irregularity, and Diameter larger than 6 mm (a pencil eraser)
- Can be best prevented by routine full body examinations by trained personnel, consistent sun protection, and prompt reporting of any suspicious or changed lesions

Pharmacologic

Topical Agents
None is indicated.

Systemic Agents
None is indicated.

Indications for Referral

- **Suspicion of malignant melanoma should always be referred to a dermatologist. Without treatment most melanomas will metastasize and cause the death of the patient.**

Molluscum Contagiosum

Overview

Pathophysiology
Molluscum contagiosum is an infection caused by a poxvirus, limited to humans and monkeys, and spread by direct skin-to-skin contact or through fomites to skin transmission. There is a 2- to 7-week incubation period with persistence of lesions for a few months, before spontaneous resolution or in association with an inflammatory reaction.

Epidemiology
Formerly the infection was found primarily in children, but now it is also seen very commonly in the pubic area and genitalia of sexually active young adults. Peak age is 20 to 29. Outbreaks centered around swimming pools have been reported. There is an increased incidence in atopic and immunosuppressed patients.

Assessment

Clinical Presentation
The lesion characteristically is a **flesh-colored firm, domed, umbilicated papule, 2 to 5 mm in diameter** (see Figure 5-28). A cheesy white material may be expressed. The lesion is

autoinoculable, as well as contagious to others, with development of further lesions occurring on contiguous sites. Lesions most commonly involve the **inner thighs, lower abdominal, and perianal areas** in young adults and the **face, eyelids, mouth, trunk, and extremities** in children. There are usually fewer than 20 lesions present, although disseminated cutaneous infection with thousands of lesions is seen in patients with atopic eczema and in the immunologically compromised. In a few patients an inflammatory dermatitis develops around the individual lesions, but most lesions are **asymptomatic** and resolve within 2 to 9 months without treatment.

Diagnostics
- Diagnosis is made clinically; a skin biopsy is optional. Skin scraping demonstrates the molluscum bodies.

Differential Diagnosis
- Dermal nevus (singular papule without central umbilication)
- Verruca plana (more keratotic; does not have central umbilication, nor is it dome-shaped)
- Condyloma acuminata (flesh-toned papules in genital, perianal, or anal location)
- Basal cell carcinoma (singular lesion with telangiectasias) (see Figure 5-4)
- Varicella (presence of blisters and vesicles) (see Figure 5-8)

MOLLUSCUM CONTAGIOSUM

- Is a viral disorder that is contagious and spread by skin-to-skin contact

Treatment

Nonpharmacologic
For a small number of lesions surgical removal with a dermal curette is appropriate.

Pharmacologic

Topical Agents
For multiple lesions **cryotherapy** with liquid nitrogen for 3 to 5 seconds may be used. Alternatively **25% podophyllin** may be painted on the lesions twice weekly for many weeks, or they may be treated on a weekly basis with a saturated **trichloroacetic acid solution. Duofilm** dressing or **Retin-A** cream applied daily may also be beneficial.

Systemic Agents
None is indicated.

Indications for Referral

- Refer immunosuppressed patients to a pulmonologist.

Nevus Sebaceus

Overview

Pathophysiology

Nevus sebaceus represents a malformation of the skin with an abundance of sebaceous glands. A basal cell carcinoma occurs in a portion of the lesion in 5% to 20% of cases.

Epidemiology

It is fairly uncommon, with an equal sexual incidence.

Assessment

Clinical Presentation

A sharply circumscribed solitary, yellow-orange oval to linear verrucous papule (see Figure 5-29), frequently present at birth, is seen. It is most commonly located on the head near the vertex of the scalp, or on the neck. It becomes more verrucous and yellow in puberty.

Diagnostics

- The diagnosis is made clinically, with a confirmatory biopsy as needed.

Differential Diagnosis

- Xanthoma (usually multiple and commonly found in the periorbital area)
- Epidermal nevus (difficult to distinguish, but usually has less of a yellow-orange tinge)
- Verruca vulgaris (usually tan-colored without the yellow-orange tinge) (see Figure 5-39, *A*)

NEVUS SEBACEUS

• Is a benign neoplasm with no malignant potential

Treatment

Nonpharmacologic

Surgical excision removes the entire growth. It is best performed before puberty, when the lesions are at their smallest size.

Pharmacologic
None is indicated.

★ | Indications for Referral |

- Refer to a dermatologist if lesions change in any way.

Sebaceous Hyperplasia

Overview

Pathophysiology
Although the exact cause is unknown, chronic sun damage is a contributing factor, particularly in fair-skinned individuals. The continued injury results in enlarged sebaceous glands.

Epidemiology
Sebaceous hyperplasia is most prevalent in fair-skinned individuals.

Assessment

Clinical Presentation
Lesions are usually *solitary* and present as *soft, yellowish papules* 2 to 3 mm in size, on the **forehead and cheeks.** Papules are **umbilicated, cauliflower-like,** and asymptomatic (see Figure 5-35). **Telangiectasias** on the surface are common but occur only in the valleys between the small, yellow lobules, rather than haphazardly, as they do in basal cell carcinoma. The condition will persist unless treated.

Diagnostics
- The diagnosis is usually made by clinical inspection but is confirmed with skin biopsy.

Differential Diagnosis
- Basal cell carcinoma (more pearllike appearance; telangiectasias present haphazardly throughout) (see Figure 5-4)
- Molluscum contagiosum (occurs on trunk and extremities, as well as face; does not have telangiectasias; usually multiple lesions) (see Figure 5-28)

SEBACEOUS HYPERPLASIA

- Is a benign neoplasm with no malignant potential

Nonpharmacologic

Because the condition is a benign disorder, no treatment is necessary unless requested by the patient for cosmetic improvement. Light electrodesiccation, liquid nitrogen cryosurgery, or shave excision is the treatment of choice for patients who are not candidates for isotretinoin (Accutane).

Pharmacologic

Topical Agents
None is indicated.

Systemic Agents
Isotretinoin (Accutane) 10 mg PO qod has been shown to be effective in patients with normal liver function study results who are not currently pregnant or planning a pregnancy for at least 1 month after the cessation of therapy.

Indications for Referral

- Refer to a dermatologist if biopsy results indicate basal cell carcinoma.

Seborrheic Keratosis

Overview

Pathophysiology
The exact cause of seborrheic keratoses (SK) is unknown; they are partially derived from the infundibular portion of the hair follicle. Additionally they represent a proliferation of epidermal keratinocytes. The development is not dependent on sun exposure and there is no malignant potential.

Epidemiology
Seborrheic keratoses are the most common skin tumors seen in the middle-aged and elderly population. They are present in 90% of people above age 50; age 30 is the average age of onset. There may be a familial, autosomal dominant trait when they appear profusely in an individual. There is an equal sex distribution and they may be associated with obesity.

Assessment

Clinical Presentation

An SK appears as a **warty,** pigmented (dirty yellow to black), sharply marginated, **greasy** papule with a **stuck-on** quality (see Figure 5-36). A cutaneous horn may develop as a keratotic, conical protuberance. Open comedones may be present in the lesions. They occur most commonly on the **back, central chest (often inframammary), face, and scalp** and may be numerous. Occasionally they are pruritic, and they may increase in number with time.

Diagnostics

- Diagnosis is usually made on the basis of clinical presentation, but if there is any doubt in differentiating from melanoma, skin biopsy must be performed.

Differential Diagnosis

- Pigmented nevus (usually smaller and more papular)
- Actinic keratosis (more erythematous and scaly; less keratotic) (see Figure 5-3)
- Malignant melanoma (irregular pigmentation, less verrucous appearance) (see Figure 5-27)
- Lentigo (flatter without induration or greasy appearance) (see Figure 6-9)

SEBORRHEIC KERATOSIS

- Is a very common cosmetic disorder with no malignant potential
- Should be removed if it becomes irritated of inflamed

Treatment

Nonpharmacologic

Removal is only done for cosmetic or diagnostic reasons. Patients should be informed that new lesions will most likely continue to appear.

Surgical treatment employs shave excision or curettage. Local anesthesia is recommended.

Cryotherapy is only appropriate when there is no doubt about the diagnosis and/or when there are hundreds of lesions. Apply liquid nitrogen for 15 to 20 seconds. Local anesthesia is not required. The lesions will crust and fall off spontaneously in a few days to a week. The cosmetic result is usually excellent.

Pharmacologic

Topical Agents
None is indicated.

Systemic Agents
None is indicated.

For Seborrheic Keratosis Patient Teaching information and materials, turn to p. 463.

Indications for Referral

- **Refer to a dermatologist if biopsy results indicate malignant melanoma.**
- Rapid onset of dozens of lesions may suggest the Leser-Trélat sign, which indicates an underlying malignancy and should be referred to a dermatologist.

Spitz Nevus (Benign Juvenile Melanoma)

Overview

Pathophysiology
Spitz nevi are benign proliferations of melanocytes, the exact cause of which is unknown.

Epidemiology
Spitz nevi are relatively uncommon, representing less than 1% of all common nevi. They occur most frequently in childhood at age 3 to 13, although up to 30% of lesions occur in adults.

Assessment

Clinical Presentation
A Spitz nevus is usually a solitary firm, slightly scaly, round, dome-shaped nodule with a pink to deep red color and sharp borders (see Figure 5-37). It may bleed easily when traumatized. Ninety-five percent of lesions are less than 1 cm in diameter and symmetric. Spitz nevi usually grow rapidly over 3 to 12 months and then stabilize in size. The face and lower extremities are the most common areas affected. The course is benign, although lesions do not regress spontaneously. They are asymptomatic, although patients may be alarmed by the sudden occurrence and rapid growth.

Diagnostics
- Although the diagnosis is usually made clinically, skin biopsy is needed for confirmation.

Differential Diagnosis

- Common melanocytic nevus (slower onset and growth; uniform color without erythema)
- Angiomas (bright red papule, usually less than 3 mm in diameter) (see Figure 12-2) Malignant melanoma (irregular borders, darker color, larger) (see Figure 5-27)

Treatment

Nonpharmacologic

Surgical excision or punch biopsy for smaller lesions is definitive therapy. Lesions may be excised by shaving, usually with an excellent cosmetic result, but recurrence is possible.

Pharmacologic

Topical Agents
None is indicated.

Systemic Agents
None is indicated.

Indications for Referral

- Referral to a dermatologist is appropriate for surgical excision or for removal of lesions in difficult or cosmetically prominent locations.

Squamous Cell Carcinoma

Overview

Pathophysiology

Squamous cell carcinoma (SCC) is a response of keratinocytes to any environmental carcinogen, but sunlight is by far the most commonly implicated. Other causes include burns, scars, chronic ulcers, and inflammatory disease. Tumors rarely arise without some previous exogenous cause. Many develop from actinic keratoses. Radiation-induced tumors or those arising at sites of previous scars or burns have a metastasis rate of 30%, whereas tumors on sun-exposed skin rarely metastasize (3% to 5%). Since metastasis occurs through the lymphatic system, lesions that occur in areas close to draining lymphatic nodes metastasize at a rate of 10% to 20%.

SPITZ NEVUS

- Is a cosmetic disorder with no malignant potential
- May be alarming because of its rapid growth rate; and if growth is rapid, should undergo biopsy

Bowen's disease is synonomous with squamous cell carcinoma in situ (confined to the epidermis). Please refer to the specific section under this heading for more information.

Epidemiology

Squamous cell carcinoma is the second most common skin cancer in whites and the most common skin cancer in blacks. The male/female ratio is 2:1. The tumor usually develops later in life, with a steep rise in incidence after age 55. It appears earlier in people with excessive sun exposure. There is up to a 35-fold increase in incidence in immunosuppressed people, who are also at greater risk of metastasis. Smokers have an increased incidence of lip involvement. One hundred thousand to 150,000 people are affected annually in the United States.

Assessment

Clinical Presentation

Squamous cell carcinoma is usually asymptomatic. Tumors appear as **firm skin-colored to reddish-brown nodules on damaged skin** (see Figure 5-38). Frequently there is a **central ulceration.** Scaling and crusting may be present. Seventy percent of lesions occur on the head and neck, although any cutaneous surface can be affected. Lesions on the lower lip appear as firm, whitish macules with possible central ulceration (leukoplakia).

Diagnostics
• A skin biopsy is required for confirmative diagnosis.

Differential Diagnosis
• Basal cell carcinoma (more pearllike) (see Figure 5-4)
• Actinic keratosis (more macular and scaly) (see Figure 5-3)
• Seborrheic keratosis (greasy, stuck-on appearance) (see Figure 5-36)
• Psoriasis vulgaris (symmetric, erythematous, scaly patch or plaque) (see Figure 3-30, *A*)

Treatment

Nonpharmacologic
Surgical excision is most appropriate since lesions commonly grow down hair follicles.

Pharmacologic

Topical Agents
None is indicated.

SQUAMOUS CELL CARCINOMA

• Is caused by cumulative sun damage to the skin over many years
• Treatment must include avoidance of the sun between 10:00 AM and 2:00 PM, consistent and liberal use of sunscreen (SPF >15), routine full body skin examinations every 6 to 12 months, and wearing protective clothing
• Should be suspected in any lesion that is scaly, red, or crusty or does not heal

Systemic Agents
None is indicated.

Indications for Referral

- Location of lesion in a cosmetically prominent location or area difficult to treat such as the eyelids, inner canthus, nose, or ears. (Refer to Mohs' surgeon.)

Verrucae (Warts)

Overview

Pathophysiology

Verrucae are caused by infection with the human papillomavirus, either by direct contact or by autoinoculation. The virus grows within the nucleus of keratinocytes, which it fills, then spills into the cytoplasm. The resulting lesion lies entirely within the stratum corneum; there are no roots penetrating into the dermis. There are numerous subtypes of the virus, all resulting in slightly varied clinical presentations. Some of the viruses may have oncogenic potential.

Epidemiology

Verrucae constitute the most common viral infection of the skin, occurring in 7% to 10% of the population. Although warts can occur at any age, they are most common between the ages of 12 and 16. The frequency of warts is believed to have increased over the past 20 years. Patients with warts may show decreased cell-mediated humoral immunity compared with that of controls. (See later sections for information regarding specific types of warts.)

Assessment

Clinical Presentation

Warts begin as minute smooth-surfaced skin-colored lesions that enlarge for a period of time. The surface becomes roughened and finely papillomatous. **Normal skin lines are obscured.** Repeated irritation may cause a wart to continue enlarging. The course is completely unpredictable. Warts may remain unchanged for years and then resolve spontaneously. Most are asymptomatic but may become tender or irritated because of their location.

There are various types of warts:

- *Verruca vulgaris (common wart):* flesh-toned or gray-brown, scaly papule of varying size, usually with visible **black dots** on the surface (thrombosed capillaries) (see Figure 5-39, *A*). May be single or multiple and is usually asymptomatic. Most frequently involves the dorsal and palmar surfaces of the hands and fingers and the area surrounding and beneath the nails. About 65% disappear spontaneously within 2 years.
- *Verruca plana (flat or juvenile wart):* smooth, flat, or slightly elevated round papule 1 to 5 mm in diameter. Usually **multiple (possibly hundreds)** and commonly located on the face, backs of hands, and shins. May coalesce in a linear arrangement in scratch marks.
- *Verruca digitata filiform (digitate or filiform wart):* a projecting lesion 1 to 10 mm in length with multiple **fingerlike projections** (see Figure 5-39, *B*). It commonly presents as a single lesion in the beard area, eyelids, neck, or scalp.
- *Verruca plantaris (plantar wart):* appears on the plantar surface of the foot like a sharply circumscribed callus (see Figure 5-39, *D*). Usually only one is present. Most warts occur beneath pressure points and thus are **tender.** The wart is frequently surrounded by a collar of hyperkeratosis. **Multiple black dots** are present (thrombosed capillaries) and bleed with removal of the surface. In some cases lateral spread of the infection results in large hyperkeratotic plaques called **mosaic** warts.
- *Condyloma acuminatum (anogenital or venereal wart):* appears as a group of moist, soft, papillary projections producing **cauliflower-like growths** on the **mucus membrane of the penis, vulva, and perianal region** (see Figure 5-39, *C*). It may also be present in the vagina and anal canal. Females are more likely to be affected than males. Eighty percent of patients are 17 to 33 years of age. Mothers with genital condylomata may infect their newborn during delivery. Cervical condylomatous changes are associated with cervical neoplasia in up to 84% of cases. Over 70% of female sexual partners of men with condyloma have condyloma themselves.

Diagnostics
- A biopsy is required to confirm the diagnosis, which is usually made on the basis of clinical presentation. The **presence of black dots and the absence of normal skin lines** help to differentiate the lesion from corns (clavi) and calluses. Plantar warts are **painful on lateral pressure,** whereas clavi are more painful on direct pressure and usually occur over bony prominences.

Differential Diagnosis

- Seborrheic keratosis (more stuck-on appearance) (see Figure 5-36)
- Molluscum contagiosum (usually has a central pore indentation) (see Figure 5-28)
- Lichen planus (usually on an erythematous or violaceous base) (see Figure 5-25)
- Callus or corn (clavus) (skin lines remain; pain is increased on direct, rather than lateral pressure; occurs over bony prominences)

Treatment

Nonpharmacologic

Sixty percent of untreated warts (in children) disappear within 2 years without treatment. Predisposing factors such as hyperhidrosis of the feet or vaginal discharge should be treated.

Surgical excision is the treatment of choice for nodular lesions (or for any in which the diagnosis is unclear), as there is a 10% incidence of its being squamous cell carcinoma in situ.

Laser therapy with the CO_2 laser may be used to remove the wart and the epidermis to a distance 2 mm from the lesion.

Pharmacologic

Topical Agents

Liquid nitrogen cryotherapy. The lesion is frozen until blanching occurs and remains for approximately 30 seconds after withdrawal of the freezing applicator. Once the skin color has returned to normal, the procedure should be repeated. If blistering occurs, the blister should be removed, with care taken not to contaminate other skin surfaces with the fluid. Cryotherapy frequently requires multiple treatments at 2- to 3-week intervals to effect a complete cure.

Keratolytic combination medications, which are various combinations of salicylic and lactic acid, podophyllin, and/or cantharidin such as **Cantharone Plus, Duofilm, and Verrusol,** applied in two coats, once nightly until resolution, are also helpful. Patients should be instructed to soak the lesion for 10 minutes in water, débride it with an emery board or pumice stone, then apply one to two drops of medication and allow it to dry. Occlusive tape should be applied over the wart (to enhance penetration) and left in place for 24 hours. The entire procedure should be repeated every 24 hours until resolution or until tenderness occurs. Combining topical at-home treatment with monthly office visits for cryotherapy often enhances resolution.

VERRUCAE

- Is a viral infection that will resolve spontaneously in time, although treatment encourages resolution
- Treatment preparations should be applied to damp, soft pared skin to allow maximum penetration of medication
- Contagion should be reduced by wearing condoms during sex if genital warts are present
- On female genitalia may be an indicator of cervical cancer; females with genital warts should therefore have annual gynecologic examinations

Potent salicylic acid preparations such as **Mediplast (40%), Duoplant gel (27%), Occlusal-HP liquid (26%), and Salonil ointment (40%)** are especially effective for plantar warts and offer the patient alternatives such as gels, plasters, and ointments. They are applied similarly to the combination products as described previously. Some patients may prefer the convenience of patches such as **Trans-Ver-Sal,** but they are slightly weaker at 15% salicylic acid. Patients should be informed that 3 to 4 months of treatment may be necessary before complete resolution of the lesion occurs.

Light electrodesiccation and curettage have a 10% recurrence rate in patients below age 18 that increases rapidly after age 25.

Twenty-five percent to 40% podophyllin in tincture of benzoin (Pod-Ben-25, Podofin) or 0.5% podofilox (Condylox) for warts on mucosal surfaces is recommended. Care should be taken to apply the solution only to the lesion itself. The surrounding normal skin can be protected with Vaseline before treatment. The application is repeated weekly (or qod in recalcitrant cases) until the wart resolves. After 6 weeks of treatment an alternative method should be tried. This method should not be used during pregnancy, in infants, or on the vagina or cervix.

Cantharidin (Cantharone) 0.7% solution is an alternative treatment for plantar warts. It is applied directly on the lesion (care should be taken to prevent contact with normal skin) and occluded under adhesive tape for 24 hours. A hemorrhagic blister will form and fall off after 7 to 14 days. Scarring is unusual. Treatment can be repeated on a weekly basis if wart tissue remains.

5-Fluorouracil cream applied qd is especially useful for vaginal and facial flat warts.

For **recalcitrant warts** the treatment regimen combines multiple approaches: freezing with liquid nitrogen, followed by electrodesiccation, concluding with cantharadin, which is occluded with moleskin tape for 24 hours.

Intralesional Agents

Bleomycin sulfate 0.5 to 1 unit/ml solution has an affinity for the epidermis, where it concentrates to produce localized necrosis. Injected intralesionally; the amount should be limited to 0.1 ml per individual site or until the lesion blanches. Treatment may be repeated weekly or monthly with only mild to moderate pain persisting up to 3 days. There is a 90% cure rate within 4 weeks for lesions on digits and a 65% cure rate for plantar warts.

Systemic Agents

Accutane 40 mg PO qd for 4 to 8 weeks may be beneficial for extensive flat warts. The same precautions apply as in the treatment of acne (see Chapter 1). **Cimetidine (Tagamet)** has also been recommended for the treatment of extensive warts. However, recent studies do not support the efficacy of this treatment, and its use is not recommended.

Indications for Referral

- The presence of vaginal or cervical warts should prompt a referral for a gynecologic exam to rule out the possibility of cancer.

For Verrucae (Warts) Patient Teaching information and materials, turn to p. 469.

Pigmentary Disorders

Figure 6-1 Café-au-Lait

Light tan macule on the lateral aspect of the thigh.

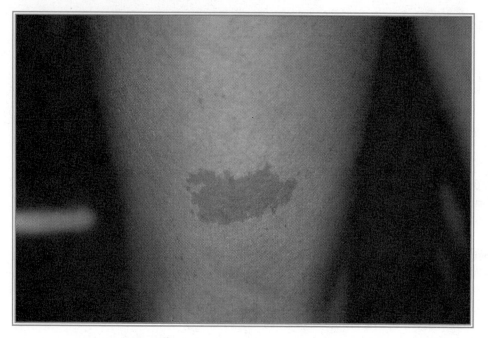

Figure 6-2 NEVUS

A, Becker's nevus: Light brown macule with overlying hair. **B,** Compound nevus: Well-circumscribed tan-brown papule on the cheek.

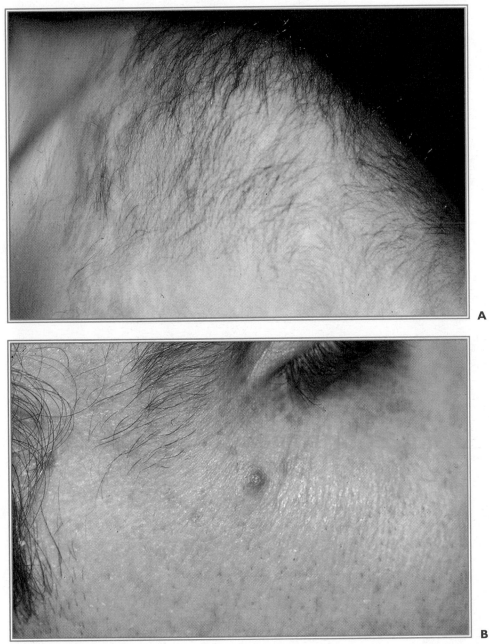

A

B

continued

Figure 6-2 NEVUS

C, Halo nevus: Pigmented, slightly irregular nevus with surrounding stark hyperpigmentation. *D,* Intradermal nevus: Well-marginated, deeply pigmented papule in the nasolabial groove.

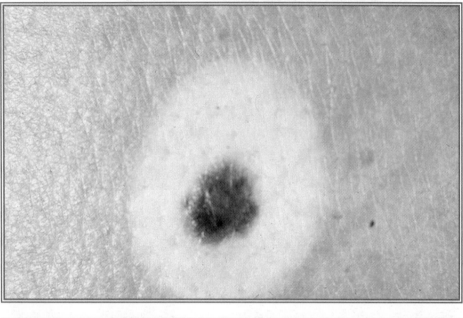

C

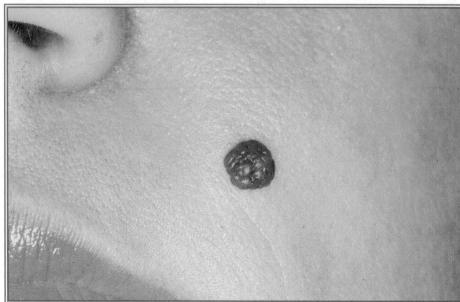

D

Figure 6-2 **NEVUS**

E, Nevus spilus: Light tan, macular lesion with multiple small black/brown macules within.

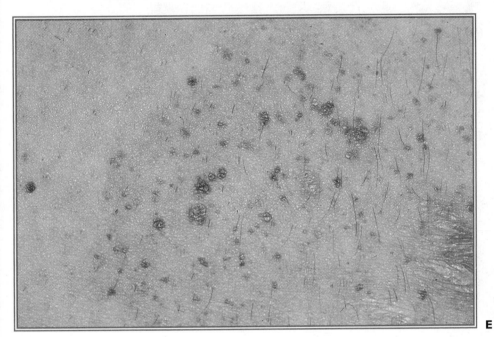

E

Figure 6-3 CONGENITAL NEVUS

Dark brown, hairy nevi on a young child, present since birth.

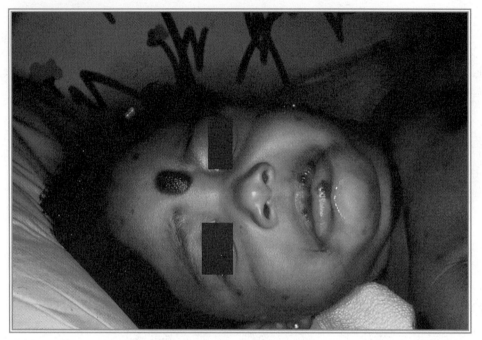

(Courtesy of Stacy R. Smith, MD.)

Figure 6-4   DYSPLASTIC NEVUS

Multiple nevi larger than 1 cm and irregularly pigmented.

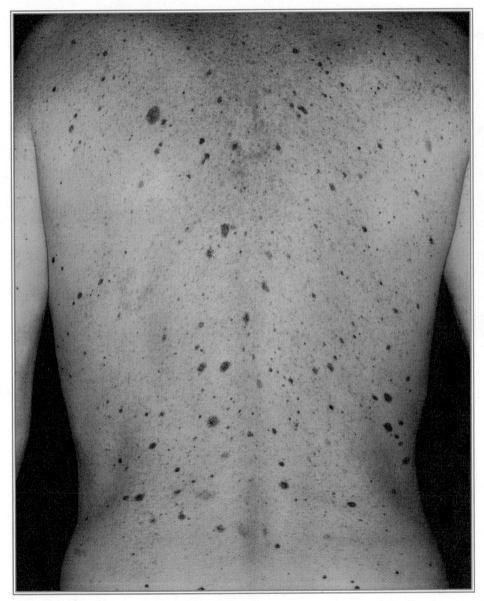

(From Habif TP: *Clinical Dermatology,* ed 3, St Louis, Mosby.)

Figure 6-5   FRECKLES

Extensive small tan to brown macules on the central aspect of the face of a 6-year-old child.

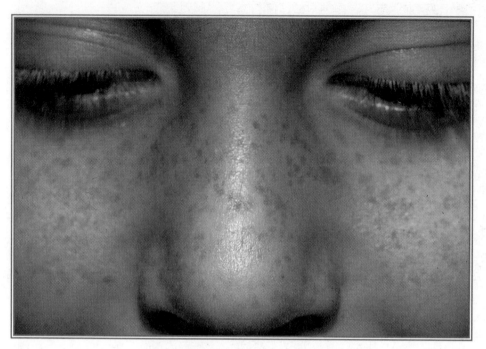

Figure 6-6   MELASMA

Blotchy dark brown macular lesions on the central aspect of the face, especially prominent on the checks and forehead.

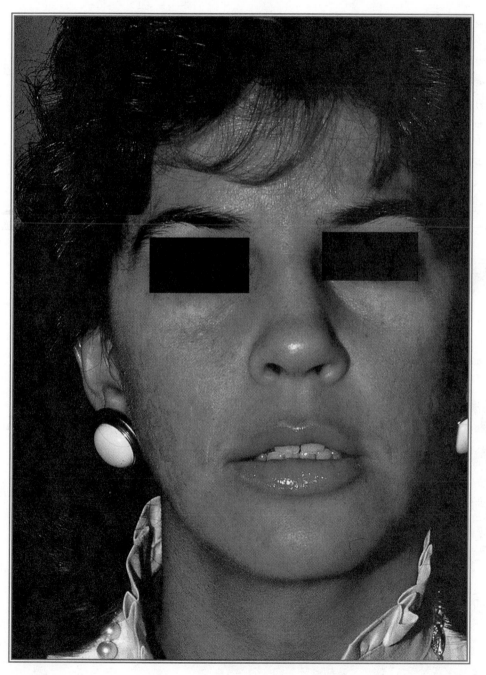

Figure 6-7 POSTINFLAMMATORY HYPERPIGMENTATION

Dark brown blotchy lesions on the lateral aspect of the forearm that developed a few weeks after the patient sustained a chemical burn.

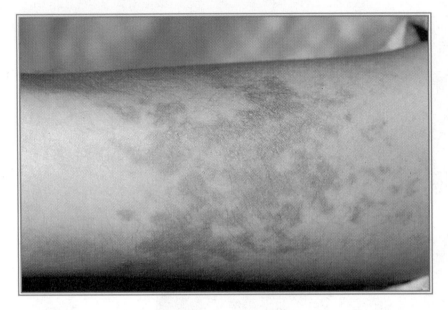

Figure 6-8 PURPURA

Erythematous to violaceous macules appearing after trauma to sun-damaged skin on the forearm of an elderly patient.

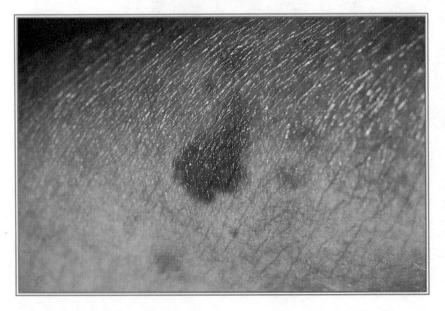

Figure 6-9 SOLAR LENTIGO

Light brown well-demarcated lesions on the dorsal aspect of the hand.

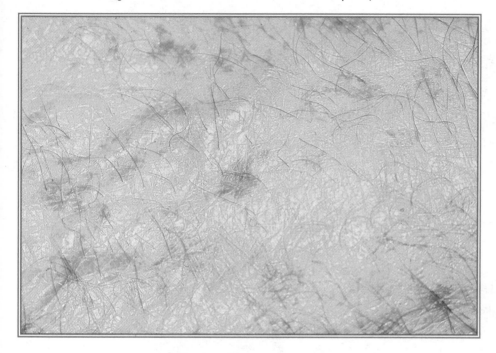

Figure 6-10 **ALBINISM**

A 4-year-old child with no pigmentation of the face, skin, or hair.

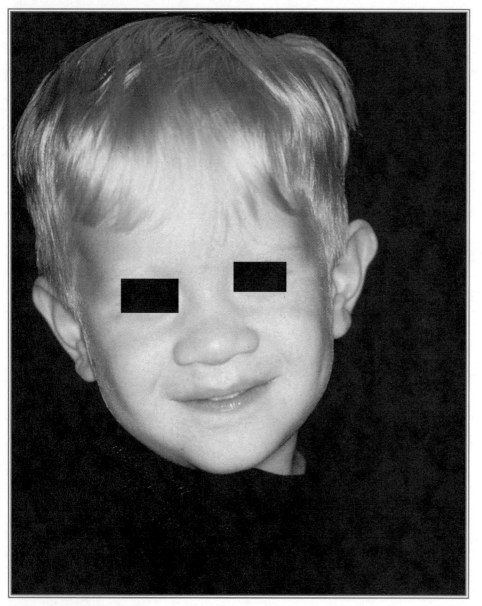

(Courtesy of Stacy R. Smith, MD.)

Figure 6-11   IDIOPATHIC GUTTATE HYPOMELANOSIS

Multiple well-demarcated hypopigmented macules on the forearm.

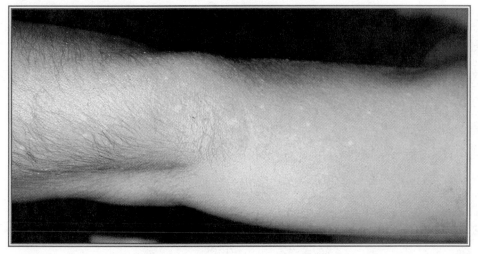

(Courtesy of Stacy R. Smith, MD.)

Figure 6-12   PITYRIASIS ALBA

Well-demarcated hypopigmented area on the lateral aspect of the cheek.

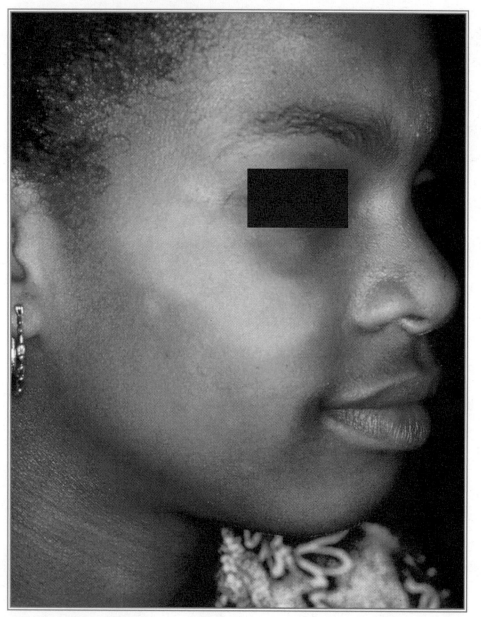

(Courtesy of Stacy R. Smith, MD.)

Figure 6-13 **POSTINFLAMMATORY HYPOPIGMENTATION**

Postinflammatory hypopigmentation after a flare of atopic dermatitis.

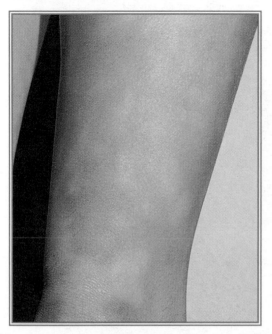

(From White G: *Levene's color atlas of dermatology,* ed 2, St Louis, 1997, Mosby.)

Figure 6-14 **TINEA VERSICOLOR**

Multiple oval tan to brown macules on the back.

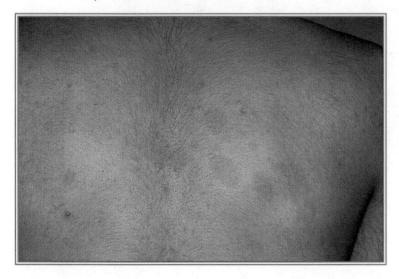

Figure 6-15   VITILIGO

Hypopigmented macular area of the axilla. Note slight erythematous hue to distal lesion, caused by patient's attempt to repigment through sun exposure.

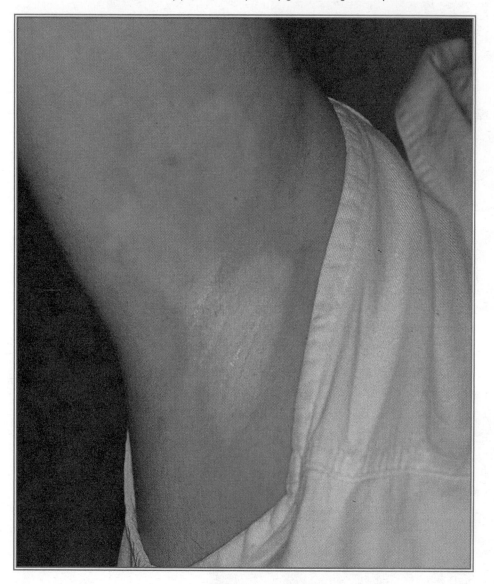

Table 6-1

Differential Diagnosis of Pigmentary Disorders: Hyperpigmentation

Disorder	Text	Keys to Diagnosis
Café-au-lait	Ch. 6, p. 285 (Figure 6-1)	Asymptomatic, tan macule, 0.5 to 20 cm in diameter
Common acquired nevus (mole)	Ch. 6, p. 286 (Figure 6-2)	Most common as a flat or slightly raised brown lesion less than 6 mm in diameter; sharp margins; may have hair or light halo; may also be flesh-toned with dark flecks of color
Congenital nevus	Ch. 6, p. 289 (Figure 6-3)	Asymptomatic, dark brown raised lesion with irregular surface and sharp border; usually has hair; present at birth
Dysplastic nevus	Ch. 6, p. 290 (Figure 6-4)	Asymptomatic red or brown macular-papular lesion with indistinct, irregular border; occurs most often on trunk and extremities; first appears in midchildhood and develops abnormal characteristics in adolescence or adulthood
Freckles (ephelides)	Ch. 6, p. 292 (Figure 6-5)	Tan to dark brown small, asymptomatic macules; increase with sun exposure and fade during winter
Melasma	Ch. 6, p. 293 (Figure 6-6)	Mottled brown, blotchy symmetric pigmentation of forehead, cheeks, upper lip, and chin
Postinflammatory hyperpigmentation	Ch. 6, p. 295 (Figure 6-7)	Asymptomatic brown or purple macule that occurs at the site of a previous lesion or trauma
Senile purpura (actinic purpura)	Ch. 12, p. 436 (Figure 6-8)	Purple macules on chronically sun-exposed skin in older adults; usually arms and hands
Solar lentigo (age spot, liver spot)	Ch. 6, p. 296 (Figure 6-9)	Macule that is darker and larger than a freckle; does not fade during winter months, and usually occurs on chronically sun-exposed skin after age 40

Table 6-2
Differential Diagnosis of Pigmentary Disorders: Hypopigmentation

DISORDER	TEXT	KEYS TO DIAGNOSIS
Albinism	Ch. 6, p. 298 (Figure 6-10)	Whitish-pink skin in whites, tan in blacks; hair is white to blond or red, eyes blue to hazel; diffuse; appears over entire body
Idiopathic guttate hypomelanosis	Ch. 6, p. 300 (Figure 6-11)	Small asymptomatic, hypopigmented guttatelike macules; most often on shins and forearms
Pityriasis alba	Ch. 6, p. 301 (Figure 6-12)	Round to oval hypopigmented patches with fine scale, occurring predominantly on face, upper arms, neck, and shoulders
Postinflammatory hypopigmentation	Ch. 6, p. 303 (Figure 6-13)	Hypopigmented macules that occur in the same location as prior inflammatory lesions
Tinea versicolor	Ch. 3, p. 141 (Figure 6-14)	Asymptomatic white-pink to brown macules with fine scale on back, chest, and upper arms
Vitiligo	Ch. 6, p. 304 (Figure 6-15)	Symmetrically distributed chalk-white, nonscaling macular patches with a complex outline

Hyperpigmentation

Café-au-Lait

Overview

Pathophysiology
These lesions are the result of an increase in the melanin pigmentation of basal cells caused by an increase in the number of basal melanocytes. There is no malignant potential.

Epidemiology
Café-au-lait spots occur in 10% of normal individuals. Presence of six or more spots indicates a 90% probability of neurofibromatosis (von Recklinghausen's disease).

Assessment

Clinical Presentation
Café-au-lait spots are asymptomatic tan macules that vary in diameter from 0.5 cm to 20 cm. (see Figure 6-1). Lesions are sharply marginated with relatively smooth borders.

Diagnostics
The diagnosis is made by clinical presentation and confirmed by skin biopsy.

Differential Diagnosis
- Solar lentigines (lesions are more numerous, less than 1 to 2 cm in diameter, and located on sun-exposed areas) (see Figure 6-9)
- Pigmented nevi (lesions are usually elevated and appear as dark brown)

CAFÉ-AU-LAIT

- Is a benign, cosmetic disorder with no malignant potential

Treatment

Nonpharmacologic
No treatment is necessary, although various pigment-specific lasers may effectively eliminate these lesions if desired for cosmetic reasons:

- Alexandrite laser, Q-switched
- Ruby laser, Q-switched
- 510 nm Pigment lesion laser
- 532 nm Q-switched YAG laser

Pharmacologic

Topical Agents
The lesions cannot be lightened by hydroquinone bleaching agents.

Systemic Agents
None is indicated.

Indications for Referral

- Referral to a dermatologist or laser surgeon is appropriate if treatment is desired.

Common Acquired Nevus (Mole)

Overview

Pathophysiology
A common nevus or mole is a benign neoplasm composed of nevus cells that are derived from melanocytes. These lesions undergo evolution, beginning as a lentigo and developing into junctional, then compound or dermal nevus as the cells migrate from the epidermis into the dermis.

Epidemiology
Moles are extremely common and appear on almost everyone, with an average number per person of 10 to 40. Some moles may be present at birth (see Congenital Nevus); most arise throughout childhood and adolescence. Children who have had painful sunburns before age 10 may have more moles than non-sunburned children. Puberty and pregnancy are times during which both the size and number of nevi increase. Very few new moles arise after age 40. Patients with an excessive number of nevi (more than 40) should be monitored closely because they are at a greater than average risk for development of malignant melanoma. Nevi occur in all races, with the vast majority not undergoing malignant change.

Assessment

Clinical Presentation
Nevi may occur anywhere on the cutaneous surface, although they appear predominantly on sun-exposed skin above the waist. The

actual clinical presentation varies, depending on the stage of evolution. Most lesions are very small (less than 1 cm in diameter).

A **junctional nevus** is the most common form, presenting as a flat or slightly raised tan-brown lesion less than 6 mm in diameter. It has sharp margins, which may be slightly irregular. The color is predominantly uniform throughout with only slight variations. Pigmented nevi of palms, soles, genitalia, and mucus membranes are almost always junctional nevi (occurring at the dermal-epidermal junction), which can be found anywhere on the skin surface. Skin furrows are preserved. Most are found in children, usually after 2 years of age.

A **compound nevus** is a slightly to markedly raised pigmented papule, which may occur on any part of the skin surface. It derives its name from the fact that histologically it occurs in both the junctional zone (dermal-epidermal junction) and the dermis. The border can be irregular (although sharp) and the surface either smooth or slightly papillary. Often there are increases in thickness and pigmentation during late childhood and adolescence with some degree of hyperkeratosis. The center of the lesion tends to be more pigmented than the periphery.

An **intradermal nevus** is an elevated, fleshy papule that appears predominantly in the dermis but may extend into the subcutaneous fat. It occurs mainly after adolescence and is pale (flesh-toned) with pigmented flecks of various shades from jet black to tan. Coarse, dark hairs may grow from the nevus (the majority of hairy nevi are intradermal nevi).

A **halo nevus** is a nevus surrounded by a ring of hypopigmentation. This lesion occurs most commonly on the backs of adolescents and gradually disappears over months to years. The halo usually repigments over time (years). Excision of the central nevus will not produce repigmentation of the hypopigmented ring. The vast majority of these lesions are benign, although multiple halo nevi may occur with melanoma.

Becker's nevus (pigmented hairy epidermal nevus) occurs predominantly on the shoulder, submammary area, or back of adolescent males. In actuality it lacks nevus cells and consists of either a brown macule, a patch of hair, or both. The size varies dramatically and may enlarge to cover the entire upper arm or shoulder. The border is irregular but sharply demarcated. There has never been a reported association with malignancy.

Diagnostics

- Clinical presentation is usually sufficient to make the diagnosis, but if any doubt exists as to the possibility of malignant melanoma, the patient should be referred to a dermatologist for surgical excision. **A possible malignant** melanoma should never be shaved because crucial indicators of metastasis (e.g., the depth of penetration) may be destroyed.

Differential Diagnosis

- Dermatofibroma (usually dimples when pinched between fingers) (see Figure 5-11)
- Lentigo (macular rather than papular, usually on sun-exposed areas) (see Figure 6-9)
- Seborrheic keratosis (appears "stuck on" with a rougher crusty, greasy surface) (see Figure 5-36)
- Malignant melanoma (rapid increase in size of lesion, diameter greater than 1 cm, multiple colors or change in color, irregular shape, bleeding, or ulceration) (see Figure 5-27).

Treatment

Nonpharmacologic

Lesions should be surgically excised by a dermatologist if there is any suspicion of malignant melanoma (see previous discussion). If the patient wishes the lesion removed for cosmetic reasons or because of discomfort from trauma by clothing, shaving, or other contact, the lesion may be shave-excised. Lesions suspected of being basal or squamous cell carcinomas may also be shaved. In selected patients who have a significant family history of dysplastic nevi and who have extensive nevi, serial pictures may be beneficial to follow the progression of individual lesions.

Pharmacologic

Topical Agents
None is indicated.

Systemic Agents
None is indicated.

COMMON ACQUIRED NEVI

- In the vast majority of cases do not become malignant
- Appear with greater frequency in sun-exposed areas
- When arising after age 40, have an increased risk of malignant melanoma
- Should be evaluated according to the ABCDs of malignant melanoma (Asymmetry of border, Border irregularity, Color variegation, Diameter larger than 6 mm)
- Should be evaluated by a professional if any change, itching, bleeding, or failure to heal occurs

Indications for Referral

- Refer to a dermatologist for surgical excision of any lesion in which malignant melanoma is suspected.

Congenital Nevus

Overview

Pathophysiology

A congenital nevus is a junctional or compound, pigmented nevus that is present at birth. The exact cause is unknown. Two thirds arise in the dermis or below; one third originate in the epidermis. Approximately 1% undergo a malignant change, although the risk appears to be related to size. In giant nevi (greater than 10 cm in diameter), there is a 10% incidence of melanoma.

Epidemiology

Congenital nevi occur equally in black and white races. No familial tendency has been identified. Approximately 1% of newborns have a congenital nevus.

Assessment

Clinical Presentation

This lesion is dark brown and raised, with an irregular surface and a sharp but irregular border (see Figure 6-3). The pigmentation remains uniform throughout. The lesions vary greatly in size, from less than 15 mm to over 10 cm in diameter, large enough to require skin grafting to repair the excision. Ninety-five percent have hair. Congenital nevi may occur anywhere on the body. The lesion itself is asymptomatic but may present a cosmetic concern.

Diagnostics
- Clinical presentation is usually sufficient to make the diagnosis, but a skin biopsy will be confirmatory.

Differential Diagnosis
- Café-au-lait spots (congenital macular lesions, lighter in color) (see Figure 6-1)
- Malignant melanoma (congenital melanoma is extremely rare) (see Figure 5-27)

Treatment

Nonpharmacologic

Because of the higher incidence of malignancy, lesions should either be surgically excised or monitored closely throughout life. Surgical excision is the treatment of choice because it removes the possibility of malignancy. Patients should be educated as to what

CONGENITAL NEVI

- Should be monitored closely throughout life because of their association with an increased incidence of malignancy

- May warrant removal, not only for cosmetic reasons, but also because of the potential for malignancy

signs and symptoms are significant and should be reported if the lesion is not removed.

Pharmacologic

Topical Agents
None is indicated.

Systemic Agents
None is indicated.

Indications for Referral

- Patients with a congenital nevus should be referred to a dermatologist for surgical excision.
- Patients with a giant nevus requiring extensive skin grafting after excision may be more appropriately referred to a plastic surgeon.

Dysplastic Nevus

Overview

Pathophysiology
The exact cause of a dysplastic nevus (DN) is unknown, but there is both a hereditary tendency (an autosomal dominant inheritance) and a relation to sunlight exposure, specifically the number of sunburns experienced during childhood. Dysplastic nevi usually occur before age 30 and almost always before age 50. They are an important indicator of persons who are at risk for development of malignant melanoma (MM) and may also be the single most important precursor of MM. Serial photographs have demonstrated the evolution of DN into MM.

Dysplastic nevus syndrome (DNS) refers to any case of dysplastic nevi. There are two types of DNS: *familial*, affecting individuals who have a family history of DN or MM, and *sporadic*, affecting those who have no family history of either DN or MM.

Epidemiology
The frequency of development of a DN without any family history (of either DN or MM) is unknown. DNS is, however, found in 90% of patients with a family history of MM. Persons with familial DNS who have both MM and DN in their family history have almost a 100% chance of development of MM.

Light-skinned persons of Celtic origin who have a positive family history for DN or MM have a greater predisposition to the development of DN.

Assessment

Clinical Presentation

Dysplastic nevi first appear in midchildhood and develop abnormal morphologic characteristics in adolescence and throughout adulthood. They are asymptomatic red or reddish-brown macular-papular lesions with an indistinct, irregular border, usually less than 10 mm in diameter but larger than common acquired nevi (see Figure 6-4). They are not common on the face and occur more often on the trunk and extremities. They also occur on areas that are rarely exposed to the sun such as the buttocks, breasts of women, and hair-bearing scalp. It is common for a DN to be asymmetric with a papular center surrounded by a lighter macular ring.

Diagnostics

- Clinical evaluation is usually sufficient, but skin biopsy should be performed if malignant melanoma is suspected.

Differential Diagnosis

- Common acquired nevi (smaller than DNs, occurring on sun-exposed areas) (see Figure 5-9, *B*)
- Malignant melanoma (blue-black color, larger than 10 mm) (see Figure 5-27)

Treatment

Nonpharmacologic

Patients should be informed of the risk of melanoma. Monthly self-examination in good lighting with a mirror to check one's back should be performed. Any changes in lesions should be reported to the practitioner. Periodic photographs and careful measurement of lesion diameter should be documented in the medical record. Total surgical excision should be performed to remove any suspicious lesions.

Pharmacologic

Topical Agents
Tretinoin (Retin-A) 0.025% to 0.1% cream has been shown to lead to regression of DNs. Consistent application of **sunscreen** is an important preventative measure.

Systemic Agents
None is indicated.

DYSPLASTIC NEVUS

- Has a higher than average risk of developing into malignant melanoma
- Should be carefully and frequently monitored by a professional or removed
- Should be monitored by the patient at least monthly (using mirrors to see the back, if necessary)

✦ | Indications for Referral |

- If any doubt exists about the possibility of malignant melanoma, the lesion should be *completely* excised and sent for pathologic evaluation. Referral to a dermatologist is appropriate.

Freckles (Ephelides)

Overview

Pathophysiology

Freckles are small benign, light tan macules. The number of melanocytes in a freckle is the same as in the surrounding skin, but they are larger and produce more melanin. Although the exact cause of this melanocytic alteration is not clearly understood, it is most likely the result of exposure to sunlight.

Epidemiology

Freckles occur predominantly in blondes, redheads, and those with blue eyes. There appears to be a genetic predisposition.

Assessment

Clinical Presentation

Freckles are tan to dark brown, small, asymptomatic superficial macules (see Figure 6-5). They first become apparent between ages 6 and 9 and are accentuated by sun exposure. A notable fading during winter months is common. The pigmentation is uniform and the borders irregular. Freckles do not occur on mucus membranes or on non–sun-exposed areas. They may increase in number and size during pregnancy.

Diagnostics

- The diagnosis of freckles is based on clinical presentation, specifically the size, distribution, and tendency of the lesions to fade during the winter months. For confirmation of the diagnosis, a skin biopsy is required but rarely necessary.

Differential Diagnosis

- Lentigo (occurs in adults and elderly persons and does not fade during winter months) (see Figure 6-9)

FRECKLES

- Are caused by exposure to sunlight
- Are a cosmetic concern only
- May be minimized through the consistent use of sunscreens and/or skin lightening preparations

- Superficial seborrheic keratosis (finely granular and slightly keratotic surface with a tendency to form larger plaques) (see Figure 5-36)
- Nevi (darker and do not fade) (see Figure 5-9, *B*)

Treatment

Nonpharmacologic

No specific treatment is necessary since the lesions are of cosmetic concern only. However patients should be educated about the importance of avoiding or limiting exposure to sunlight, as well as the conscientious application of sunscreen, both of which are effective preventive therapy.

Pharmacologic

Topical Agents

Bleaching creams such as **4% hydroquinone (Melanex, Solaquin Forte, Eldoquin Forte)** applied bid will slowly fade freckles over a period of weeks to months. A **light trichloroacetic (TCA) acid peel** or light **liquid nitrogen** application will also decrease pigmentation. Caution must be exercised to prevent hypopigmentation of the surrounding skin. **Tretinoin (Retin-A)** applied qhs has also been used successfully for this condition.

Systemic Agents

None is indicated.

Indications for Referral

- None, unless the diagnosis is in doubt.

Melasma (Chloasma, Mask of Pregnancy)

Overview

Pathophysiology

The most important factors in the pathogenesis of melasma are a genetic predisposition and exposure to ultraviolet (UV) radiation. There are three types of melasma:

1. *Epidermal:* 70% of cases. An increased amount of pigmentation, visible under a Wood's light, is diagnostic.
2. *Dermal:* 15% of cases. There is no change in pigment under a Wood's light.
3. *Indeterminant:* Occurs primarily in deeply pigmented persons.

Epidemiology

Melasma is more prevalent in women than in men, and in persons of Hispanic origin. It occurs in 20% of women during the childbearing ages, and in 10% to 30% of women taking birth control pills or hormonal supplements. When present during pregnancy, melasma begins during the third or fourth month and fades slowly after delivery, although it may never resolve completely. In up to 30% of cases there may be a familial relationship. When it occurs after hormonal supplementation or birth control pills, it may be permanent.

Assessment

Clinical Presentation

Mottled brown, blotchy symmetric pigmentation, primarily of the forehead, cheeks, upper lip, and chin (see Figure 6-6), melasma frequently occurs in conjunction with darkening of the nipples and moles. It is asymptomatic.

Diagnostics

- The diagnosis is based on clinical presentation and history. Skin biopsy will confirm the diagnosis if necessary.

Differential Diagnosis

- Postinflammatory hyperpigmentation (history of preceding inflammatory process) (see Figure 6-7)
- Tar melanosis (patchy hyperpigmented areas on sun-exposed regions of the face caused by photo contact dermatitis from cosmetics, perfumes, or other products containing tar)

Treatment

Nonpharmacologic

Discontinuation of oral contraceptives or hormonal supplements is mandatory. Limiting the amount of exposure to sunlight is strongly recommended.

Pharmacologic

Topical Agents

Consistent use of a **sunscreen** with a sun protection factor (SPF) of at least 30 is essential. Topical depigmentation agents such as

MELASMA

- Occurs primarily in females who are pregnant, use birth control pills, or have hormone replacement therapy
- Is exceptionally difficult to treat, especially as long as the hormonal alterations persist
- May be minimized through the consistent use of sunscreen and skin lightening preparations

hydroquinone 4% (Solaquin Forte, Melanex) will help promote fading of the lesions. These agents do not actually bleach the skin but rather reduce the amount of pigment produced by the melanocytes. Their use must be continued for months. Depigmentation may be enhanced when hydroquinones are used in conjunction with **tretinoin (Retin-A 0.1% cream). Azelaic acid (Azelex)** cream applied qhs may also be effective.

Systemic Agents
None is indicated.

Indications for Referral

- Refer to a dermatologist skilled in laser therapy for consideration of laser treatment to minimize pigmentation.

Postinflammatory Hyperpigmentation

Overview

Pathophysiology
Postinflammatory hyperpigmentation (PIP) is due to epidermal cell damage caused by an acute or chronic inflammatory process, such as acne.

Epidemiology
Persons with darker skin are at higher risk for development of PIP.

Assessment

Clinical Presentation
The disorder presents as a brown or purple macule occurring at the site of a previous inflammatory lesion. The pigmentation persists after the inflammatory process has resolved. The lesions are asymptomatic and are of cosmetic concern only.

Diagnostics
- The diagnosis is based on history and clinical presentation. A confirmatory skin biopsy to exclude other disorders may be required.

Differential Diagnosis

- Melasma (blotchy light to dark brown areas on face, occurring without preceding inflammation) (see Figure 6-6)
- Café-au-lait (a single, well-circumscribed lesion approximately 2 to 3 cm in diameter, occurring without a preexisting inflammation) (see Figure 6-1)

Treatment

Nonpharmacologic

Prevention of new lesions through resolution of the underlying inflammatory process will stop the development of hyperpigmentation. Spontaneous improvement, although slow, is expected.

Pharmacologic

Topical Agents

Retinoic acid (Retin-A creme 0.05%) and azelaic acid (Azelex) applied qhs will hasten resolution. **Hydrocortisone and alpha hydroxyacids** applied bid will also help reduce inflammation and itching.

Systemic Agents

None is indicated.

> **POSTINFLAMMATORY HYPERPIGMENTATION**
>
> - Is a cosmetic disorder only, with no malignant potential
> - Can be prevented through prevention of new inflammatory lesions
> - Can be minimized through the consistent use of sun protection agents

Indications for Referral

- Physician consultation may be appropriate either to confirm the diagnosis or to assist with the resolution of the underlying inflammatory process.

Solar Lentigo (Age Spot, Liver Spot)

Overview

Pathophysiology

Lentigines are common benign skin lesions whose exact cause is unknown, although there is both a familial tendency and a direct relationship to chronic sun exposure.

Epidemiology

Lentigines occur in adult and elderly individuals and are rare before the age of 40. Those with skin type I (those who are fair, burn easily, and tan poorly) are at greatest risk. These lesions occur in 90% of whites after age 70.

Assessment

Clinical Presentation
Lentigines are macules that are darker and larger than freckles (see Figure 6-9) and do not characteristically fade during winter months. They show a predilection for sun-exposed areas such as the backs of the hands, forearms, shoulders, and forehead. Occasionally they may coalesce and become more numerous and larger with advancing age.

Diagnostics
- Lentigines are diagnosed clinically, but a biopsy specimen should be taken from any lentigo that develops an irregular border, uneven pigmentation, or thickening to rule out lentigo maligna melanoma.

Differential Diagnosis
- Freckle (develops in children and adolescents and fades during winter months) (see Figure 6-5)
- Superficial seborrheic keratosis (finely granular and slightly keratotic surface with a tendency to form larger plaques) (see Figure 5-36)
- Nevus (darker, may be larger, and does not fade) (see Figure 5-9, *B*)
- Lentigo maligna (more variable color; larger lesion that continues to grow)

SOLAR LENTIGINES

- Are caused by chronic, long-standing exposure to sunlight
- Are a cosmetic concern only
- May be minimized through the consistent use of sunscreens and/or skin lightening preparations

Treatment

Nonpharmacologic
No specific treatment is necessary since the lesions are of cosmetic concern only. However, patients should be educated about the importance of avoiding or limiting exposure to sunlight, as well as the conscientious application of sunscreen, both of which are effective preventive therapy.

Pharmacologic

Topical Agents
Bleaching creams such as **4% hydroquinone (Melanex, Solaquin Forte, Eldoquin Forte)** applied bid will slowly fade freckles over a period of weeks to months. A light **trichloroacetic acid peel** or light **liquid nitrogen** application will also decrease pigmentation. Caution must be exercised to prevent hypopigmentation of the sur-

rounding skin. **Tretinoin (Retin-A),** applied qhs, has also been used successfully to treat this condition.

Systemic Agents
None is indicated.

Indications for Referral

- Consultation may be appropriate to confirm the diagnosis.

Hypopigmentation

Albinism

Overview

Pathophysiology
Albinism is a recessively inherited congenital disorder of melanin synthesis. There are two types of albinism; in both types, melanocytes are present but do not produce melanin normally:

    1. Tyrosinase-negative: There is an inability to synthesize tyrosinase, a necessary precursor to the formation of melanin. Consequently there is no production of melanin at any time during the life of the individual and hypopigmentation is permanent.
    2. Tyrosinase-positive: These patients, although possessing measurable amounts of tyrosinase, have only a minimal, abnormal ability to produce pigment. The exact pathophysiologic mechanism is unknown.

Epidemiology
The general incidence of albinism is 1:20,000. Tyrosinase-positive albinism is more common then tyrosinase-negative albinism in most racial groups.

Assessment

Clinical Presentation
Onset at birth and a **diffuse presentation** of hypopigmentation over the entire body are characteristic hallmarks of albinism. The skin is whitish pink in whites and tan in blacks. Hair is white to

blond or red; eyes are blue to hazel. Photophobia, visual defects, and nystagmus are common, although patients are otherwise healthy. Because of the skin's inability to protect itself from solar radiation, patients commonly have multiple actinic keratoses or other manifestations of photo damage.

Diagnostics
- Diagnosis is usually made on the basis of clinical presentation and history. If the diagnosis is in doubt, a skin biopsy is confirmatory.

Differential Diagnosis
- Vitiligo (areas of hypopigmentation are macular rather than diffuse and are not present at birth) (see Figure 6-15)

Treatment

Nonpharmacologic
There is no treatment to correct the defect of melanin production. Patients should be advised, however, of the importance of protecting their eyes and skin from the sun to prevent secondary changes resulting from chronic solar exposure. Avoidance of the sun between the hours of 10:00 AM and 3:00 PM is recommended. An annual full body cutaneous examination should be performed to identify any premalignant or malignant skin changes. Genetic counseling may also be appropriate.

Pharmacologic

Topical Agents
Sunscreens with an SPF of 15 or greater should be used consistently.

Systemic Agents
None is indicated.

ALBINISM

- Is caused by a genetic defect in melanin production
- Cannot be cured
- Renders a patient defenseless against sun; radical sun protection efforts should therefore be implemented
- May be appropriate to refer for genetic counseling

Indications for Referral

- For patients desiring genetic counseling, appropriate referrals are essential.
- Referrals to a dermatologist are appropriate for patients with cutaneous carcinomas.

Idiopathic Guttate Hypomelanosis

Overview

Pathophysiology
The basic cause of this disorder is unknown, but it may be the result of repeated injury or trauma, ultraviolet exposure, or an age-related mutation of melanocytes.

Epidemiology
It is more common in individuals above the age of 40; 70% of patients are in their fifties. A very common disorder, it is present in 50% to 68% of the population. Women are affected more regularly than men, and there appears to be a familial tendency.

Assessment

Clinical Presentation
As the name suggests, lesions are small, asymptomatic hypomelanotic droplike (guttate) macules with sharply defined borders (see Figure 6-11). The surface of the lesion is smooth, without scaling, scarring, or atrophy. They most commonly occur on sun-exposed skin, particularly the shins and forearms, but never on the face or trunk. It is rare for the lesions to become numerous, although they do increase in number with age. The size of individual lesions does not change and they do not spontaneously repigment.

Diagnostics
- The diagnosis is made by clinical presentation and confirmed by skin biopsy.

Differential Diagnosis
- Vitiligo (lesions are larger and may continue to increase in size, sometimes fusing with neighboring lesions) (see Figure 6-15)
- Tinea versicolor (lesions are scaly and are frequently found on the chest and back) (see Figure 6-14)
- Chemical depigmentation (history will reveal chemical contact)
- Postinflammatory hypopigmentation (occurs after an eczematous inflammation) (see Figure 6-13)

Treatment

Nonpharmacologic
No treatment is necessary since the condition is of only minor cosmetic significance. If treatment is demanded by the patient,

IDIOPATHIC GUTTATE HYPOMELANOSIS

- Is a cosmetic defect with no malignant potential
- May be accentuated by tanning, because the surrounding areas darken, thus increasing the contrast in skin tone
- May be minimized through the use of self-tanning preparations, which do not rely on the body's production of melanin and thus result in a more even tan

however, Psoralen used in conjunction with ultraviolet A (UVA) light therapy (PUVA) may be an option. It has been tried with limited effectiveness, but the results are lost at discontinuation of therapy.

Patients should be advised that tanning may accentuate the disorder rather than minimizing it, by creating a greater contrast between the normal and hypopigmented skin. An avoidance of tanning may thus help minimize the disorder.

Minigrafts have not been effective in restoring the lost pigment.

Pharmacologic

Topical Agents
Self-tanning lotions, which do not depend on the production of melanin but rather act by staining the epidermis, may help to even the pigmentary irregularities.

Systemic Agents
Recent studies have shown encouraging results from the intralesional injection of **triamcinolone (Kenalog)** 2.5 mg/ml on a monthly basis, resulting in repigmentation.

Indications for Referral

- No referral is necessary, because of the benign nature of the condition.
- Patients finding the disorder cosmetically unacceptable may be referred to a dermatologist for more innovative and/or unconventional therapy trials.

Pityriasis Alba

Overview

Pathophysiology
The exact cause is unknown, although it is believed that exposure to sunlight and resultant tanning may accentuate the hypopigmented lesions. The hypopigmentation results primarily from a reduction in the number of active melanocytes in the affected skin. The disorder may also be a form of atopic dermatitis that results in postinflammatory hypopigmentation.

Epidemiology

Pityriasis alba occurs primarily in preadolescent children. There is an increased incidence in persons with atopic dermatitis.

Assessment

Clinical Presentation

Lesions are initially slightly erythematous and then become hypopigmented. They are round to oval, fine, scaly patches occurring predominantly on the face, upper arms, neck, or shoulders. They are usually asymptomatic but occasionally are slightly pruritic.

Diagnostics

- The diagnosis is made by clinical presentation and can be confirmed by skin biopsy if necessary.

Differential Diagnosis

- Tinea versicolor (KOH preparation result is positive; lesions are usually on the back and chest, sparing the face) (see Figure 6-12)
- Vitiligo (lesions do not scale) (see Figure 6-15)
- Postinflammatory hypopigmentation (always a history of previous inflammation) (see Figure 6-13)
- Pityriasis rosea (begins with herald patch; lesions form Christmas tree pattern; collarette scale) (see Figure 3-28)
- Nummular eczema (lesions usually on legs, arms, and neck) (see Figure 2-1)

PITYRIASIS ALBA

- Is a cosmetic defect, whose cause is not clear
- Is temporary and will resolve in time
- Can be accentuated by sun exposure and minimized by self-tanning products

Treatment

Lesions spontaneously resolve in months and/or with puberty.

Nonpharmacologic

Reassurance that the disorder is a temporary, cosmetic condition that will resolve in time is necessary.

Pharmacologic

Topical Agents

Lac-Hydrin 12% cream applied to affected areas bid will help remove scale and prevent dryness, making the skin more receptive to sunlight and repigmentation. **LactiCare HC 2$^1/_2$%** helps relieve dryness and decreases inflammation. Low-potency corticosteroids such as **desonide (DesOwen)** and **hydrocortisone (Hytone)** applied bid may also help decrease inflammation.

Systemic Agents
None is indicated.

Indications for Referral

- None.

Postinflammatory Hypopigmentation

Overview

Pathophysiology
Postinflammatory hypopigmentation is an inflammation of the skin that causes depigmented lesions after the inflammation has resolved. Occasionally the pigmented variation is permanent.

Epidemiology
The disorder occurs most commonly in deeply pigmented persons and in those with chronic eczema.

Assessment

Clinical Presentation
The diagnostic hallmark is the presence of macular, hypopigmented lesions that occur in the same location as prior inflammatory lesions (see Figure 6-13). There is no other abnormality of the skin surface.

Diagnostics
- The diagnosis is made by clinical presentation but can be confirmed by skin biopsy.

Differential Diagnosis
- Pityriasis alba (hypopigmented macules with very fine scale, usually on the face, neck, and upper arms) (see Figure 6-12)
- Idiopathic guttate hypomelanosis (scaly lesions less than 2 to 3 mm in diameter that occur on sun-exposed areas) (see Figure 6-11)

POSTINFLAMMATORY HYPOPIGMENTATION

- Is a cosmetic disorder
- Can be minimized by controlling eczema and keeping the skin well hydrated, to prevent future and/or continued outbreaks

Treatment

Nonpharmacologic

Treatment should be directed to correction of the underlying disorder and thus to prevention of future lesions. Appropriate hydrosis of the skin is always important.

Pharmacologic

Topical Agents

Those products indicated for the treatment of the underlying disorder will help in the prevention of future lesions.

Systemic Agents

Systemic therapy is only indicated if necessary for the treatment of the underlying disorder.

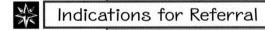

Indications for Referral

- None.

Vitiligo

Overview

Pathophysiology

Vitiligo is an acquired localized loss of melanocytes from skin and hair. There are three hypotheses as to the exact cause: (1) it is an autoimmune disorder, (2) there are toxic compounds that inhibit melanogenesis, and (3) the melanocytes self-destruct as a result of a defect in the natural protective mechanism that removes the toxic compounds.

Epidemiology

Vitiligo occurs in 1% of the United States and world population. It is a major worldwide cause of disfigurement, especially in darkly pigmented people. Fifty percent experience its onset before age 20. In 25% to 40% of patients there is a positive family history. Approximately 10% of patients also have an autoimmune disorder (such as diabetes, hypothyroidism, or Addison's disease), and 50%

of patients have a halo nevus (a nevus encircled by a lighter colored ring).

Assessment

Clinical Presentation

Vitiligo may occur spontaneously after severe emotional or physical stress or in association with localized cutaneous trauma. The lesions are **symmetrically distributed** and present as **nonscaling, macular patches** with a convex outline (see Figure 6-15). They increase in irregularity and size until they fuse with neighboring lesions to form complex patterns. Although the lesions themselves are chalk-white, hairs in the patches may or may not be hypopigmented. The disorder is rapidly progressive, especially in the first few months. Approximately 10% of patients experience spontaneous repigmentation in sun-exposed areas. The loss of pigment occurs predominantly in exposed areas, in intertriginous areas, over bony prominences, and around the mouth.

Diagnostics

- Diagnosis is based on clinical presentation and confirmed by biopsy.

Differential Diagnosis

- Piebaldism (hypopigmented patches present at birth, usually on the chest, abdomen, and limbs)
- Tinea versicolor (lesions pinker, scaling, and primarily on upper back and chest) (see Figure 6-14)
- Pityriasis alba (hypopigmented macules with fine scale, usually appearing on face, neck, and upper arms) (see Figure 6-12)
- Idiopathic guttate hypomelanosis (lesions scaly, less than 2 to 3 mm in diameter, and occurring on sun-exposed areas) (see Figure 6-11)

VITILIGO

- Is a cosmetic disorder
- Spontaneously repigments in 15% of cases
- Patients are at a greater risk of sunburn because of their lack of natural skin pigment

Treatment

Spontaneous repigmentation occurs in only about 15% of cases and is usually spotty with a "salt and pepper" appearance. With therapy, 30% to 40% of patients may experience some improvement.

Nonpharmacologic

Camouflage with various dyes and cosmetics may help minimize the pigmentary irregularities. If the lesions are in sun-exposed areas, patients should be advised to use sunscreen consistently since they are at a higher risk of burning.

Pharmacologic

Topical Agents

Topical **psoralen** with sun exposure is helpful in certain cases. Alternatively, a 1 : 10,000 dilution of **tincture of methoxsalen** is painted on the affected areas once or twice a week. The concentration is increased by a factor of 10 every month until repigmentation occurs. If it does occur, it is slow and takes place over months to years. Children have a quicker response than adults. Therapy is continued for 6 months to several years. At best it is 60% successful.

Group I topical corticosteroids (**clobetasol propionate [Temovate]** 0.05% cream) applied bid are recommended. Therapy should not continue more than 2 weeks because of possible systemic absorption of steroid.

Systemic Agents

Oral **PUVA** therapy may be initiated in patients unresponsive to topical applications (see the section on Psoriasis).

Indications for Referral

- Patients requiring the administration of oral PUVA therapy should be followed by a physician or an experienced phototherapist.

Pruritic Disorders

Figure 7-1 **ACUTE NUMMULAR ECZEMA**

Multiple coinlike hyperkeratotic erythematous lesions on the medial aspect of the thigh, with surrounding erythematous papules.

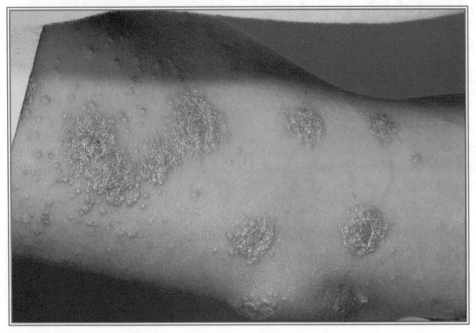

(Courtesy of Stacy R. Smith, MD.)

Figure 7-2 ALLERGIC CONTACT DERMATITIS

A, *Well-demarcated erythematous macule caused by contact with the undersurface of a nickel-plated watch.* *B,* *Rhus variety: Linear vesicular lesions on the thigh and knees are characteristic of poison ivy exposure.*

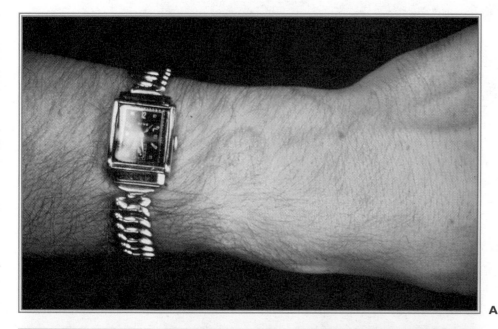

A

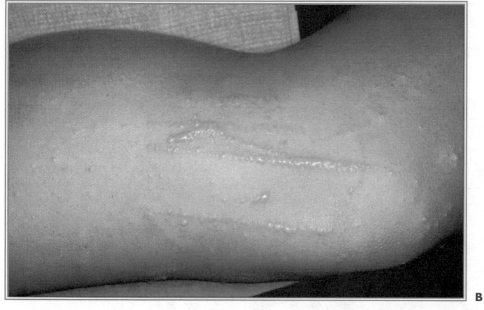

B

Figure 7-3 ATOPIC DERMATITIS

Blotchy erythematous lesions on the face with accentuation in the central facial area.

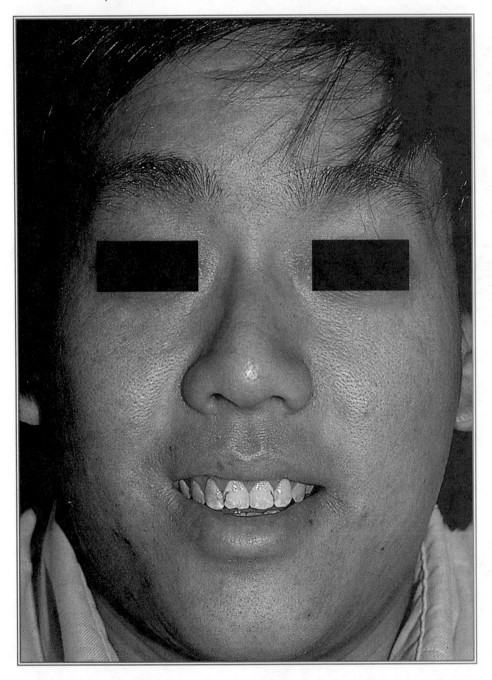

Figure 7-4 ACUTE CANDIDA INTERTRIGO

Note peripheral fringe of scale and satellite lesions.

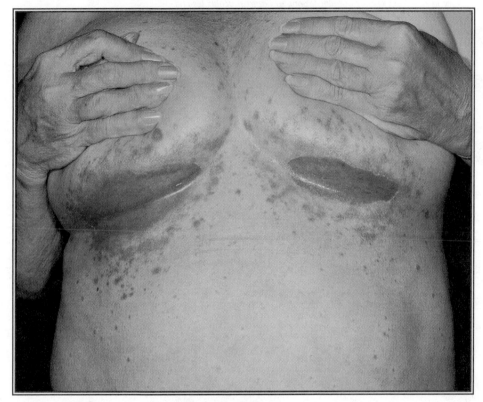

(From Habif TP: *Clinical dermatology*, ed 3, St Louis, 1996, Mosby.)

Figure 7-5 CHICKENPOX

Small vesicles on an erythematous macular base, in a generalized distribution on the back. Lesions vary in size from (early) papular lesions to (later) macular lesions.

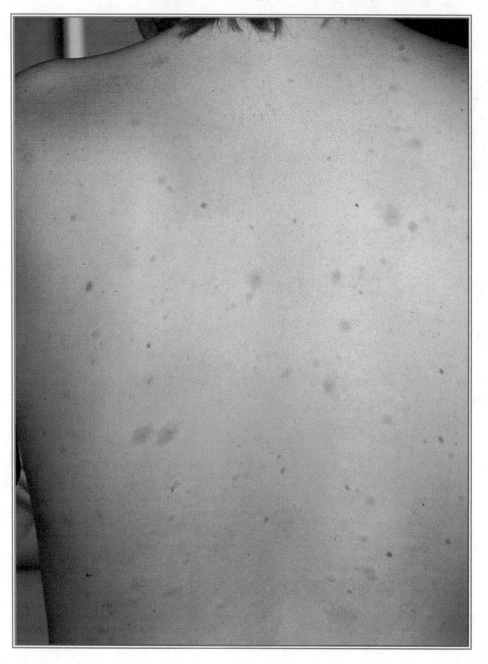

Figure 7-6

A, Tinea capitis: Thick scale and crust on the apical aspect of a child's head.
B, Tinea corporis: Annular lesion with a sharply marginated erythematous border. Note central clearing with appearance of normal skin.

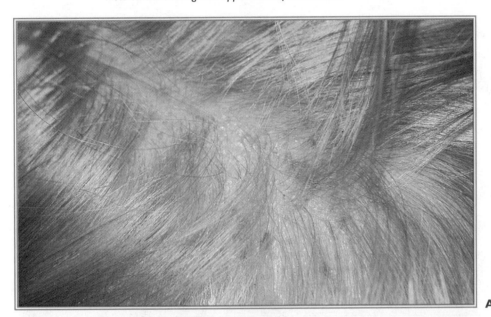

A

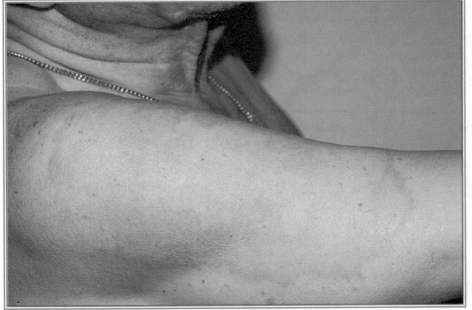

B

(**C through F,** From Habif TP: *Clinical dermatology,* ed 3, St Louis, 1996, Mosby.)   *continued*

Figure 7-6—cont'd

C, *Tinea cruris: Half-moon shaped erythematous plaque with a slightly scaling border. Note sparing of the scrotum.* **D,** *Tinea manus: Tinea of the palm. Note thickened, dry, scaly skin.*

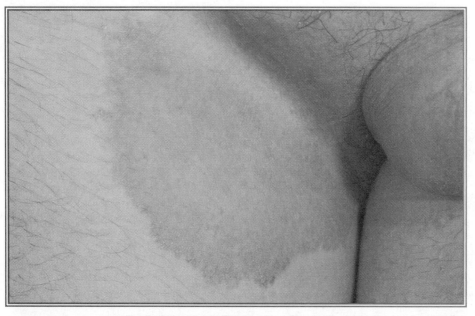

C

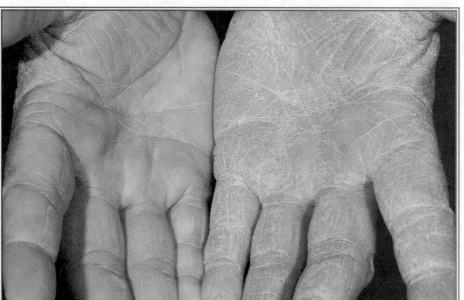

D

Figure 7-6—cont'd

E, Tinea pedis: Inflammation of the sole and lateral edges of the foot, giving it a moccasin-like appearance. *F,* Tinea pedis: The infection has macerated the skin in the toe web. Inflammation extends to the dorsum of the foot.

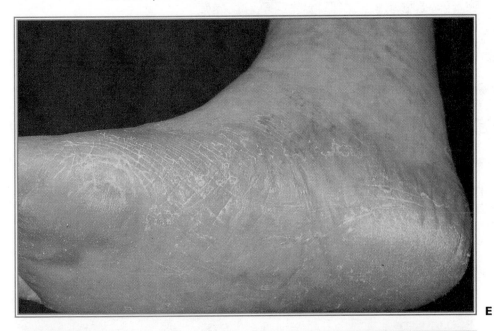

E

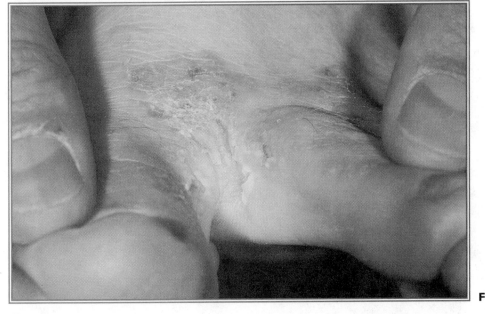

F

Figure 7-7 DYSHIDROTIC ECZEMA

Erythematous palms with only small areas of normal skin. Many areas are hyperkeratotic.

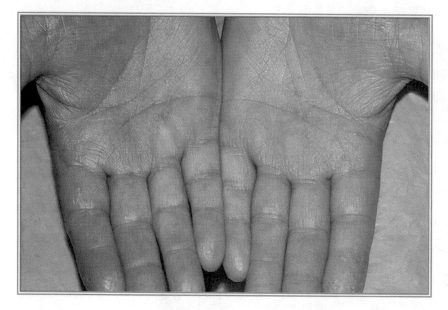

Figure 7-8 FOLLICULITIS

Extensive inflammatory closed comedones centered around hair follicles on the cheek of a male electrical worker exposed to fluorocarbons.

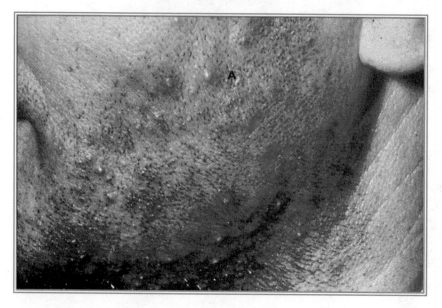

Figure 7-9 ICHTHYOSIS VULGARIS

Polygonal scalelike lesions of brown hyperkeratotic skin of the lower extremities.

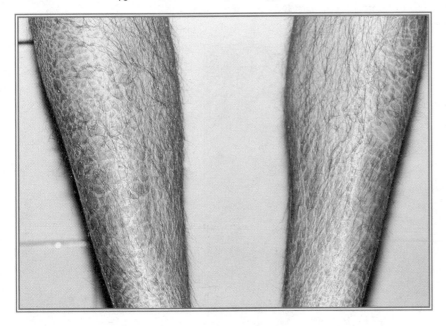

Figure 7-10 IMPETIGO

Erythematous lesions with honey-colored crust on the posterior thigh and buttock regions.

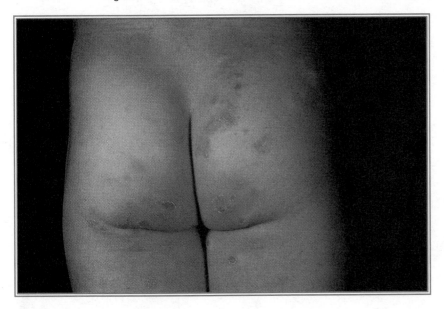

Figure 7-11 **INSECT BITES**

> **A,** *Papular flea-bite reaction at typical site above the top of the sock. Note grouping of lesions.* **B,** *Insect bites with characteristic purpuric spots in center of papule. A central punctum is typical.*

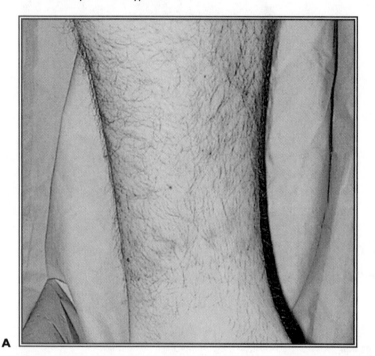

A

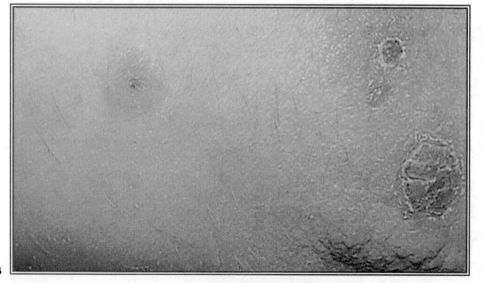

B

(From Cox N, Lawrence C: *Diagnostic problems in dermatology,* St Louis, 1997, Mosby.)

Figure 7-12

A, *Pediculosis capitis: Heavy infestation of lice and nits is present in scalp hair.*
B, *Pediculosis pubis: Multiple dark arthropods adhering to hair follicles are visible.*

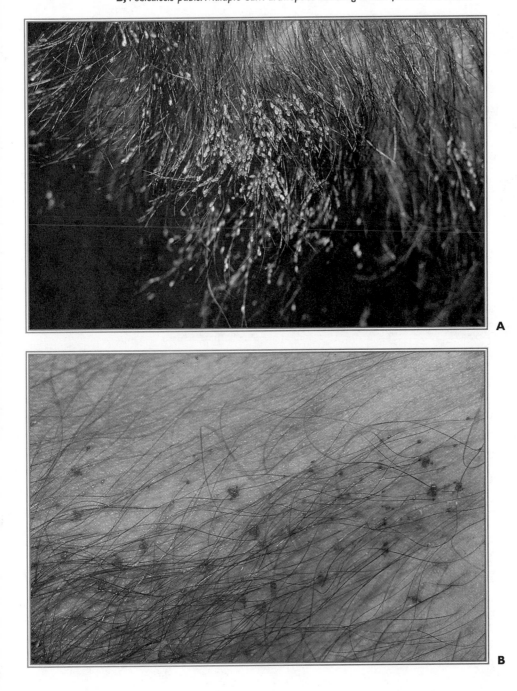

A

B

Figure 7-13 LICHEN PLANUS

Erythematous to violaceous, flat-topped polygonal papules on the dorsal and lateral aspect of the foot.

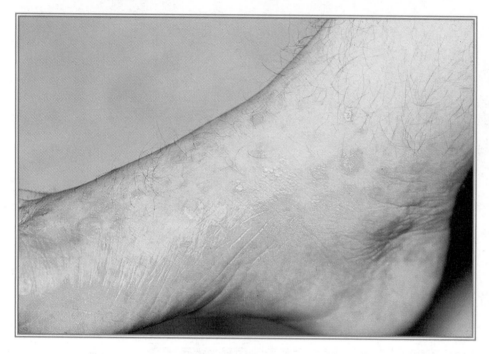

Figure 7-14 LICHEN SIMPLEX CHRONICUS

Thick eczematous hyperkeratotic plaque with accentuated skin lines, created by rubbing with the opposite heel.

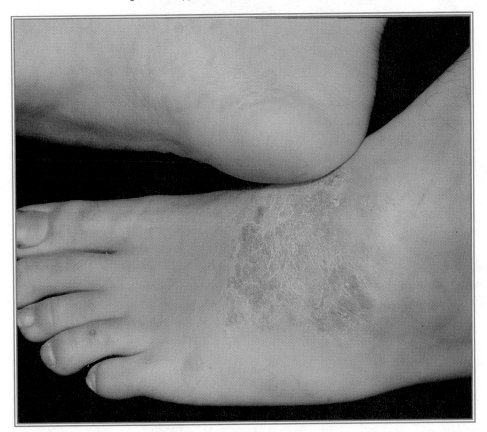

(From Habif TP: *Clinical dermatology,* ed 3, St Louis, 1996, Mosby.)

Figure 7-15 Rubeola

Erythematous macules on the lateral aspect of the neck.

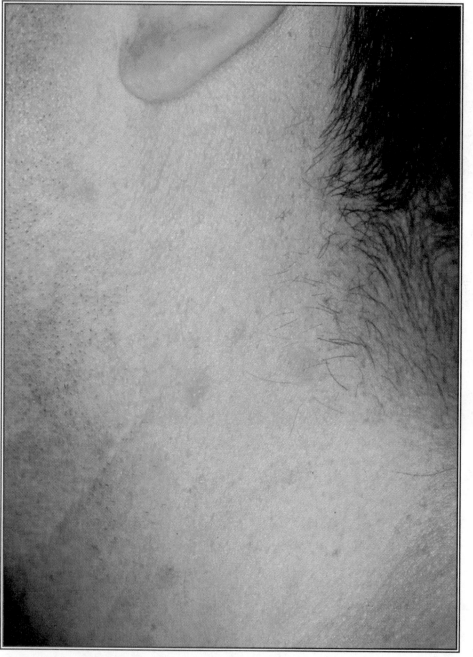

Figure 7-16   **PERIORAL DERMATITIS**

Inflammatory closed comedones and generalized inflammation in a perioral distribution.

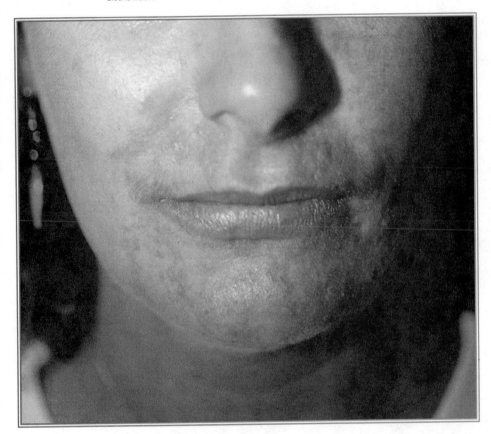

Figure 7-17 PHOTOALLERGIC REACTION

Erythematous to violaceous dermatitis on the dorsal aspect of the hand of a photographer who uses multiple chemicals to develop film.

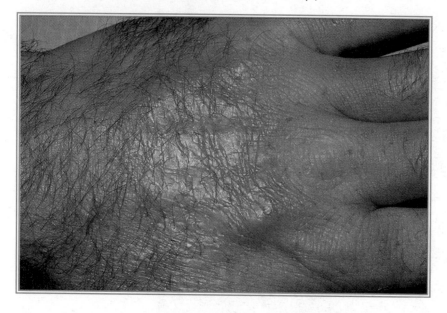

Figure 7-18 POLYMORPHOUS LIGHT ERUPTION

Diffuse erythematous eruption, noted predominantly over sun-exposed areas.

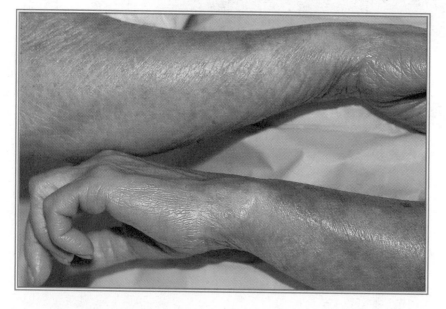

Figure 7-19 PRURITIC URTICARIAL PAPULES AND PLAQUES OF PREGNANCY (PUPPP)

Erythematous macular eruption with multiple urticarial and papular lesions on the central aspect of the abdomen in a pregnant woman.

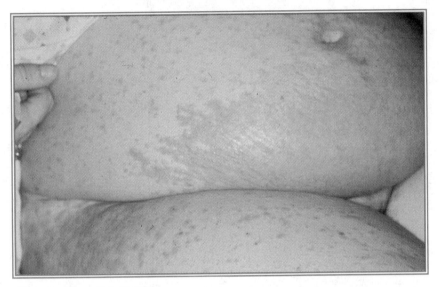

(Courtesy of Stacy R. Smith, MD.)

Figure 7-20 PSEUDOFOLLICULITIS

Inflammatory lesions with some pustules in the mandibular angle. Note curled hairs, some of which are embedding back into the skin.

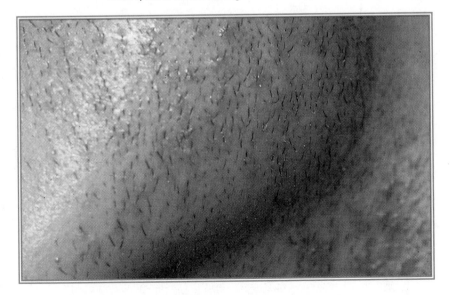

Figure 7-21 SCABIES

Black linear tract with surrounding erythema.

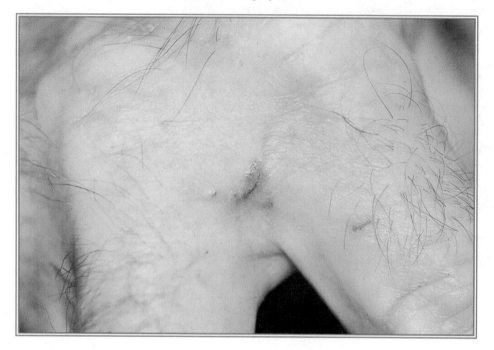

Figure 7-22   SEBORRHEIC DERMATITIS

Erythematous patches with some evidence of scale in the usual facial distribution.

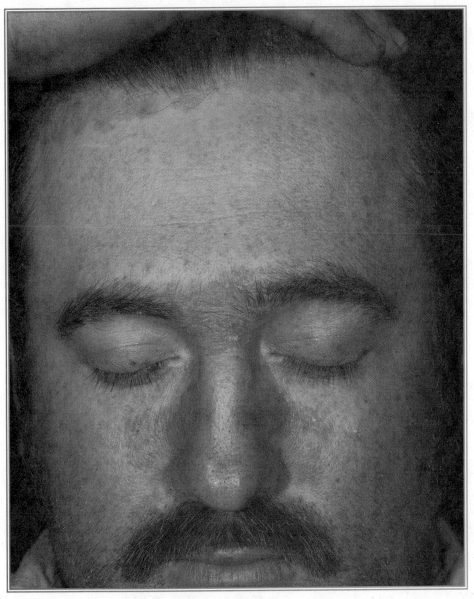

(From Habif TP: *Clinical dermatology,* St Louis, 1996, Mosby.)

Figure. 7-23

A, Urticaria: Typical urticarial lesions, showing edematous macules over slightly erythematous skin. **B,** Dermatographism: Erythematous urticarial lesions that appeared within 1 to 2 minutes after drawing on the patient's back with a blunt object.

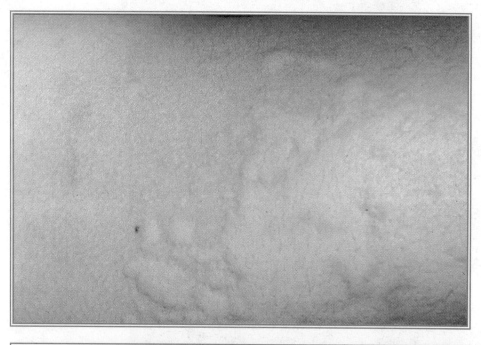

A

B

Figure 7-24   XEROSIS

Parchmentlike skin with overlying scales on a background of erythema.

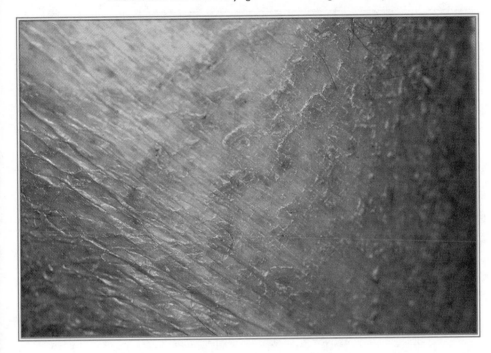

Table 7-1 *continued*

DISORDER	TEXT	KEYS TO DIAGNOSIS
Measles (rubeola)	Ch. 4, p. 189 (Figure 7-15)	Prodrome of cough, coryza, conjunctivitis, and high fever with cervical lymphadenopathy; erythematous pruritic macules that become papular on face, neck, trunk, and extremities
Perioral dermatitis	Ch. 1, p. 44 (Figure 7-16)	Pruritic, burning discrete erythematous or flesh-colored papules and pustules around mouth and in nasolabial folds
Photoallergic reaction	Ch. 4, p. 190 (Figure 7-17)	Erythematous papular rash in sun-exposed areas; no sharp borders; pruritus; occurs 24 hours or more after sun exposure
Polymorphous light eruption	Ch. 4, p. 192 (Figure 7-18)	Pruritic erythematous papules, widely scattered over sun-exposed areas; occurs within a few hours of sun exposure
Pruritic urticarial papules and plaques of pregnancy (PUPPP)	Ch. 7, p. 345 (Figure 7-19)	Tiny erythematous pruritic papules and plaques; occurs late third trimester in primigravidas; usually begins on abdomen and spreads to buttocks, arms, and hands
Pseudofolliculitis	Ch. 1, p. 46 (Figure 7-20)	Erythematous papules and pustules on shaved areas, especially beards of men with coarse, curly hair; may be asymptomatic or painful and pruritic
Scabies	Ch. 7, p. 346 (Figure 7-21)	Crusted papules or burrows on genitals, wrists, finger webs, belt line; intensely pruritic
Seborrheic dermatitis	Ch. 3, p. 138 (Figure 7-22)	Sharply marginated yellowish-red patches with sharp borders and greasy scales; scalp, central face, eyebrows, eyelids, nasolabial folds, and external ear most commonly affected; may be pruritic
Urticaria (hives)	Ch. 4, p. 198 (Figure 7-23)	Intense pruritus; primary lesion is the wheal; migration of lesions; angioedema; dermatographism
Xerosis (dry skin)	Ch. 7, p. 349 (Figure 7-24)	Dry, slightly scaly skin with variable erythema and superficial fissuring; pruritus common; most prominent on extremities

Acute Nummular Eczema

Overview

Pathophysiology

Pathophysiologic characteristics of the condition are unknown. It may be induced or perpetuated by a variety of factors, including emotional stress, heat, and moisture, probably differing in their relative importance in different age groups. It is not genetic or allergic in nature.

Epidemiology

Peak incidence for women is in the twenties and for men is between ages 40 and 80. There is an approximately equal sex distribution. Emotional stress is usually present. Palmar and plantar lesions of dyshydrotic eczema are commonly associated.

Assessment

Clinical Presentation

Pruritic, chronic coin-shaped plaques 1 to 5 cm in diameter or closely set papulovesicles occur on an erythematous base (see Figure 7-1). Plaques often become acutely exudative and crusted. Involvement usually begins on the dorsa of the hands or the trunk and may include the posterior or lateral neck, thighs, buttocks, and legs with single or multiple lesions. Chronic lesions are usually lichenified. Most lesions occur in the winter with remissions in the summer. All forms are chronic with partial remissions and relapses.

Diagnostics

• Biopsy may be necessary to confirm the diagnosis.

Differential Diagnosis

• Dermatophyte infection (scaly, erythematous lesions with central clearing) (see Figure 3-9, *B*)
• Contact dermatitis (lesions are usually distributed in areas where contact with the offending agent occurs) (see Figure 7-2)
• Dyshydrotic eczema (grouped tapiocalike vesicles on lateral fingers) (see Figure 7-7)
• Psoriasis vulgaris (symmetric erythematous lesions with gray-white scale) (see Figure 3-30, *A*)
• Drug eruption (usually presents with overlying scale; history of drug ingestion)
• Atopic dermatitis (distribution of lesions in antecubital and popliteal areas) (see Figure 7-3)

ACUTE NUMMULAR ECZEMA

• Can be minimized by wearing nonirritating clothing, using gentle cleansers and moisturizers, and reducing stress

- Stasis dermatitis (lesions on lower extremities)
- Impetigo (honey-colored crusts on lesions usually less than 1 cm in diameter) (see Figure 2-12)
- Mycosis fungoides (usually associated with widespread lesions)

Treatment

Nonpharmacologic

Decrease or control of stress is essential. Soft, nonirritating clothing is recommended to minimize itch.

Pharmacologic

Topical Agents

Potent topical corticosteroids **Temovate, Psorcon, Diprolene, Ultravate)** are used bid. Liquid nitrogen cryotherapy may be useful in minimizing pruritus.

Systemic Agents

Antihistamines **(Atarax** 25 to 50 mg tid to qid) to control pruritus. Systemic antibiotics **(Dicloxacillin or Erythromycin** 250 mg PO q6h for 10 days) are prescribed to treat or prevent secondary infection.

Indications for Referral

- Ineffective response to treatment, requiring systemic corticosteroids.

Allergic Contact Dermatitis

Overview

Pathophysiology

The disorder is a manifestation of cell-mediated hypersensitivity, which causes a delayed reaction on first exposure. The allergens are first sequestered in Langerhans' cells, which migrate to regional lymph nodes, where they stimulate antibody production.

The incubation period after initial exposure to an antigen is 5 to 21 days; on reexposure a patient will react within 12 to 48 hours. Exposure to toxicodendrons such as the *Rhus* genus of plants (poison oak, ivy, and sumac), mango, and cashews will result in a clinical eruption within 12 to 72 hours on first exposure and within minutes on reexposure. Once acquired, contact sensitivity usually persists without repeated exposure. Other common allergic sensitizers include nickel (often used in jewelry), rubber compounds (in gloves, shoes, elastic bands), benzocaine (in antipruritic creams), formaldehyde (in permanent-press clothes), perfume, hair dyes, and other cosmetics.

Epidemiology

An estimated 1% to 18% of the U.S. population is sensitive to an environmental or occupational chemical. Among North Americans 25% to 60% are sensitive to plants of the *Rhus* genus, and 10% of women are allergic to nickel. A bricklayer's or cement worker's sensitivity to chromium often requires more than 10 years to develop and is the most common industrial exposure in males. There appears to be some familial tendency, with an increased frequency of positive patch test results in siblings and children of patients. The incidence of clinical manifestation in adults is eight times that in children.

Assessment

Clinical Presentation

An initial erythema may progress to an **intense inflammatory pruritic papulovesicular eruption** (see Figure 7-2, *A*). Ruptured vesicles drain serous fluid and the surface becomes moist and crusted. Large bullae, fever, lymphadenopathy, and malaise may occur if the reaction is severe. Chronic, less vehement reactions may be dry and scaly.

The distribution is often suggestive of the diagnosis. The palms are rarely affected; dermatitis more often occurs on the lateral aspect of the fingers and the dorsal hand. A **linear eruption,** caused by dragging the allergen over the skin while scratching, is the hallmark of most plant dermatoses (see Figure 7-2, *B*). A pattern of eruption under a piece of jewelry or clothing or only on exposed areas is another clue. Photosensitizers cause erythematous patches in areas of contact after exposure to sunlight or on areas exposed to sunlight if the allergen is systemic.

An acute reaction usually resolves in days to weeks after the allergen has been removed. If the reaction continues, a search for another offending substance should occur. The eruption is usually **very pruritic** and secondary bacterial infection from excoriation is common.

Diagnostics
- **Patch testing** with suspected allergens may be helpful in difficult cases, but more often careful history taking and observation will be sufficient to make the diagnosis.

Differential Diagnosis
- Irritant contact dermatitis (patch testing is the only method for differentiation between the two; the clinical presentation is similar)
- Atopic dermatitis (distribution is in popliteal and antecubital areas) (see Figure 7-3)
- Seborrheic dermatitis (occurs mostly in facial, scalp, and central chest locations) (see Figure 3-34)
- Stasis dermatitis (distribution is on lower legs)
- Herpes simplex (lesions are usually smaller areas of grouped vesicles) (see Figure 2-10, *A*)
- Herpes zoster (lesions are painful and usually unilateral) (see Figure 2-11)
- Photodermatitis (lesions are only in areas exposed to sunlight)

Treatment

Nonpharmacologic
Avoidance of allergens can prevent allergic reactions.

Pharmacologic

Topical Agents
Cold compresses of **Burow's solution** or a 1:10 dilution of vinegar and water for 20 minutes every 4 to 6 hours is soothing. Potent topical corticosteroids **(Ultravate, Temovate, Diprolene, Psorcon)** may be used twice daily for no more than 2 weeks except in intertriginous areas or on the face. Ointments may be more soothing than creams. For the face and intertriginous areas midpotency steroids such as **Cutivate, Aclovate, Elocon,** or **Westcort** may be used twice daily for no more than 2 weeks.

Systemic Agents
Antihistamines such as **diphenhydramine (Benadryl) or hydroxyzine (Atarax)** 25 to 50 mg PO tid to qid, **loratadine (Claritin)** 10 mg PO qd, or **cetirizine (Zyrtec)** 10 mg PO qd will help relieve pruritus; the latter two are nonsedating. For severe cases a single IM injection of **triamcinolone (Kenalog) 40 mg and betamethasone (Celestone) 6 mg,** or a 3-week course of oral

---

ALLERGIC CONTACT DERMATITIS

- Can be prevented by avoiding precipitating factors/allergens
- Can be minimized with the use of cool soaks, antihistamines, and steroids
- When treated with sedating antihistamines, precludes patients from engaging in activities that require mental alertness
- Is not spread by the fluid in the resulting blisters
- When caused by plants, is contagious only through continued contact with the plant resin, which may remain in clothing and on animal fur

prednisone (60 mg qAM for 1 week, then 40 mg qAM for 1 week, then 20 mg qAM for 1 week) may be necessary.

Indications for Referral

- Persistent or recurring reactions.
- Progression of secondary infection or deteriorating systemic condition.
- Evaluation of positive patch testing results.

Atopic Dermatitis

Overview

Pathophysiology

Patients have several abnormal physiologic responses (including those to temperature, low humidity, stress, trauma, sweating, and common environmental allergens), as well as immunologic abnormalities. The characteristic dry skin may result from increased transepidermal water loss or decreased sebaceous gland lipid levels.

The acute phase appears to result from mast cell release of mediators including histamine, leukotrienes, prostaglandins, and proteases in response to allergic, physical, and/or neural stimuli. Serum immunoglobulin E (IgE) levels may be increased in proportion to the extent or severity of the dermatitis.

A high carriage rate for *Staphylococcus aureus* is found in these patients and may play a role in exacerbations and prolongation of cutaneous disease. Breast feeding may reduce the incidence and delay the appearance of eczema and atopy in childhood.

Epidemiology

There is a genetic predisposition to atopic dermatitis. Patients usually have a **family history of asthma or hay fever.** There is an increased frequency of bacterial, fungal, and viral infections. Patients with allergic rhinitis or bronchial asthma have a worse prognosis for remission.

Seventy-five percent of patients have an initial onset before 12 months of age; spontaneous improvement is common throughout childhood. The more severe and widespread the disease is in infancy and childhood, the fewer remissions occur over time. Relapses may occur in adult life.

Assessment

Clinical Presentation

Patients report being allergic to "everything." Their chief complaint is itching, which leads to scratching and the resultant dermatitis (see Figure 7-3). **Pruritus** may be so severe as to distract them from their daily activities or wake them at night. Scratching will produce white **dermatographism** (see Figure 4-37, *B*). The skin is characteristically erythematous and weeping during acute flares but dry, hyperkeratotic, and lichenified with chronic disease. Infants display the disorder as bright red cheeks, whereas the sides of the neck and flexural surfaces are the most commonly affected areas after age 12. Ichthyosis vulgaris and keratosis pilaris are common. **Palmar markings** increase in number. An **infraorbital fold** just beneath the lower eyelid margin is usually present. A thinning or **absence of the lateral eyebrows** may occur. Pityriasis alba (white, scaling patches on the face) is common. Severe cases may have a generalized exfoliative dermatitis. A visible superimposed bacterial infection is common, as is irritant contact dermatitis.

Reactions resulting from ingestion of foods usually occur within 15 to 90 minutes after ingestion and may be associated with gastrointestinal (GI) symptoms of loose stools and abdominal pain.

During infancy lesions are most prominent on the face and scalp **(red cheeks)**. With crawling the knees are especially involved. Associated diaper dermatitis is common. Later (age 12) there is more localization to the sides of the **neck and flexural surfaces.**

Diagnostics

- Diagnosis is made on the basis of a detailed personal and family history, factors likely to trigger flares, and the distribution of the lesions. Patch testing may be helpful to rule out allergic contact dermatitis.

Differential Diagnosis

- Allergic contact dermatitis (lesions are usually distributed in areas where contact with the offending agent occurs) (see Figure 7-2, *A*)
- Irritant contact dermatitis (lesions are usually distributed in areas where contact with the offending agent occurs)
- Seborrheic dermatitis (distribution is on the scalp, face, and central chest) (see Figure 3-34)
- Lichen simplex chronicus (usually a single, larger lesion) (see Figure 7-14)
- Acute nummular eczema (lesions usually appear on arms, legs, and neck) (see Figure 7-1)

ATOPIC DERMATITIS

- Is a chronic condition that cannot be cured
- Can be minimized through the avoidance of irritating or precipitating factors
- May flare if patients wear wool clothing, bathe more than once daily, use harsh soaps, or do not moisturize regularly
- May result in a secondary bacterial infection if skin is allowed to dry and crack

Treatment

Nonpharmacologic

- Frequent bathing should be avoided. Tepid water and mild, unscented **soap (Dove, Cetaphil, Basis, Oil of Olay)** should be used.
- Moisturization is key, especially after bathing and as often as needed.
- Aggravating factors should be controlled.
- New clothes should be laundered before wearing to wash out formaldehyde resins that are added to clothing to maintain freshness.
- Clothing should be soft, light, and preferably made of cotton or another natural fiber *except* wool.
- Activity that produces sweating should be reduced and the environment kept cool and well ventillated.
- Dietary manipulation may help prevent flares but is not curative.
- Biofeedback may help control pruritus.

Pharmacologic

Topical agents

Urea creams such as **U-Lactin** have a hydrating, anesthetic, and antibacterial effect on the stratum corneum. For acute, wet, or crusted lesions soaking with **Burow's solution** will hydrate the stratum corneum, remove the crusts, and facilitate the penetration of topical steroids, which are helpful in reducing inflammation and pruritus. Low-potency steroids **(Hytone, DesOwen)** bid are safe for use on the face for periods of up to 6 months. Midpotency steroids **(Cutivate, Elocon, Westcort)** bid will provide better relief for other areas of the body but should not be used for longer than 2 weeks at a time. High-potency steroids **(Ultravate, Psorcon, Temovate)** should be reserved for use during extreme flares and for use on the acral skin of hands and feet, but for no longer than 2 weeks at a time and no more frequently than bid. Substitution of emollients and moisturizers should occur as soon as possible. Tar compounds, which have vasoconstrictive, antipruritic, and antibacterial properties, may be applied alternately with steroids, at night or in the bath.

Systemic Agents

Erythromycin or **dicloxacillin** 250 mg PO q6h for 10 days should be started at the first sign of a bacterial infection. Tricyclic antidepressants such as **doxepin (Sinequan)** 25 mg PO qhs have been shown to decrease the itch-scratch-itch cycle and provide sedative effects. Antihistamines such as **hydroxyzine (Atarax, Vistaril)** 25 to 50 mg PO tid also help to relieve itching. Some studies have shown that tricyclic antidepressants, such as **doxepin (Sinequan)** 25 mg PO qhs, is helpful in significantly decreasing itching. **PUVA** is effective in 75% of recalcitrant patients. Exposure three to four times a week is needed, with a slow increase in joules of 0.5 J per treatment. After clearance one treatment per month is needed for 6 months. A short course of **prednisone** 60 mg PO qd for 1 week, then 40 mg PO qd 1 week, and then 20 mg PO qd for 1 week can be helpful in difficult cases.

Indications for Referral

- Unremitting discomfort despite treatment as outlined.
- Secondary infections unresponsive to therapy.

Dyshidrotic Eczema (Pompholyx)

Overview

Pathophysiology
Dyshidrotic eczema is an inflammation of the palms and soles and occasionally sides of the fingers. The cause is largely unknown.

Epidemiology
Onset is unusual before puberty, as most cases occur between **ages 20 and 40.** About half of patients have a positive family history or an **atopic background.** The incidence increases in warm weather. Emotional **stress** is a frequent provocative factor.

Assessment

Clinical Presentation
Pruritus is followed by the outbreak of **bilateral symmetric vesicles on the soles and palms,** which may be chronic or acute (see Figure 7-7). The vesicles on the sides of the fingers may resemble **tapioca.** Hands may be erythematous and **sweaty.** Within a month the vesicular eruption subsides with peeling of the affected skin. Lesions may progress to lichenification, fissures, and/or erosions. Hyperhydrosis may or may not be present.

Diagnostics
- Diagnosis is made by clinical presentation and history.

Differential Diagnosis
- Pustular psoriasis (lesions are usually generalized over large areas and there is a prior history of psoriasis) (see Figure 3-30, *C*)
- Allergic contact dermatitis (lesions are usually distributed in areas where contact occurs with the offending agent) (see Figure 7-2, *A*)
- Id reaction to dermatophyte infection (generalized, eczematous nummular lesions)
- Acute nummular eczema (lesions usually occur on arms, legs, and neck) (see Figure 7-1)
- Viral exanthems (e.g., hand-foot-mouth disease) (distribution of lesions usually occurs on lateral aspects of fingers and feet)

DYSHIDROTIC ECZEMA

- Can be controlled by reducing precipitating factors, especially stress
- Is less pruritic if skin is kept well moisturized and supple, but not wet

Treatment

Nonpharmacologic
Controlling stress is essential. Cool footwear with nonirritating powders (cornstarch) may be helpful.

Pharmacologic

Topical Agents
Soak affected areas three to four times a day in normal saline solution or apply a compress of **Burow's solution** for 20 minutes qid. High-potency topical corticosteroids **(Diprolene, Ultravate, Temovate, Psorcon)** are usually necessary to penetrate the thicker skin of the palms and soles. Patients should be encouraged to use ointment formulations at night, but may prefer creams during the day. Applications twice a day for up to 2 weeks may be necessary.

Systemic Agents
For severe and/or recalcitrant cases **PUVA** therapy qod, in either a topical or systemic modality, may be helpful. Systemic steroids are rarely required for severe or recalcitrant cases.

Indications for Referral

- If a secondary pyoderma is suspected and does not respond to systemic antibiotics.

Lice (Pediculosis)

Overview

Pathophysiology

Pediculosis is an infestation of the skin caused by lice. Females lay four eggs per day, which incubate over 8 to 9 days and may then lie dormant for up to 35 days. Symptoms may thus develop well after infection occurred. Lice feed four or five times a day, injecting saliva when feeding. It is the saliva that causes an allergic reaction leading to pruritus, a mild fever, myalgias, and occasionally swelling of the cervical lymph glands. There are three main types, defined by the body part affected:

Pediculosis capitis (head lice) is caused by *Pediculus humanus capitis*, approximately 1.5 mm in length. The scalp is usually infested with about 10 insects.

Pediculosis corporis (body lice) is caused by *Pediculus humanus corporis*, approximately 2 mm in length. The female louse lays eggs in the seams of clothing. The lice live in clothing that is in contact with the skin. They are only found on the skin when they are taking a meal.

Pediculosis pubis (pubic lice or crabs) is caused by *Pthirus pubis*, approximately 1 mm in length. The female lice lay 10 to 12 eggs per day, producing large populations within a few months.

Epidemiology

Pediculosis capitis occurs most commonly in children and in adults with poor hygiene. Epidemics may occur in schools and playgrounds. It is very rare in blacks because the lice cannot hold onto black, curly hair. Infestation may be transmitted by shared hats and combs.

Pediculosis corporis generally occurs in patients with poor hygiene. Infestation is usually transmitted by clothing or bedding.

Pediculosis pubis is transmitted 95% of the time through sexual exposure with an infected person.

Assessment

Clinical Presentation

Pediculosis capitis: Pruritis is most severe around the back and sides of the scalp. Nits (eggs) are found most easily when attached to the hair shafts of the occiput and above the ears, about $1/4$ inch from the scalp (see Figure 7-12, *A*). The condition may be misdiagnosed as seborrhea. Erythematous papules and excoriations are common.

Pediculosis corporis: Bites by the louse provoke pruritic, red papules with a characteristic central punctum that crust and may become secondarily infected with bacteria.

Pediculosis pubis: Itching in the genital region is the characteristic symptom, but the eyebrows, eyelashes, chest, beard, or legs may be infested. Small yellow-brown to gray dots in infested areas represent either ingested blood in the adult lice or their excreta (see Figure 7-12, *B*). Occasionally with heavy infestation a bluish macular eruption (maculae ceruleae) on the inner thighs or lateral trunk results from altered blood pigments.

Diagnostics
Culture may be necessary if excoriations are impetiginized.

- *Pediculosis capitis:* Identification of the nits attached to the hair shaft confirms the diagnosis. Microscopic examination may be necessary to differentiate the nit from dandruff.
- *Pediculosis corporis:* Diagnosis is made by thoroughly searching the seams of clothing in close contact with skin to detect the presence of lice.
- *Pediculosis pubis:* Identification of nits or the lice themselves attached to the pubic hair shaft or on the eyebrows, eyelashes, chest, beard, or legs confirms the diagnosis.

Differential Diagnosis
- Seborrheic dermatitis (distribution of lesions occurs primarily on the scalp, face, and central chest) (see Figure 3-34)
- Flea bites (lesions are located on the lower legs and are usually in a linear pattern of three to four "bites") (see Figure 4-24)
- Folliculitis (lesions are all associated with hair follicles) (see Figure 1-6)

PEDICULOSIS

- Is very contagious; good hygiene is essential
- Can be spread through personal contact or sharing of hats, combs, clothing, and linen
- Treatment requires that all members of the household be treated simultaneously

Treatment

Nonpharmacologic
- *Pediculosis capitis:* Avoid sharing hats and combs. Treat all contacts and family members.
- *Pediculosis corporis:* Assure hygienic standards when multiple persons share clothing or bedding.
- *Pediculosis pubis:* All sexual contacts should be treated.

Pharmacologic
Pediculosis capitis: **Lindane (Kwell)** shampoo is applied and massaged into the scalp for 4 to 5 minutes. Wash off completely. Retreat in 1 week. Do not use on pregnant or nursing mothers.

Pyrethrins (A-200, RID) are the least toxic to humans: Apply to dry scalp until saturated. Leave on for 10 minutes and shampoo out. Repeat the treatment in 1 week. Saturate hair and scalp with **Permethrin (NIX);** rinse out after 10 minutes. A single treatment is sufficient. This treatment is safe for children above 2 years of age but should not be used by nursing mothers. A **creme rinse** is effective in the removal of nits by loosening the bond attaching the nit to the hair. Apply to wet hair after pediculicidal shampoo is washed out with water. Leave on 10 minutes and comb with metal nit removal comb. Re-treat in 1 week. Topical corticosteroids will be helpful in relieving pruritus. Gels **(Lidex 0.05%, Topicort 0.05%)** or solutions **(Halog 0.1%, Lidex 0.05%)** used qd are more acceptable in the scalp.

Pediculosis corporis: See Pediculosis capitis. Corticosteroid creams or lotions **(Elocon 0.1%, Halog 0.025%)** used bid are helpful in relieving pruritus.

Pediculosis pubis: See Pediculosis capitis. Pruritus is best relieved in the genital area with a mild corticosteroid cream **(Hytone 1.0%)** used bid.

In all cases of pediculosis systemic antihistamines **(hydroxyzine [Atarax] 25 to 50 mg)** at bedtime may be useful in relieving pruritus and inducing sleep.

Indications for Referral

- Condition unresponsive to treatment.
- Development of severe secondary bacterial infection.

Lichen Simplex Chronicus (Neurodermatitis)

Overview

Pathophysiology

The actual cause is unknown. Any number of factors (xerosis, emotional stress) may cause itching that leads to rubbing and/or scratching. In time the epidermis lichenifies and causes continued pruritus, scratching, and lichenification. There appears to be some familial predisposition in patients with atopic conditions. The extreme pruritus associated with this condition may be due to an increase in the number of dermal nerves.

Epidemiology

The disorder is more common in **women** than in men with a peak incidence at **ages 30 to 50.** It is infrequent in children. There is a sevenfold increased incidence in **Asian races.**

Assessment

Clinical Presentation

Pruritus is the predominant symptom. It is severe and paroxysmal and most often occurs just **before or during sleep. Lichenified plaques** are located most frequently **on the ankles and anterior tibial and nuchal areas,** inner thighs, lateral neck, extensor surfaces, and anogenital region (see Figure 7-14). Plaques are thickened, scaly, erythematous, and frequently excoriated. Sites may be singular or multiple. With persistent rubbing and excoriation lichenified nodules may develop. Follicular papules may be seen in blacks.

Diagnostics

- Skin biopsy is indicated when symptoms do not respond to appropriate treatment.

Differential Diagnosis

- Atopic dermatitis (distribution of lesions primarily in popliteal and antecubital areas) (see Figure 7-3)
- Psoriasis vulgaris (symmetric, erythematous lesions with gray-white scale) (see Figure 3-30, *A*)
- Stasis dermatitis (distribution of lesions on lower legs)
- Allergic contact dermatitis (lesions usually distributed in areas of contact with the offending agent) (see Figure 7-2, *A*)
- Irritant contact dermatitis (lesions usually distributed in areas of contact with the offending agent)
- Dermatophyte infection (scaly, erythematous lesion with central clearing) (see Figure 3-9, *B*)
- Lichen planus (multiple violaceous flat-topped papules, usually less than 15 mm in diameter) (see Figure 3-22)

LICHEN SIMPLEX CHRONICUS

- Is a chronic condition in which the "itch-scratch-itch" cycle must be broken
- Can be controlled by reducing precipitating factors, especially stress
- Is less pruritic if skin is kept well moisturized and supple, but not wet

Treatment

Nonpharmacologic

Bland creams or ointments **(Cetaphil, Aquaphor)** lubricate the skin.

Pharmacologic

Topical Agents

Emollients containing menthol **(Sarna** lotion) may be soothing. High-potency steroids (Class I or II, such as **Temovate-E,**

Ultravate, Psorcon, Diprolene) should be used as necessary, avoiding the face, axillae, and groin. Moist compresses before steroid use will facilitate penetration through plaques. Steroid-impregnated tape **(Cordran)** is useful for its occlusive and protective properties. **Liquid nitrogen cryotherapy** may deaden sensory nerves and relieve the associated pruritus.

Intralesional Agents
Triamcinolone (Kenalog) 5 mg/ml IL produces the most rapid response and is helpful if topical agents are ineffective.

Systemic agents
Antihistamines **(hydroxyzine [Atarax]** 25 to 50 mg PO tid and qhs) may help to relieve pruritus and induce sleep.

Indications for Referral

- Failure to respond to therapy.

Pruritic Urticarial Papules and Plaques of Pregnancy (PUPPP)

Overview

Pathophysiology
The cause is thought to be a sensitization to placental hormones.

Epidemiology
PUPPP occurs late in the **third trimester** in **primigravidas** and rarely recurs with subsequent pregnancies. It is the most common eruption of pregnancy and resolves with delivery. There is no danger to either mother or child.

Assessment

Clinical Presentation
This disorder begins with the eruption of **tiny erythematous papules and plaques in the abdominal striae.** The lesions may coalesce and spread within days to the **entire abdomen,** buttocks, thighs, and arms (see Figure 7-19). **Itching** is moderate to severe. Excoriations are rare.

Diagnostics
- Laboratory test results are normal, and the diagnosis is made clinically.

Differential Diagnosis
- Herpes gestationis (lesions are more vesicular)
- Urticaria (lesions are more generalized) (see Figure 7-23)
- Allergic contact dermatitis (lesions are usually distributed in areas of contact with the offending agent) (see Figure 7-2, *A*)

Treatment

Nonpharmacologic
Ice water compresses help to relieve itching. Mild, unscented soaps **(Dove, Cetaphil, Basis, Oil of Olay)** and soft, nonirritating clothing may be useful. Moisturization helps prevent dry skin (winter itch).

Pharmacologic
Group V topical corticosteroid creams or ointments **(Aclovate, Westcort)** applied bid to the affected areas will help reduce pruritus and erythema. In severe cases **prednisone** 20 mg PO qAM for 4 days, followed by tapering doses of 15 mg, 10 mg, and 5 mg, each for 4 days, may be used.

PRURITIC URTICARIAL PAPULES AND PLAQUES OF PREGNANCY

- Will resolve spontaneously after delivery
- Does not pose any danger to either mother or child

Indications for Referral

- For histologic confirmation of the diagnosis

Scabies

Overview

Pathophysiology
Infestation with the mite *Sarcoptes scabei humani* commonly results from prolonged personal contact with an infected person but may result from transmission through clothing, linens, or towels since the female can survive for 2 to 3 days off the human host. The fertilized female excavates a burrow in the stratum corneum into

which she deposits 10 to 25 eggs. The larvae emerge from the eggs after 3 to 7 days, mature over 30 days, and travel on the skin surface. After an incubation period of from 1 to 2 months an acquired sensitivity to the organism or to fecal pellets develops, leading to intense pruritus. Symptoms with reinfection occur within 24 hours and the pruritus is more intense. The disorder can persist indefinitely unless treated.

Epidemiology

Scabies epidemics persist for 15 years and occur every 30 years. Most cases occur in individuals who are in close contact with others. The occurrence of scabies in the black population is rare.

Assessment

Clinical Presentation

Classically pruritic **crusted papules** are found on the **genitals** (penile lesions are common), **wrists,** buttocks, **finger webs,** axilla, and breasts and around the umbilicus. Burrows appear as 5 to 20 mm S-shaped ridges or dotted lines resembling black thread (most commonly found on the wrists) (see Figure 7-21). Often the burrow is indistinguishable as a result of scratching and excoriation. Pruritus is most intense at night. The **belt line** is commonly involved. A secondary skin infection may result from scratching and excoriation. In infants and young children vesicles are frequently present, and the distribution of the disease may include the **palms, soles,** head, neck, or face.

Diagnostics

Mites and ova may be identified in skin scrapings obtained with a no. 15 blade dipped in oil. The sample is obtained through vigorous scraping (to open the burrow) and then placed in a drop of oil on a glass slide. It should be examined under low power. **Avoid** using **KOH** because it dissolves the feces and immobilizes the female.

Differential Diagnosis

- Lichen simplex chronicus (no evidence of burrows; distribution of lesions is not typically on wrists or finger webs) (see Figure 7-14)
- Atopic dermatitis (distribution of lesions occurs on antecubital and popliteal areas) (see Figure 7-3)
- Flea or insect bites (lesions are usually single or multiple papules) (see Figure 2-13)
- Pruritus of systemic disease (usually associated with maculopapular eruption of generalized xerosis)

SCABIES

- Is contagious with prolonged personal contact with an infected person
- May be transmitted through clothing, linens, and personal items
- Will persist indefinitely unless treated
- May continue to cause itching for days to weeks after treatment
- Is best eliminated by treating the entire household simultaneously

Treatment

Nonpharmacologic

All contacts should be treated at the same time, including the entire family. Clothing and bedding used over the past week should be laundered.

Pharmacologic

Lindane (Kwell) 1% cream or lotion is rubbed over the entire body below the neck, with special attention to brushing it under the fingernails. Only 1 to 2 oz. should be used to cover the entire body. It is left on for 6 hours and then washed off. The entire process is repeated in 1 week. It should not be used in children below age 5 or in pregnant women because of possible central nervous system (CNS) toxicity. An irritant contact dermatitis may result, intensifying the itching.

Crotamiton 10% cream or **lotion (Eurax)** is a safer alternative to **lindane** (especially in young children and pregnant women) and has some antipruritic properties. It is massaged into the skin of the entire body from the neck down, especially in skin folds. A second coat is applied in 24 hours without removing the first. The patient should bathe 48 hours after the second treatment.

For children less than 2 years old and pregnant women a 10% precipitated **sulfur** ointment may be preferred. It is applied from the neck down on 3 consecutive nights and washed off with soap and water on day 4 of the treatment.

Hydroxyzine (Atarax) 25 to 50 mg PO qhs may be extremely beneficial in relieving the pruritus that intensifies at night and precludes sleep. Nonsedating antihistamines such as **loratadine (Claritin)** 10 mg PO qAM or **cetirizine (Zyrtec)** 10 mg PO qAM may provide relief during waking hours. Midpotency topical corticosteroids (**Elocon** cream or lotion 0.1%) applied bid for 2 weeks also helps in reducing pruritus.

Indications for Referral

- The development of nodular lesions in the groin, axilla, or buttocks.
- Norwegian scabies (infestation with large numbers of mites) producing a total erythroderma.

For Scabies Patient Teaching information and materials, turn to p. 461.

Xerosis (Dry Skin)

Overview

Pathophysiology

Xerosis is caused by dehydration of the epidermis. It occurs in those with naturally dry skin (most have a genetic predisposition) and is exacerbated by reduced epidermal lipid production (which occurs with increasing age, illness, hormonal decline, malnutrition, low-cholesterol diet, and use of lipid lowering drugs) and factors that decrease skin hydration (low humidity; diuretics; excessive bathing, especially with hot water and harsh soap; and incomplete drying with resultant evaporation).

Xerosis may be associated with atopic and contact dermatitis, the ichthyoses, and hyperthyroidism.

Epidemiology

Xerosis is more common in the elderly and in conditions of low environmental humidity.

Assessment

Clinical Presentation

The chief complaint is usually generalized or localized **pruritus.** The involved area is dry and **slightly scaly** with variable **erythema** and **superficial fissuring** (see Figure 7-24). Coin-shaped areas of eczema may be present (nummular eczema). Involvement is **most prominent on the extremities,** especially the anterior tibial region, dorsa of hands, and forearms.

Diagnostics

- Diagnosis is made by clinical presentation. A thorough history taking is essential, including both personal and family history, as well as current methods of skin care (frequency of bathing, types of skin care products used, etc). Because xerosis may be associated with various systemic diseases (hypothyroidism, contact dermatitis, ichthyoses, atopic dermatitis), an evaluation of possible underlying medical conditions is also essential.

Differential Diagnosis

- Acute nummular eczema (lesions usually on arms, legs, and neck) (see Figure 7-1)
- Irritant contact dermatitis (lesions are usually distributed in areas where contact occurs with the offending agent) (see Figure 7-2, *A*)
- Stasis dermatitis (distribution is on lower legs)

XEROSIS

- Is a chronic condition
- Can be minimized by taking no more than one bath per day and keeping the use of soap to a minimum
- Necessitates the application of emollients immediately after bathing on still-damp skin

- Psoriasis (symmetric erythematous lesions with gray-white scale) (see Figure 3-30, *A*)
- Dermatophyte infection (lesions are usually localized) (see Figure 3-9, *B*)

Treatment

Nonpharmacologic

Restrict number of baths to one per day (no longer than 10 minutes). Keep the use of soaps to a minimum. Soaps, preferably fatted or soap substitutes such as **Cetaphil** or **Aquanil,** should only be used in the axillae and groin. Skin should be patted dry and immediately lubricated with oils or ointments. Water temperature should be tepid. Patients may consider having soft water installed in their hot water system at home.

Pharmacologic

Topical Agents

Products containing urea **(U-lactin)** attract and hold water on the surface of the skin. **Sarna** anti-itch lotion provides lubrication while soothing itching. Another soothing lotion consists of **Cetaphil** lotion, 1% **hydrocortisone,** and 1% **menthol. A 1% hydrocortisone cream** or **0.025% triamcinolone ointment** used bid may also reduce inflammation and pruritus. **Lac-Hydrin** cream or lotion will help to exfoliate the thicker layers of dried skin, allowing greater penetration of moisture to the deeper layers.

Systemic Agents

For severe pruritus or pruritus resulting in insomnia, **hydroxyzine (Atarax)** 25 to 50 mg tid and qhs may provide much needed relief.

Indications for Referral

- Subtherapeutic response to treatment.

For Pruritic Disorders Patient Teaching information and materials, turn to p. 457.

Hair Disorders

Figure 8-1   ALOPECIA AREATA

Localized bald area of the scalp. Note short hairs within the lesion.

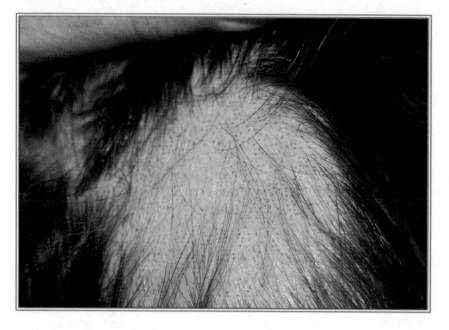

Figure 8-2   ANDROGENETIC ALOPECIA

Frontotemporal and midfrontal recession of scalp hair. Note decreased density of hair over the vertex and top of scalp.

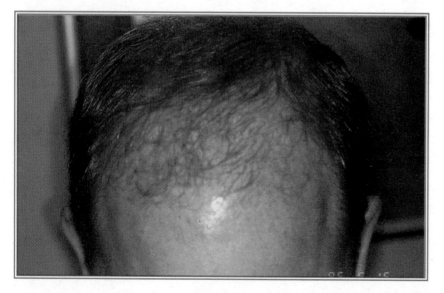

Figure 8-3 FOLLICULITIS

Extensive number of inflammatory closed comedones centered around hair follicles on the cheek of a male electrical worker exposed to fluorocarbons.

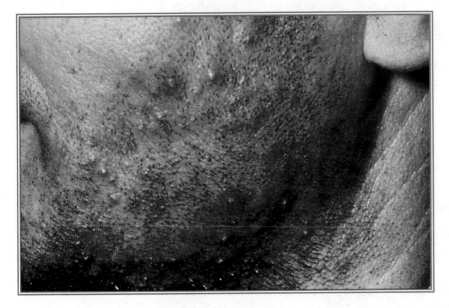

Figure 8-4 PSEUDOFOLLICULITIS

Inflammatory lesions with some pustules in the mandibular angle. Note curled hairs, some of which are embedding back into the skin.

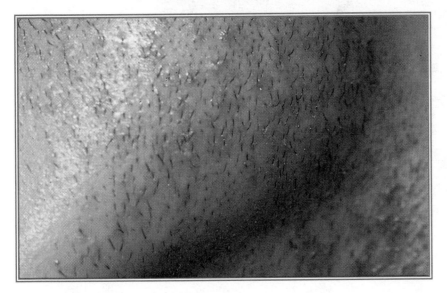

Figure 8-5 Seborrheic Dermatitis

Erythematous patches with some evidence of scale in the usual facial distribution.

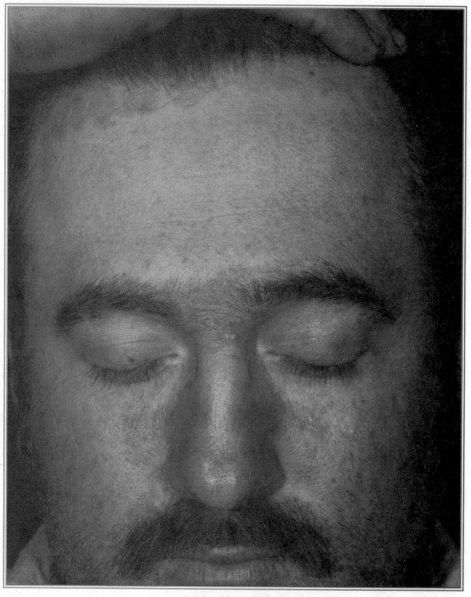

(From Habif TP: *Clinical dermatology,* ed 3, St Louis, 1996, Mosby.)

Figure 8-6   TINEA CAPITIS

Thick scale and crust on the apical aspect of a child's head.

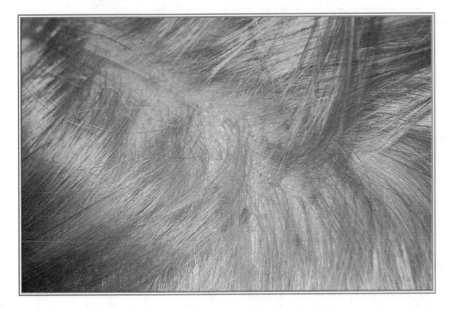

Figure 8-7   TRICHOTILLOMANIA

Multiple areas of partially alopecic skin within the scalp. Note that some of the hairs are growing within the bald area.

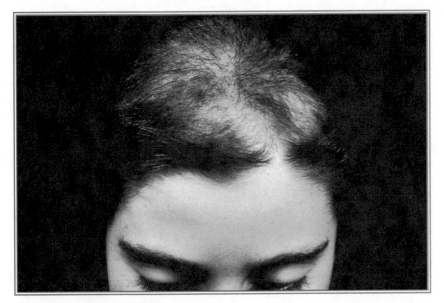

(Courtesy Stacy R. Smith, MD.)

▎Table 8-1

Differential Diagnosis of Hair Disorders

DISORDER	TEXT	KEYS TO DIAGNOSIS
Alopecia areata	Ch. 8, p. 357 (Figure 8-1)	Asymptomatic, nonscarring patches of complete hair loss, which appear suddenly
Androgenetic alopecia	Ch. 8, p. 359 (Figure 8-2)	Normal scalp surface; gradual diffuse thinning of hair on vertex (females) or bitemporal and anterior (males)
Folliculitis	Ch. 1, p. 36 (Figure 8-3)	Follicular erythematous papules and pustules on any hair-bearing surface; *Pseudomonas* folliculitis occurs 1 to 3 days after use of a hot tub
Pseudofolliculitis	Ch. 1, p. 46 (Figure 8-4)	Erythematous papules and pustules on shaved areas, especially beards of men with coarse, curly hair; may be asymptomatic or painful and pruritic
Seborrheic dermatitis (scalp)	Ch. 3, p. 138 (Figure 8-5)	Diffuse, poorly marginated erythematous areas of scale; known as "cradle cap" in infants, "dandruff" in adults; may also occur in the beard, mustache, and hairy areas of the chest
Telogen effluvium	Ch. 8, p. 362	Diffuse shedding of hairs at an above average rate; scalp is normal; hair loss follows mental or physiologic stress by 6 weeks to 4 months
Tinea capitis	Ch. 3, p. 116 (Figure 8-6)	Asymptomatic patchy loss of hair; numerous broken hairs, inflammation, and scaling also occur
Trichotillomania	Ch. 8, p. 364 (Figure 8-7)	Single or multiple patches of alopecia; normal hairs interspersed among short, broken hairs; scalp is normal; alopecia more pronounced on patient's dominant side

Alopecia Areata

Overview

Pathophysiology

Alopecia areata (AA) is an idiopathic noninflammatory, nonscarring patchy loss of hair. There is an immunologic cause (dysfunction of suppressor T cells) and an association with autoimmune disorders including vitiligo, pernicious anemia, diabetes mellitus, Addison's disease, atopic dermatitis, and thyroid disease. It may also develop as a temporary condition 2 weeks after psychologic trauma.

Epidemiology

A relatively common disorder, AA occurs in 1 in 200 people in the United States. There is an equal sex distribution, but a positive family history in 10% to 30% of patients. Most cases occur between ages 5 and 40. If the disorder occurs before age 10, the probability of permanent hair loss is increased. Over 20% of pediatric patients have evidence of a thyroid hormone abnormality.

Assessment

Clinical Presentation

Well-defined single or multiple patches of **asymptomatic non-scarring complete loss of hair** (see Figure 8-1) occur. New lesions may be slightly erythematous. The **patches appear suddenly,** frequently almost overnight. The classic lesion occurs on the scalp, although the eyebrows, eyelashes, or beard may also be affected. (Nail changes, specifically pitting in regular rows, may occur but are most often associated with extensive alopecia.) The skin surface is normal. One patch may be regrowing as another new area of hair loss occurs. The lesion margins may have broken-off hair stumps **("exclamation-mark hairs")** in which the diameter of the hair shaft tapers to a small point. The condition may progress. With small limited lesions 80% of patients regrow hair. Only 5% of patients with alopecia totalis (complete absence of scalp hair) and 1% of patients with alopecia universalis (complete absence of all body hair) will have spontaneous hair regrowth.

Diagnostics

- The diagnosis is usually based on clinical presentation; punch biopsy will confirm the diagnosis.
- A TSH should be performed in patients whose history and physical examination results suggest hypothyroidism.

- A fungal culture may be appropriate if there is significant scaling, to rule out tinea capitis.
- A psychologic evaluation may be appropriate if trichotillomania (an uncontrollable impulse to pull out one's own hair) is a possibility.

Differential Diagnosis

- Syphilitic alopecia (more ragged with incomplete hair loss within the patch: a moth eaten appearance)
- Androgenetic alopecia (slow, progressive male hair loss in a characteristic pattern) (see Figure 8-2)
- Trauma to the scalp (history of pressure, traction or trichotillomania)
- Tinea capitis (scaling, positive fungal culture result) (see Figure 3-9, *A*)
- Hypothyroidism (low TSH level; coarse, sparse, dry hair; flat affect; slow speech; hoarse voice; weight gain)

ALOPECIA AREATA

• Can be reduced or eliminated by treating the underlying cause

Treatment

Nonpharmacologic

Treat the underlying cause if possible: reduce pressure or traction on the scalp; provide psychologic intervention for trichotillomania. Because of the psychologic distress that may be caused by the condition, referral to an alopecia support group may be beneficial.

Pharmacologic

Topical Agents

Minoxidil topical solution (Rogaine) applied bid to the diseased area is beneficial in about 30% of cases. However, treatment must be continued or hair loss will resume. A superpotent corticosteroid cream such as **clobetasol (Temovate), betamethasone (Diprolene) or diflorasone (Psorcon)** may be used bid for a persistent single disfiguring patch. Some regrowth should occur in 4 to 6 weeks but the treatment should be continued until either hair growth or skin atrophy occurs. Alternatively **anthralin (Dritho-Scalp)** gel 1% to 2% may be applied to the affected areas qhs until the hair regrows or irritation becomes intolerable. Topical sensitization with **dinitrochlorobenzene (DNCB)** or another allergen qd until hair growth is stimulated is also effective.

Intralesional Agents

Triamcinolone acetonide (Kenalog) 5 mg/ml injected into the affected area with a 30-gauge needle, 0.05 to 0.1 ml per site for a total injected volume of 1 to 2 ml, can halt and reverse AA. Injections can be repeated at 4- to 6-week intervals for up to three treatments. Local atrophy is a potential side effect.

Systemic Agents

Systemic **prednisone** (40 mg PO qd tapered over 4 to 6 weeks) may stimulate a remission but will not prevent the eventual progression to baldness. Repeated or prolonged courses of systemic steroids produce more risks than benefits and should be avoided. **Psoralen with ultraviolet A (PUVA)** therapy may be considered as a final treatment option but is both expensive and time-consuming with treatments needed two or three times weekly. **Spironolactone (Aldactone)** 25 to 50 mg PO bid may also be helpful. Doses may be increased up to 100 mg bid, but potassium levels should be checked at 2-month intervals since it is a potassium-sparing diuretic and may cause hyperkalemia. Therapy should be continued for 9 to 12 months. Patients should be informed that it has been known to cause breast cysts in laboratory animals; mammography is therefore recommended every 2 years.

Indications for Referral

- A dermatologist should be consulted if PUVA therapy is desired.
- Referral to a psychologist or psychiatrist may be appropriate if mental distress is severe.

Androgenetic Alopecia (Male Pattern Baldness)

Overview

Pathophysiology

Androgenetic alopecia (AGA) occurs in both men and women and is defined as genetically influenced hair loss on the top of the scalp (vertex) in which the production of androgens is normal. This disorder is not to be confused with androgenic alopecia (AG), which is hair loss in women caused by excessive amounts of androgens. In women AGA may be caused by abrupt hormonal shifts such as those that result from childbirth, menopause, anovulation, or use of oral contraceptives. In men both the age of onset and the degree of balding are genetically determined. In both sexes AGA is further stimulated by elevated dihydrotestosterone (DHT) production.

The mechanism of hair thinning is the gradual shrinkage of hairs from terminal (the type of hair found on the scalp, eyebrows, and eyelashes) to vellus (the fine, unpigmented hair found over most of the body). The hairs become finer and thinner and the size of the hair bulbs become progressively smaller.

Epidemiology

Approximately 50% of white females, aged 50 and over, are affected to some degree by AGA. Severe degrees of alopecia are rare. In men, although all races are affected, it is most common in whites with Asian and black races less frequently and less severely affected. Approximately 20% of white males show some degree of balding by age 20, and 50% are affected by age 50. By age 70, 80% of males show some degree of alopecia.

Assessment

Clinical Presentation

In females there is a more diffuse and generally less severe pattern of hair loss, with the thinning most marked on the vertex. Additionally the scalp may become increasingly greasy. Bitemporal recession is more characteristic in men and is associated with a slow recession of the anterior hairline. In both sexes the scalp surface is normal.

Diagnostics

- In females routine lab work should include TSH level (to rule out hypothyroidism), serum iron level and total iron-binding capacity, and complete blood count (all to rule out anemia). If hair loss is accompanied by the development of male characteristics (deepening of the voice, hair growth in areas of the body other than the scalp, etc.) lab studies should also include serum testosterone (free and total), serum prolactin, and dehydroepiandrosterone sulfate (DHEAS) levels. Total testosterone levels higher than 2 ng/ml and DHEAS levels higher than 9,000 ng/ml are suggestive of an adrenal tumor for which the patient should be referred to a specialist.
- In males the characteristic pattern of hair thinning over a normal scalp makes the diagnosis clear, especially if there is a positive family history.

Differential Diagnosis

- Alopecia areata (hair loss occurs rapidly rather than gradually) (see Figure 8-1)
- Traction alopecia from styling aids or hair style (thinning occurs in areas of greatest traction)

ANDROGENETIC ALOPECIA

- Is a common condition in genetically predisposed individuals
- Cannot be cured but can be treated cosmetically through topical, oral, and/or surgical methods
- May necessitate psychologic reassurance and support

- Telogen effluvium (hair loss occurs in a diffuse pattern over the entire scalp)

Treatment

In most cases the disorder follows its genetically programmed course and therapy is not effective to a satisfactory degree.

Nonpharmacologic

Hair transplantation from occipital and parietal regions to the bald areas, with or without scalp reduction, is effective but may require repeated procedures to maintain coverage as the balding progresses. Treatment is also quite expensive.

Pharmacologic

Topical Agents
Minoxidil topical solution (Rogaine) stimulates the growth of vellus, as well as terminal hairs. Additionally it increases the diameter of hairs in the androgen (growth) phase and prevents hairs from entering the telogen (resting) phase. A 2% concentration is applied in 1-ml doses bid to the scalp. A 5% solution shows increased efficacy. **Progesterone 4% lotion** applied bid and usually combined with monthly intradermal injections of **triamcinolone acetonide (Kenalog),** 2.5 to 10 mg/ml with injection of just enough solution to blanch the skin, may slow the loss of hair. **Nicotinic acid topical solution** applied qhs may be helpful in up to 75% of patients, to prevent further hair loss.

Systemic Agents
Spironolactone (Aldactone) 25 to 50 mg PO bid is an androgen antagonist and a blocker of peripheral androgen receptors. It may be helpful in up to 85% of young women with severe baldness who have normal menstrual cycles. Results may not be evident for 9 months, however. Patients should be informed that doses of 100 mg per day may cause irregular menses. Additionally the drug has been shown to cause tumors when administered in toxic doses to rats and should therefore be avoided in patients with a positive family history of breast cancer. Intermittent evaluation of electrolytes should also occur, since it is a potassium-sparing diuretic.
Finasteride (Propecia) 1 mg PO qd taken by men with mild to moderate hair loss in the vertex and anterior midscalp maintained the hair count in 83% of study patients and regrew hair in 66%. Stopping treatment leads to gradual reversal of the beneficial

effects. Continued treatment is unlikely to be of benefit if the drug has not worked within 12 months.

Cimetidine (Tagamet) 300 mg PO five times daily acts as a peripheral androgen blocking agent. Hair regrowth is noted within 10 to 18 weeks in up to 70% of women.

An alternative approach to blocking androgen production in women may be the administration of oral contraceptives with relatively high levels of estrogen and low androgenic potential **(Demulen, Desogen, Ortho Tri-Cyclen).**

Indications for Referral

- For diffuse hair thinning in females, accompanied by the development of male characteristics and elevated total testosterone and DHEAS levels, the patient should be referred to an endocrinologist.
- Women being treated by hormonal adjustment should be followed concomitantly by a gynecologist.

Telogen Effluvium

Overview

Pathophysiology

Scalp hair goes through repetitive cycles throughout the life of an individual. The growth phase is called *anagen* and is followed by a brief transitional phase called *catagen*, which in turn is followed by a resting or *telogen* phase. At the end of telogen the hair is shed and replaced by a new hair in the anagen phase, thus completing the cycle. Approximately 90% of hairs are in the anagen phase at any one time, 1% in catagen, and the remaining 9% in telogen. Anything that upsets this delicate balance can cause an increase in the number of hairs lost daily, a pathologic state called *telogen effluvium*, literally a "flood of resting hairs." Causes include acute or chronic illnesses, emotional stress, surgery, childbirth, rapid weight loss, poor diet, hepatitis, febrile illness, iron deficiency, and thyroid abnormalities. Various medications, including beta blockers, allopurinol, warfarin, heparin, gold, retinoids, vitamin A, and birth control pills, should also be considered potential causative agents. Characteristically the inciting event occurs 6 weeks to 4 months before the first noticeable loss of hair. It is common for the loss to continue for 2 to 5 months.

Epidemiology

No sexual preponderance has been identified, but those persons experiencing any of the stressors mentioned are at higher risk of development of the disorder.

Assessment

Clinical Presentation

The only symptom is *diffuse* shedding of hairs at a daily rate much above the normal rate of 50 to 100 hairs per day. Loss of over 30% of the total number of hairs rarely occurs. (Over 25,000 hairs, approximately 25% of the total number, need to be shed before unmistakable thinning is apparent.) Bitemporal recession is common. The scalp appears normal. An examination of the shed hairs will reveal a greater than normal percentage of hairs in the telogen phase (greater than 25%). Telogen hairs are characterized by a bulbous, nonpigmented tip (club-shaped, like a Q-tip), whereas hairs in the anagen phase have a tapered tip that is darkly pigmented.

Diagnostics

- A thorough history may reveal an emotional or physical "trauma" that occurred 6 weeks to 4 months before the noticeable hair loss.
- The patient should be asked to collect and count all shed hairs for 3 consecutive days, and the counts should be greater than 100 hairs per day for telogen effluvium to be considered.
- An evaluation of the telogen/anagen ratio may prove beneficial. If under microscopic evaluation more than 25% of the hairs are in telogen (bulbous, nonpigmented tip), then telogen effluvium is suggested.
- Thyroid-stimulating hormone (TSH) level, complete blood count, serum iron level, and total iron-binding capacity are indicated to rule out other systemic causes.

Differential Diagnosis

- Alopecia areata (very rapid onset) (see Figure 8-1)
- Acute syphilitic alopecia (patchy hair loss)
- Drug-induced alopecia (almost all lost hairs are in the anagen phase)

TELOGEN EFFLUVIUM

- Will resolve spontaneously when the causative stress is identified and eliminated
- Requires psychologic support and reassurance that the patient will not become bald and that the thinning of hair is temporary

Treatment

Nonpharmacologic

Unless the causative stress continues, spontaneous and complete regrowth takes place within 6 months. Emotional support is often necessary.

Pharmacologic

Topical Agents

Minoxidil topical solution (Rogaine) will promote more rapid hair regrowth and stabilize or minimize further hair loss. A 2% concentration is applied in 1-ml doses bid to the scalp. A 5% solution shows increased efficacy.

Indications for Referral

- None is indicated.

Trichotillomania

Overview

Pathophysiology

Trichotillomania is a form of alopecia caused by an uncontrollable urge to pull out one's own hair. In adults it is usually the manifestation of a psychologic disorder or an unconscious habit.

Epidemiology

The disorder is most common in children, as a manifestation of stress.

Assessment

Clinical Presentation

Trichotillomania presents with single or multiple patches of alopecia in which normal hairs are interspersed among short, broken hairs. The scalp is usually normal. The frontal, parietal, and temporal areas of the scalp are most commonly involved. If the patient is right-handed, more alopecia may be detected on the right side of the scalp than on the left, and vice versa. The condition continues until the causative abnormality is corrected. With chronic trichotillomania the follicles may become permanently damaged, resulting in permanent hair loss.

Diagnostics

- The diagnosis is made clinically and can be confirmed by protecting the head from further trauma. Such action will result in normal regrowth of hair if the diagnosis is correct.

- A fungal culture should be performed if there is any concern as to the presence of tinea capitis.

Differential Diagnosis
- Alopecia areata (affected areas have complete hair loss without any broken hairs) (see Figure 8-1)
- Tinea capitis (scalp itself may be scaling, inflamed, and/or characterized by broken-off hairs) (see Figure 3-9, *A*)

Treatment

Removal of the causative disorder will correct the condition. Psychologic intervention may be indicated.

| Indications for Referral |

- In adults with uncontrollable and severe trichotillomania referral to a psychologist or psychiatrist may be appropriate.

TRICHOTILLOMANIA

- Will persist until the psychologic abnormality is corrected
- May result in permanently damaged hair follicles
- Is best treated through psychologic intervention

Nail Disorders

Figure 9-1 **INGROWN TOENAIL**

Swelling, inflammation, and exudate occur at the medial fold of the great toe.

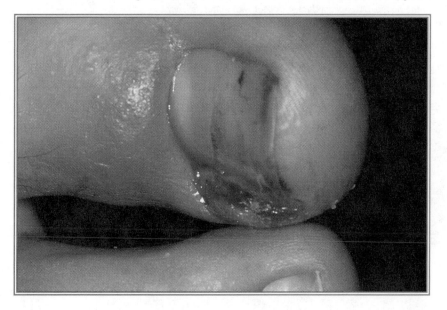

Figure 9-2 **LICHEN PLANUS OF THE NAIL**

Ridging of the distal aspect of the nail occurs in conjunction with an accentuated widening and separation from the nail bed.

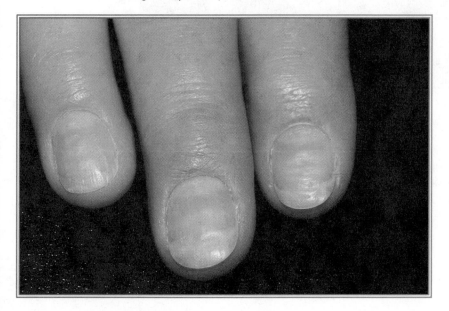

Figure 9-3 Nail Manifestations of Internal Disease

A, Melanoma: Linear pigmentation of the full thickness of the nail, with some pigmentation extending to the nail fold. **B,** Koilonychia: In patient with iron deficiency thin nails that curl upward.

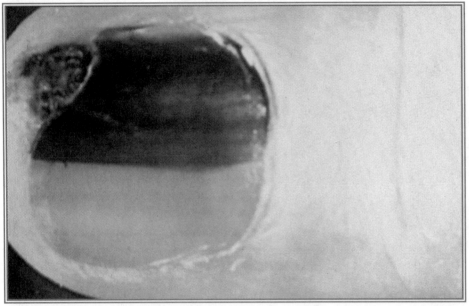

A

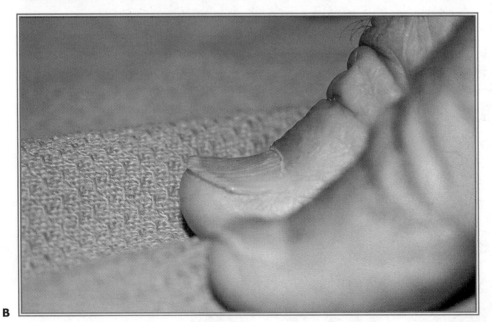

B

Figure 9-3   **NAIL MANIFESTATIONS OF INTERNAL DISEASE**

C, Bronchitis and bronchiectasis: Yellow nail syndrome apparent in a 64-year-old male with a 2-year history of bronchitis. Nails cleared after pulmonary symptoms were treated. *D,* Finger clubbing: Distal phalanges are enlarged and rounded; angle between the nail and the proximal nail fold increases; nail enlarges and curves downward.

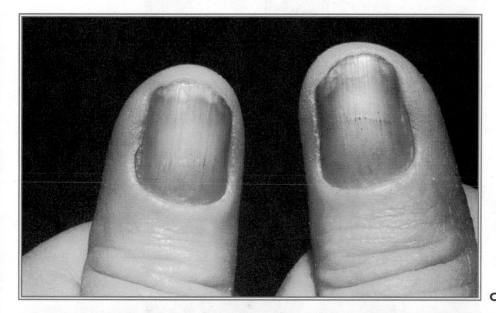

C

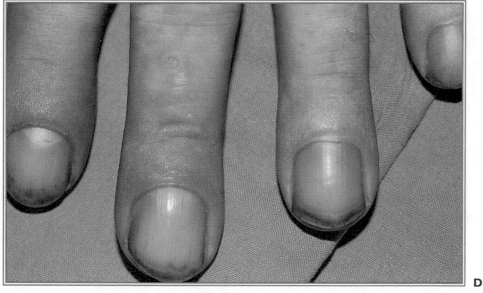

D

continued

Figure 9-3   **NAIL MANIFESTATIONS OF INTERNAL DISEASE**

E, Beau's lines: All nails show a linear white line associated with exacerbation of Raynaud's phenomenon, which occurred approximately 2 months previously. *F,* Terry's nails: Note white nail bed with only a narrow zone of pink at the distal end.

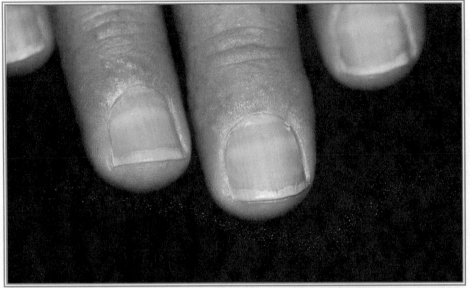

E

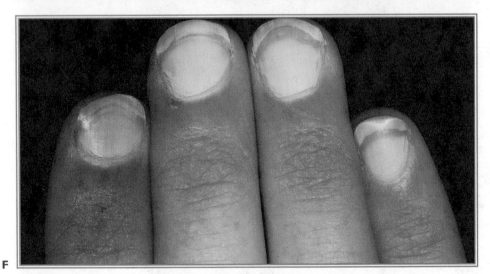

F

(**F,** From Habif TP: *Clinical dermatology,* ed 3, St Louis, 1996, Mosby.)

Figure 9-4 NAIL TRAUMA

*A, Onycholysis: Shortly after skiing in uncomfortably tight ski boots, this patient noticed multiple pigmented lesions on the nails, consistent with trauma. **B,** Nail biting: Several nails have been bitten almost as far as the lunula. Note distal finger inflammation caused by strips of skin that have been peeled away.*

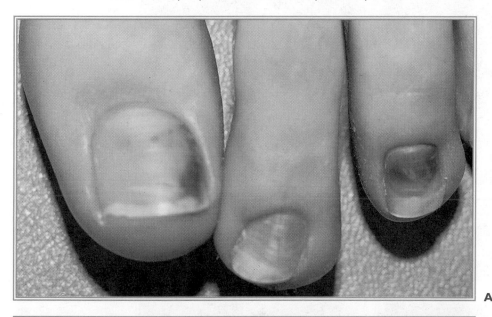

A

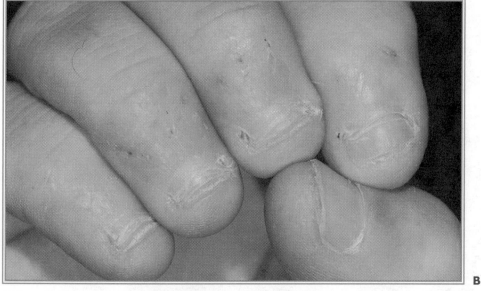

B

(**B through G,** From Habif TP: *Clinical dermatology*, ed 3, St Louis, 1996, Mosby.) *continued*

Figure 9-4   NAIL TRAUMA

C, Hematoma: The blood or dark discoloration may remain under the nail plate until it grows out. *D,* White spots: Spots may resolve or grow out with the nail.

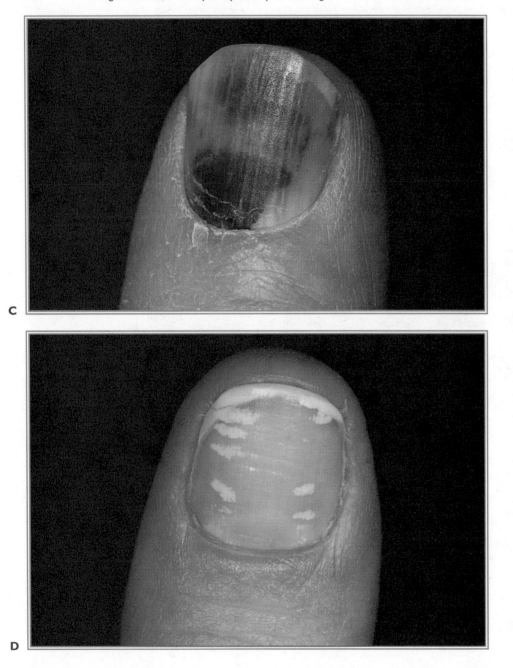

Figure 9-4 **NAIL TRAUMA**

E, Brittle nails: The distal nail plate splits, causing the remaining nail to become dry and brittle. **F,** Habit-tic deformity: the medial thumb nail is deformed due to constant picking of the proximal nail fold with another finger.

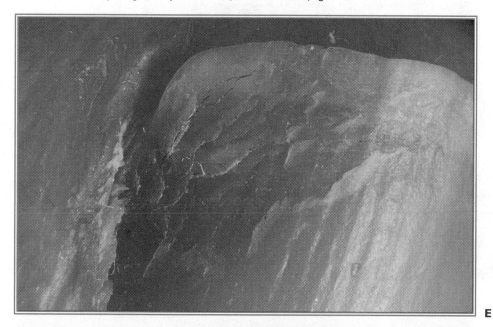

E

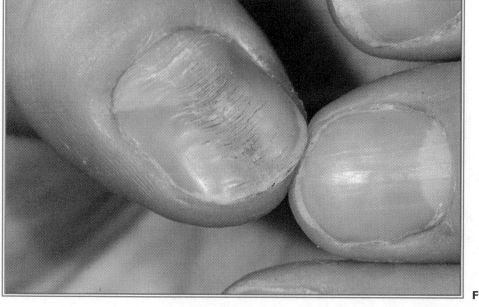

F

continued

Figure 9-4 NAIL TRAUMA

G, *Pincer nails: Over-curvature of the lateral edges of the nail results in a pincer-shaped deformity.*

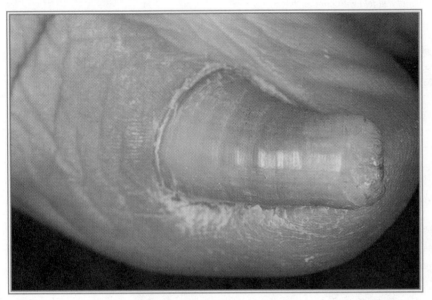

G

Figure 9-5 ONYCHOMYCOSIS

White superficial onychomycosis of the right great toe and both second toes. Subungual onychomycosis involves the lateral nail plate of the left great toe.

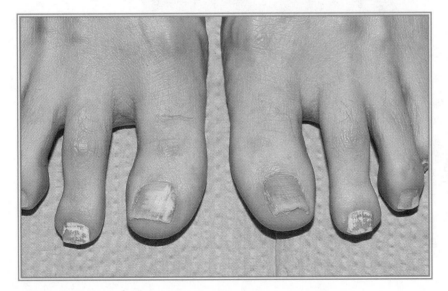

Figure 9-6   PARONYCHIA

Erythema and purulent material at the proximal nail fold.

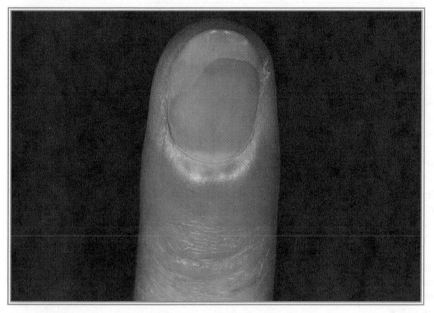

(From Habif TP: *Clinical dermatology*, ed 3, St Louis, 1996, Mosby.)

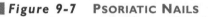

Figure 9-7   **PSORIATIC NAILS**

Yellowish nail with multiple pits in a patient with psoriasis.

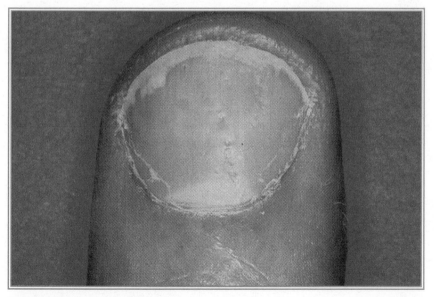

(Courtesy of Stacy R. Smith, MD.)

Table 9-1

Differential Diagnosis of Nail Disorders

Disorder	Text	Keys to Diagnosis
Ingrown toenail	Ch. 9, p. 377 (Figure 9-1)	Pain, erythema, swelling, and pus formation
Lichen planus of the nail	(Figure 9-2)	Longitudinal ridges and adhesion of the proximal nail fold to the nail may occur; nail may become thin or absent
Nail manifestations of internal disease	Ch. 9, p. 378 (Figure 9-3)	*Beau's lines:* transverse depression on all of internal nails; *yellow nail syndrome:* nail yellow, curved, and ridged; *spoon nails:* elevation of lateral edges; *clubbed fingers:* distal phalanges enlarged, nail thickened and curving downward; *Terry's nails:* normal-colored band at distal edge; elsewhere nail white or light pink
Nail trauma	Ch. 9, p. 380 (Figure 9-4)	*Onycholysis:* distal portion of nail opaque white, yellow, or black; *nail biting:* nails excessively short with surrounding skin usually inflamed or cracked; *subungual hematoma:* dark discoloration under nail that grows out as nail grows; *white spots:* spots at the lunula, which may remain or grow out with the nail; *brittle nails:* distal portion of the nail split into layers and peeling; *habit-tic deformity:* series of horizontal grooves along medial portion of nail; *pincer nails:* lateral edges that curve in and under
Onychomycosis	Ch. 9, p. 383 (Figure 9-5)	Nail becomes brown, then thickens, and separates from bed with debris between nail and nail bed
Paronychia	Ch. 9, p. 386 (Figure 9-6)	Nail fold red, edematous, and tender; a bead of pus may be expressed from one corner or from the cuticle
Psoriatic nails	Ch. 9, p. 388 (Figure 9-7)	Pitting, white or yellow discoloration, malformation of nails, and splinter hemorrhages evident

Ingrown Toenail

Overview

Pathophysiology

Penetration by the nail plate into the lateral nail fold and on into the dermis causes a foreign body reaction. The condition is frequently caused by poorly fitting shoes (causing compression of the toe from the side), improper nail trimming, or trauma.

Epidemiology

Ingrown toenail is common, and the lateral aspect of the great toe is the most commonly affected.

Assessment

Clinical Presentation

Pain, erythema, swelling, and pus formation (resulting from subsequent infection with bacteria, fungi, or yeast) are evident (see Figure 9-1). Eventually granulation tissue develops.

Diagnostics

- Diagnosis is based on clinical presentation.

Differential Diagnosis

- Nail trauma (no evidence of paronychia, but a positive history of trauma) (see Figure 9-4)
- Paronychia (nail not involved) (see Figure 9-6)

INGROWN TOENAIL

- Is frequently caused by improperly fitting shoes or improperly trimmed nails
- Can be discouraged by trimming nails straight across and by wearing footwear that fits properly and is sufficiently wide that it does not crowd toes

Treatment

Nonpharmacologic

Prevention consists of trimming the nails straight across and wearing properly fitting wide, pliable footwear. Because it is a mechanical problem, treatment consists of removal of the affected nail plate with destruction of the associated nail matrix. The lateral nail fold is infiltrated with 2% **lidocaine (Xylocaine).** Nail-splitting scissors are inserted under the ingrown nail, parallel to the lateral nail fold, and a wedge-shaped portion of nail is cut and removed. The nail matrix proximal to the ingrown nail is then excised, vaporized with a CO_2 laser, or chemically destroyed. Soaks with cool **Burow's solution** several times a day are soothing for a few days after treatment.

Pharmacologic

Topical Agents
None is indicated.

Systemic Agents
Antibiotics will treat the infection caused by the foreign body reaction. **Dicloxacillin** 250 mg PO qid usually provides appropriate therapy. If a penicillin allergy exists, **erythromycin** 250 mg PO qid may be substituted.

Indications for Referral

- Referral to a dermatologist may be appropriate for avulsion of all or part of the nail in addition to destruction of the lateral nail matrix.

Nail Manifestations of Internal Disease

Overview

Pathophysiology
Melanoma: The tumor metastasizes aggressively.

Beau's lines: The disorder is caused by any stressful event that interupts normal nail formation and growth, such as severe illness, including peripheral vascular disease, zinc deficiency, or disorders that cause high fevers.

Yellow nail syndrome: Diseases reported to be associated with this disorder are lower extremity or facial edema and respiratory tract disorders including pleural effusion, bronchiectasis, sinusitis, bronchitis, and chronic respiratory infections. It has also been reported in some cases of patients with acquired immunodeficiency syndrome (AIDS).

Spoon nails: Spoon nails may be a variation of normal and appear in healthy children. A spontaneous onset of spoon nails has been reported to occur in patients with iron deficiency anemia, hemochromatosis, and polycythemia vera.

Clubbed fingers: Clubbing may be a normal variant or be associated with a number of diseases, including lung, cardiovascular, or thyroid disease; cirrhosis; and colitis.

Terry's nails: Frequently associated with cirrhosis, chronic congestive heart failure, adult-onset diabetes mellitus, and age.

Epidemiology

Melanoma: Melanoma occurs most frequently in blacks and Asians.

Beau's lines: The disorder may occur in anyone at any age, several weeks after a stressful event.

Yellow nail syndrome: The syndrome occurs predominantly before, during, or after certain respiratory diseases or dseases associated with lymphedema as listed.

Spoon nails: The abnormality may occur naturally or in association with disorders as described above.

Clubbed fingers: Clubbing may be a normal variant or occur in conjunction with diseases, as described. There does not appear to be a correlation with hypoalbuminemia or anemia.

Terry's nails: The disorder occurs in association with various systemic illnesses, as described.

Assessment

Clinical Presentation

Melanoma (see Figure 9-3, *A*): A pigmented longitudinal band, originating in the proximal nail fold (Hutchinson's sign), suggests melanoma. It must be differentiated from pigmented bands that are a normal variation in the majority of blacks.

Beau's lines (see Figure 9-3, *E*): A transverse depression on the surface of all nails, which progresses distally with normal nail growth and eventually disappears without permanent abnormality.

Yellow nail syndrome (see Figure 9-3, *C*): Patients report a spontaneous appearance of yellow nails, accompanied by a definite slowing of normal nail growth. The nail plate may become excessively curved and the surface ridged with transverse delineations. Partial and in some cases total separation of the nail plate may occur.

Spoon nail (see Figure 9-3, *B*): Elevation of the lateral edges accompanied by depression of the central portion results in the appearance of a spoon-shaped nail.

Clubbed finger (see Figure 9-3, *D*): The distal phalanges of the fingers and toes enlarge to form a bulbous shape. The nail enlarges, curves downward, and thickens. The angle between the proximal nail fold and the nail plate flattens.

Terry's nails (see Figure 9-3, *F*): Nails appear white or light pink except at a thin, normal-colored band at the distal edge.

Diagnostics

- Diagnosis is made on the basis of history and clinical presentation.

Differential Diagnosis
- Self-induced trauma (elicited by careful history)
- Nail pigmentation from nail polish (elicited by careful history)

Treatment

There is no specific treatment other than that of the underlying disease. In most cases the nails spontaneously improve when the associated disease resolves. The changes associated with clubbed fingers are permanent, even after correction of the underlying disease.

Indications for Referral

- Because the presence of dark longitudinal bands extending from the proximal nail fold to the distal edge may indicate melanoma, the patient should be referred to a dermatologist for further investigation.

Nail Trauma

Overview

Pathophysiology
Onycholysis: Asymptomatic separation of the nail plate from the nail bed. Causes include psoriasis, trauma (usually resulting from long nails striking objects in the course of daily activities and being "lifted" off the nail bed), fungal infections, prolonged immersion in water, and allergic contact dermatitis in response to nail products.

Nail biting: A habit usually resulting from nervousness.

Subungual hematoma: Caused by trauma to the nail, finger, or toe.

Brittle nails: Splitting or peeling of the distal portion of the nail plate, usually caused by continual or prolonged immersion in water. Some patients appear to have a genetic predisposition; the condition may be associated with dry skin.

Habit-tic deformity: Caused by the continual biting or picking of the proximal nail fold by another finger.

Pincer nails: Compression of both sides of a toenail that results from tight-fitting shoes is thought to be the most common cause; the exact cause is unknown.

NAIL MANIFESTATIONS OF INTERNAL DISEASE

• The underlying systemic disorder (precipitating factor) must be corrected in order for the nail disorder to resolve

White spots (leukonychia punctata): Results from manipulation of the cuticle or other forms of mild trauma such as overzealous manicuring.

Epidemiology

Onycholysis: Usually seen in women with long fingernails, or in the absence of other skin diseases.

Nail biting: Usually begins in childhood but may persist into adulthood or until the drive for aesthetically pleasing nails overpowers the habit. It is frequently exacerbated during periods of physical inactivity.

Subungual hematoma: May occur in anyone at any age, but is most frequent in persons involved in manual labor, either as a vocation or as a hobby.

White spots: A common finding in those who treat their hands and nails roughly.

Brittle nails: A normal variant in about 20% of the adult population.

Habit-tic deformity: A common finding, occurring most often as a nervous habit similar to nail biting. Patients are usually not aware that they are the cause of the deformity.

Pincer nails: Toe nails are most commonly involved. The condition is most prevalent in women who wear pointed-toe shoes and/or high heels that squeeze the toes together.

Assessment

Clinical Presentation

Onycholysis (see Figure 9-4, *A*): The distal portion of the nail, which is lifted from the nail bed, becomes an opaque white or yellow. A green tinge that represents either the primary cause of onycholysis (fungal infection) or a secondary fungal infection resulting from the separation of nail from plate allowing the entrance of pathogens, may be present.

Nail biting (see Figure 9-4, *B*): One or all of the nails may be affected. Occasionally the nails are bitten down as far as the lunula (crescent-shaped white area at proximal edge of nail). Strips of skin on the lateral and proximal edges of the nails may be peeled away, leaving inflamed or bleeding skin.

Subungual hematoma (see Figure 9-4, *C*): Hematoma is usually caused by trauma to the nail that causes bleeding and bruising. The quantity of bleeding may be sufficient to cause a separation of the nail plate. The blood or dark discoloration may remain under the nail plate until it grows out.

White spots (see Figure 9-4, *D*): Spots occur at the lunula or arise spontaneously anywhere. They may resolve or grow out with the nail.

Brittle nails (see Figure 9-4, *E*): The process appears similar to the scaling of dry skin, as the distal portion of the nail splits into layers and peels away.

Habit-tic deformity (see Figure 9-4, *F*): A series of horizontal grooves or depressions grow out along the median portion of the nail plate, extending from the proximal nail fold to the distal tip. There may be a concomitant yellowish discoloration.

Pincer nails (see Figure 9-4, *G*): The lateral edges of the nail curve in and under, resulting in a tubelike or pincerlike appearance.

Diagnostics

- Diagnosis is made on the basis of history and clinical presentation.

Differential Diagnosis

- Onychomycosis (positive culture or KOH result) (see Figure 9-5)
- Chronic paronychia or chronic eczematous inflammation of the proximal nail fold (smooth rippling of the medial portion of the nail) (see Figure 9-6)

Treatment

Nonpharmacologic

Onycholysis: All of the separated nail is removed. Fingers should be kept dry to discourage secondary infection. Manicures should be gentle or omitted.

Nail biting: The desire to stop biting is the only cure.

Subungual hematoma: Avoidance or prevention of trauma is obviously the most effective treatment. Puncturing the nail to relieve accumulated blood is effective treatment.

White spots: Prevention of trauma and patience while the nail grows out are needed.

Brittle nails: Wearing gloves while hands are immersed in water is excellent protection and prevention. Daily or bid massaging of heavy lubricants or oils into the nail and surrounding skin produces improvement.

Habit-tic deformity: Awareness of the cause and a strong desire to stop are the only cures.

NAIL TRAUMA

- Can be prevented by gentle manipulation of nails and cuticles during manicures and use of gloves as necessary to protect nails and prevent trauma
- Can be minimized by using moisturizing oils to keep nails and surrounding skin supple rather than brittle, and therefore better able to withstand the effects of the environment

Pincer nails: Properly fitting shoes are essential, especially those with flat heels and rounded toes. If pain is significant, surgical removal of the nail may be a viable option.

Pharmacologic

Topical Agents
Chemical preparations that are painted on the nails and produce a bitter taste are helpful reminders to the patient who unconsciously bites nails.

Systemic Agents
None is indicated.

Indications for Referral

- Referral to a psychiatrist may be appropriate in cases in which nervousness or another psychologic aberration is prolonging the resolution of the nail deformity.
- Referral to a dermatologist for nail avulsion is appropriate when more conservative methods of treatment are unsuccessful.

Onychomycosis (Tinea Unguium)

Overview

Pathophysiology
Onychomycosis represents 30% to 50% of all nail disorders. It is a common fungal infection of the nails that occurs to some extent in 90% of all elderly people. *Trichophyton rubrum* and *Trichophyton mentagrophytes* are the two most common dermatophytes that infect the nails. *T. rubrum* is associated with deep infections and occurs most commonly on the fingernails. *T. mentagrophytes* is usually superficial and remains localized to one portion of the nail.

Epidemiology
The disorder is common in adults but rare in children except when a parent has a *T. rubrum* infection. It is commonly associated with tinea pedis.

Assessment

Clinical Presentation

At first a brownish discoloration occurs at the edge of the distal nail or along the lateral edge and spreads to the entire nail. The nail becomes thickened, separates from its bed, crumbles, and develops characteristic white diffuse or speckled patches (see Figure 9-5). The paronychium is usually not affected. It is unusual for all 10 nails to be affected simultaneously. The condition itself is usually asymptomatic.

There are four patterns of nail infection:

1. *Distal subungual onychomycosis:* In this most common presentation the distal nail plate turns yellow or white and begins to lift off the nail bed, as a result of an accumulation of debris under the nail.

2. *White superficial onychomycosis:* The surface of the nail plate is invaded by *T. mentagrophytes,* leaving it soft and powdery.

3. *Proximal subungual onychomycosis:* Fungi invade the cuticle area and spread to the nail bed from below, leaving the surface of the nail intact. As hyperkeratotic debris begins to accumulate, the nail plate separates from the nail bed, leaving transverse white bands that grow distally within the nail.

4. *Candida onychomycosis:* Seen primarily in patients with chronic mucocutaneous candidiasis, this disorder is caused by *Candida albicans* and usually involves all 10 fingernails. The nail plate thickens and becomes yellow-brown.

Diagnostics

- A KOH examination of subungual debris may show hyphae. If the result is negative, a sample of the nail itself should be tested.
- A fungal culture will confirm the diagnosis, although less than 50% of clinically suspected cases are culture-positive.

Differential Diagnosis

- Psoriasis (usually has evidence of psoriatic lesions elsewhere on the body) (see Figure 9-7)
- Lichen planus (longitudinal grooving and ridging, and adhesion of the proximal nail fold to the matrix [pterygium], resulting in a thinned or absent nail plate) (see Figure 9-2)
- Trauma (usually history of a sports or related injury) (see Figure 9-4, *A*)
- Defective peripheral circulation (other symptoms of peripheral vascular disorders usually also present, such as clubbing and cyanosis of the extremities, venous or arterial insufficiency)

ONYCHOMYCOSIS

- Is better prevented than treated; prevention is key

- May become a chronic or frequent problem in the presence of artificial nails; if so, the nails should be removed

- Although treatable, it permanently damages the nail; affected nail will not repair but must grow out and be replaced by healthy nail

- May remain visible without obvious signs of improvement for weeks to months after treatment

- Nail dystrophy caused by eczema (no crumbling of the nail plate and no subungual debris)

Treatment

The cure rate for toenails is 75% and for fingernails is virtually 100% with use of newer systemic antifungal agents. Topical therapy is usually ineffective. Patients should be told that improvement may not be noted for 6 to 8 months as the destroyed nail must grow out; it will not "clear."

Nonpharmacologic

Prevention is most effective. Patients with frequent fungal infections of the nails should be cautioned against the use of artificial nails. Nails should be kept short so as not to catch and "lift," allowing organisms to penetrate under the nail plate.

Pharmacologic

Topical Agents

Topical therapy is frequently less effective than systemic therapy because of the difficulty of applying the medication directly to the fungus (i.e., under the nail). Topical lotions and creams do not penetrate the nail plate. Nevertheless, if patients are not good candidates for systemic therapy or prefer a more conservative approach, antifungal lotions may be dripped under the nail plate bid. After nail avulsion treatment with topical agents is more likely to be successful. Medications include **ciclopirox (Loprox)** lotion and **Exelderm** solution, both massaged gently into the affected area bid. Improvement should be noticed within 4 weeks.

Systemic Agents

Terbinafine (Lamisil) 250 mg PO qd, taken 6 weeks for fingernail infection and 12 weeks for toenail infection, is an effective treatment. Pulsed therapy with **itraconazole (Sporanox)** 200 mg bid 1 week per month for 2 months for fingernails, 3 to 4 months for toenails, is an alternative. **Ketoconazole (Nizoral)** 200 mg PO qd for 1 month past complete clearing of the nails is successful in 75% of patients who fail griseofulvin therapy; **Griseofulvin Ultramicrosize (Gris-PEG)** 250 to 500 mg PO qd for 6 months (fingernails) to 18 months (toenails) is an alternative but is usually ineffective.

⬢ Indications for Referral

- Refer to dermatologist for nail avulsion when more conservative approaches are unsuccessful.
- If avulsion is not an option, a cream compounded by the pharmacist consisting of **40% urea, 40% white petrolatum, 15% lanolin, and 5% beeswax** in a volume of 60 g applied under occlusion to the nails qhs until the dystrophic nail falls off (5 to 10 days), is an option. This procedure may be quite painful if significant inflammation of the surrounding skin occurs.

Paronychia

Overview

Pathophysiology
Paronychia is an inflammation of the nail fold that may be either acute (caused by *Staphylococcus aureus*) or chronic (caused by *Candida albicans*) and usually is the result of improper manicuring. Loss of the cuticle allows the space between the posterior nail fold and nail plate to become colonized with pathogens. Foreign material passes through the epidermis of the nail fold and acts as a foreign body to set up a chronic inflammation in the adjacent dermis.

Epidemiology
Paronychia is the most common nail complaint seen in a medical office. Persons whose hands are cold or frequently in water are at greatest risk. The disorder may occur at any age but usually occurs between ages 30 and 60. It is also common in diabetics. Occasionally children who are thumb-suckers may be affected.

Assessment

Clinical Presentation
Initially the cuticle is lost from all or part of the nail. The nail fold becomes red, edematous, and tender. A small bead of pus (frequently containing *Candida* spp.) may be expressed from one corner of the nail fold (see Figure 9-6). Edges of the nail plate may become irregular and discolored, and the nail may appear smaller as a

result of the surrounding edema. The infection often remains confined to one or two fingers.

Diagnostics
- Culture of pus or of scrapings from the underside of the nail will help determine pathogen sensitivities if the condition is unresponsive to therapy.
- KOH of pus will demonstrate hyphae.

Differential Diagnosis
- Onychomycosis (the nail itself is involved, rather than the nail fold) (see Figure 9-5)
- Psoriasis (nail pitting, onycholysis, discoloration, subungual thickening, and nail plate alterations are evident) (see Figure 9-7)
- Dermatitis (inflammation is usually not limited to only one or two nail folds)

Treatment

Nonpharmacologic
Patients should be encouraged to keep hands as dry as possible, although soaking the affected digit(s) for 20 minutes in warm water tid may be soothing and promotes drainage of pus. Gloves should be worn for wet work. Incision and drainage may be necessary if an abscess is present.

Pharmacologic

Topical Agents
Clotrimazole (Lotrimin) 1% lotion or cream applied bid is a conservative initial treatment option. If it is ineffective, other antifungals **(ciclopirox [Loprox], oxiconazole [Oxistat], econazole [Spectazole])** should be tried. A solution of **3% thymol in 95% ethanol,** compounded by a pharmacist, may be applied to the affected area tid if antifungal creams fail.

Systemic Agents
In the early stages of paronychia with erythema and discomfort, **dicloxacillin** 250 mg PO qid or **cephalexin (Keflex, Duricef)** 500 mg bid is first-line therapy. **Erythromycin** 333 mg PO tid is an alternative. A 1-week course of oral antifungals **(ketoconazole [Nizoral] or terbinafine [Lamisil])** may be considered for recalcitrant cases. Single-dose therapy with **fluconazole (Diflucan)** 400 mg PO is also effective.

PARONYCHIA

• Can be minimized by careful manicures and by a conscious effort to keep hands as dry as possible

---

✦ | Indications for Referral |

> • Consultation with a dermatologist is appropriate if there is concern about hepatotoxicity either before or during oral antifungal therapy.

Psoriatic Nails

Overview

Pathophysiology

Psoriasis affects nails in a similar fashion to the way it affects skin: part of the nail is shed more rapidly than other parts, leading to pitting, thickening, and discoloration.

Epidemiology

Nail involvement in the patient with psoriasis occurs in 10% to 50% of cases. It may occur with or without signs of skin disorder.

Assessment

Clinical Presentation

The most common characteristic of psoriatic nails is **pitting,** or sharp, ice-pick depressions in the nail plate (see Figure 9-7). Onycholysis, or separation of the nail plate from the nail bed, is also common. It begins at the distal edge and moves proximally, appearing as an opaque **white or yellow discoloration.** All or several nails may be involved. If psoriasis occurs in the hyponychium (distal portion of the undersurface of the nail bed), yellow debris may accumulate, elevating the nail plate and mimicking onychomycosis. Severe psoriasis of the nail bed results in **malformed nails** and **splinter hemorrhages** (longitudinal streaks of blood under the nail plate caused by the rupture of small blood vessels in the nail bed).

Diagnostics

• Culture of underlying debris, nail scrapings, or fragments is taken to rule out onychomycosis.

Differential Diagnosis

• Onychomycosis (positive culture or KOH result) (see Figure 9-5)
• Trauma (negative culture or KOH result, history of trauma to nails, or presence of long nails) (see Figure 9-4)

PSORIATIC NAILS

• Are a chronic condition for which there is no cure
• May occur even without signs of a psoriatic skin disorder

Treatment

Nonpharmacologic
None is indicated

Pharmacologic

Topical Agents
None is indicated.

Systemic Agents
Intralesional injections of **triamcinolone acetonide (Kenalog)** 2.5 to 5 mg/ml with a 30-gauge needle is painful but produces the most satisfactory results. Treatments are repeated every 3 to 4 weeks.

Indications for Referral

- Consultation with a dermatologist for severe or recalcitrant psoriasis.

Ulcers

Figure 10-1   CHANCRE

Well-demarcated primary chancre with clean base.

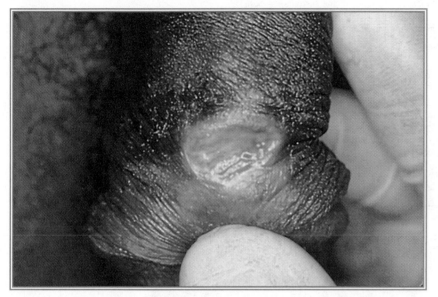

(From Goldstein BG, Goldstein AO: *Practical dermatology,* ed 2, St Louis, 1997, Mosby.)

Figure 10-2   DECUBITUS ULCER

A pressure sore in a typical location (tailbone) that developed after a CVA.

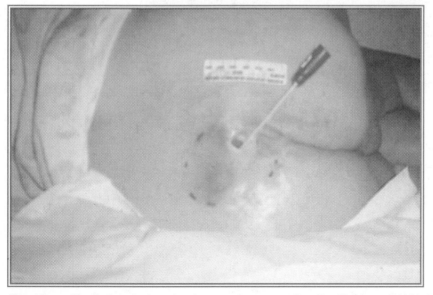

(From Morison M, and others: *A color guide to the nursing management of wounds,* ed 2, St Louis, 1998, Mosby.)

Figure 10-3 **ISCHEMIC ULCER (ARTERIAL INSUFFICIENCY)**

Arterial ulcer in a typical dorsal foot site. Note punched-out appearance of lesion. There is no pigmentation or dermatitis of the surrounding skin.

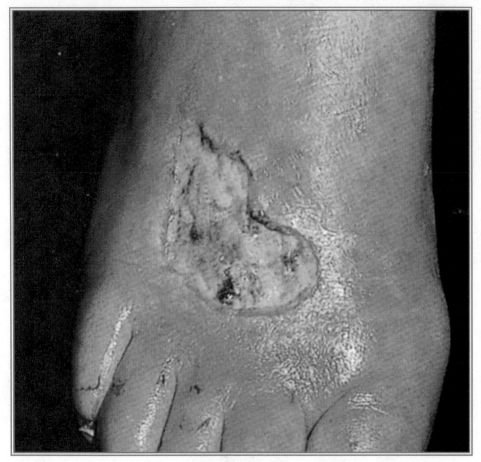

(From Cox N, Lawrence C: *Diagnostic problems in dermatology,* St Louis, 1998, Mosby.)

Figure 10-4 SQUAMOUS CELL CARCINOMA

Firm elevated mass with central crust, occurring on sun-damaged skin of the lower lip.

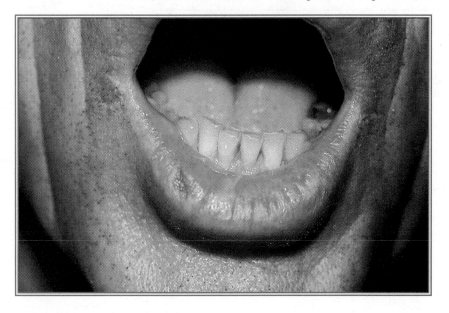

Figure 10-5 VENOUS STASIS ULCER

Ulceration within a diffuse area of erythematous, thickened skin in a woman with venous insufficiency

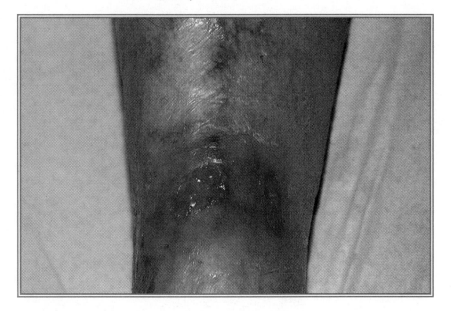

▌ *Table 10-1*

Differential Diagnosis of Ulcers

DISORDER	TEXT	KEYS TO DIAGNOSIS
Chancre (primary syphilis)	Ch. 10, p. 395 (Figure 10-1)	Base of the lesion is clean and smooth; edges are raised and well circumscribed; usually occurs in genital region or on lips
Decubitus ulcer	Ch. 10, p. 397 (Figure 10-2)	Occurs over pressure points and bony prominences, usually in elderly, debilitated, and/or bedridden patients
Ischemic ulcer (arterial insufficiency)	Ch.10, p. 399 (Figure 10-3)	Occurs on lateral aspect of lower extremities; history of arteriosclerosis or chronic hypertension
Squamous cell carcinoma	Ch. 5, p. 260 (Figure 10-4)	Firm skin-colored or reddish-brown nodule on sun-damaged skin; ulceration, scaling, and crusting frequently present
Venous stasis ulcer	Ch. 10, p. 401 (Figure 10-5)	Usually occurs on the medial aspect of lower extremities; rolled borders, cobblestone appearance; history of venous incompetence, varicose veins, congestive heart failure

Chancre (Primary Syphilis)

Overview

Pathophysiology

Syphilis is an infectious disease caused by the sexual transmission of *Treponema pallidum*. Once the pathogens enter the body, they multiply and invade the blood stream and lymphatics. The body's reaction to the invasion leads to an erosion at the site of inoculation, the characteristic chancre.

Epidemiology

Peak incidence occurs at age 20 to 24 but can occur in any sexually active adult at any age. The male/female ratio in the United States is 2:1. The U.S. incidence has been steadily decreasing since 1941. Over 50% of syphilis cases of less than 1 year's duration are detected as a direct result of serologic tests. The number of cases of congenital syphilis has also decreased since the 1940s.

Assessment

Clinical Presentation

The first sign of a syphilitic chancre is an eroded papule that becomes ulcerated (see Figure 10-1). Without treatment the chancre will heal in 2 to 4 weeks but may relapse for up to 4 years. All lesions are contagious. The base is characteristically clean and smooth, although a serous discharge may be produced by exerting pressure on the lesion. The edges of the ulcer are raised, firm, and well circumscribed. Most lesions occur in the genital area and are painless. In males they are seen on the penis and occasionally the scrotum; in females they are often intravaginal and asymptomatic, and therefore undetected. Regional adenopathy is common. The nodes draining the area of the chancre are discretely enlarged, hard, and nontender. They never coalesce or suppurate unless there is a mixed infection. Extragenital chancres are painful and may occur on any area of the body but are usually present on the lips: upper lip in males and lower lip in females. Other sites include the tongue, tonsil, uvula, rectum, fingers, and breasts.

Diagnostics

- **Darkfield microscopy:** Specimens must be taken from moist, nonbleeding lesions, placed on a saline solution slide, and examined promptly. Specimens require experience with preparation and reading; they must be sent to an appropriately equipped lab. The local county public health authority may be helpful in obtaining an acceptable specimen.

- Serologic tests include the **Venereal Disease Research Laboratories (VDRL)** and **rapid plasma reagent (RPR)** tests. The RPR is most useful as a screening test. The VDRL is the test of choice for following the therapeutic response to treatment. Results of these tests are negative 50% of the time in the initial stages of syphilis, becoming positive 1 to 3 weeks after the chancre appears. The **fluorescent treponemal antibody absorption (FTA-ABS)** test combined with the other two serologic tests makes an early presumptive diagnosis possible; none of the tests is sufficient alone. For sequential serologic testing it is recommended that the same test and the same laboratory be used.
- **Biopsy** of the chancre helps to confirm the diagnosis.

Differential Diagnosis

- Herpes simplex (grouped multiple painful vesicles; prodrome is common) (see Figure 2-10, *B*)
- Carcinoma of the penis (lesions may be painful; the ulcer does not spontaneously resolve)
- Bacterial ulcer (usually associated with perilesional erythema and lymphatic spread)
- Chancroid (painful, vague border, exudative)

Treatment

Nonpharmacologic

All patients should be screened for human immunodeficiency virus (HIV) and other sexually transmitted diseases. They should be advised to abstain from sexual intercourse until the lesions have completely healed. Use of condoms should be emphasized and sexual partners must be notified.

Pharmacologic

Topical Agents
None is indicated.

Systemic Agents
Benzathine penicillin G 2.4 million U, IM, is prescribed in a single dose or once per week for 2 weeks. In nonpregnant patients who are allergic to penicillin, one of the following is recommended: **doxycycline** 100 mg PO bid for 2 weeks *or* **tetracycline** 500 mg PO qid for 2 weeks *or* **erythromycin** 500 mg PO qid for 2 weeks.

CHANCRE

- Is contagious: patients should abstain from sexual intercourse or use a condom until lesion has completely healed
- Should prompt a human immunodeficiency virus (HIV) test to rule out acquired immune deficiency syndrome (AIDS)
- Should be reported to all sexual partners

Patients should be followed at 3- and 6-month intervals for clinical and serologic improvement. If the VDRL titer has not decreased fourfold in 3 months, an HIV test and cerebrospinal fluid (CSF) examination are indicated.

Indications for Referral

- Referral to the hospital pathologist or local county health department is appropriate to ensure accuracy of diagnosis.
- Consultation with a dermatologist or infectious disease specialist is recommended.

Decubitus Ulcer (Bedsore)

Overview

Pathophysiology

Decubitus ulcers arise when external pressure exceeds the pressure in localized blood vessels, causing them to collapse. Without blood flow tissues are not oxygenated and cell death occurs. Ischemic pallor is followed by reactive erythema, the first stage of decubitus development. Six hours of unrelieved pressure, even in normal, healthy skin, will lead to ulcer formation. Secondary infection in patients who are already debilitated may lead to rapid spread of the ulcer. In addition to immobility, contributing factors include malnutrition, decreased sensation, advanced age, decreased mental status, and incontinence.

Epidemiology

These ulcers occur primarily in older, bedridden patients but can occur in patients of any age who cannot voluntarily move to relieve pressure.

Assessment

Clinical Presentation

Lesions begin as red macules. The four stages of decubitus ulcer development include the following:

1. Skin is unbroken, but red
2. Epidermis is broken by either a blister or a superficial ulcer that may extend into but not through the dermis

3. A break in the epidermis involves the dermis and subcutaneous tissue

4. Breakdown penetrates epidermis, dermis, subcutaneous tissue and may extend into muscle and bone.

Lesions occur most commonly over pressure points in bedridden patients, specifically the presacral (see Figure10-2) and scapula areas, ischial tuberosities, heels, and sometimes pinna of ears. Patients report a dull, aching, or boring sensation. A sense of burning may occur if the wound becomes secondarily infected. If the ulcer deepens to involve the bone, pain may be excruciating. The size of the ulcer may be quite variable, ranging from less than 1 cm to over 20 cm.

Diagnostics
- The diagnosis of decubitus ulcers is based on clinical presentation. A culture of exudate may be indicated to determine the presence of infection and to determine the appropriate antibiotic.

Differential Diagnosis
- Venous stasis ulcer (usually lower extremity, not over pressure point) (see Figure 10-5)
- Pyoderma gangrenosum (predilection for lower extremities; exudative with sharply demarcated border)

Treatment

Nonpharmacologic
Prevention is essential. Adequate blood flow must be maintained at all times by **relieving pressure.** Patients on bed rest should be turned at least every 2 hours, and bony prominences cushioned to distribute pressure. One body part should not be allowed to lie against another. Heels should be lifted entirely off the bed by placing a pillow under the lower legs. **Sheepskin** placed under bony prominences is also helpful in prevention. **Special mattresses** that circulate air, water, or special "beads" are ideal preventive measures.

Ulcers that have already developed should be soaked (ideally in a whirlpool bath) for 15 minutes bid to aid in wound débridement. Wounds may then be covered with nonstick dressing **(Telfa)** to prevent disruption of new granulation tissue when the dressing is removed. Alternatively a **Duoderm** dressing may be applied; it should remain in place for several days or until fluid under the dressing begins to leak out around the edges.

DECUBITUS ULCER

- Is much easier to prevent than to treat; prevention is key
- Can be prevented by relieving pressure (especially over bony prominences) at least every 2 hours to assure adequate blood flow to all areas
- Sheepskin and/or special mattresses are helpful in distributing pressure evenly and preventing skin breakdown

Pharmacologic

Topical Agents
Antibiotic ointment **(Polysporin)** applied directly on the ulcer b.i.d. is helpful in preventing infection, but secondary allergic contact dermatitis may occur.

Systemic Agents
Antibiotics are indicated to treat secondary bacterial infections and should be selected on the basis of culture results. Common choices include **dicloxacillin** 250 mg PO q6h or **erythromycin** 250 to 500 mg PO q6h for patients allergic to penicillin. As a further adjunct to therapy **pentoxifylline (Trental)** 400 mg PO tid for a minimum of 6 to 8 weeks may encourage wound healing by stimulating blood flow to ischemic areas and modulating inflammatory mediators.

Indications for Referral

- Referral to a dermatologist is appropriate if the ulcer shows no signs of healing after 3 to 4 weeks of therapy, or if the ulcer is very large and skin grafting is a consideration.
- Consultation with a dermatologist may be appropriate if a severe secondary infection develops.

Ischemic Ulcer (Arterial Insufficiency)

Overview

Pathophysiology
Occlusion of the arterial blood supply to the skin results in necrosis. As the necrotic tissue is sloughed, an ulcer is formed. The occlusion can be caused by various factors, including constriction of the vessel (Raynaud's phenomenon), blockage in the vessel (embolism), or thickening of the vessel wall (atherosclerosis). Ischemic ulcers may also develop in conjunction with various systemic disorders affecting the vasculature. Scar tissue, secondary infection, or chronic edema of the lower extremity may delay healing or contribute to the chronicity of the ulcer.

Epidemiology
Ischemic ulcers occur primarily in persons with arteriosclerotic disease or in those with chronic hypertension.

Assessment

Clinical Presentation

Ischemic ulcers usually present on the lateral aspect of the lower extremities. Edges of the ulcer are sharp and defined, and the base is pale (see Figure 10-3). Yellowish exudate may be present. Patients describe an intense, boring pain made worse by elevation of the extremity (especially at night). Pain may be somewhat lessened by keeping the legs dependent. Feet feel cold, and patients may complain of cold intolerance and claudication on exercise. On physical examination peripheral pulses in the lower extremities may be weak or absent and capillary refill delayed. Feet become pale with elevation and ruddy when dependent. Shiny skin and a lack of hair on the affected extremity are also usually noticed.

Diagnostics

- The diagnosis is based on clinical presentation and history of arterial disorders. Doppler ultrasound may help to determine the extent of arterial insufficiency. If physical examination and Doppler results suggest significant arterial compromise, the patient should be referred to a vascular surgeon for arteriographic studies and possible surgery. A culture of wound exudate will help establish the presence of secondary infection and guide the selection of antibiotic.

Differential Diagnosis

- Venous stasis ulcer (usually on the medial aspect of the lower extremity; pain is increased with dependency rather than decreased) (see Figure 10-5)

Treatment

Nonpharmacologic

Treatment involves recognition and treatment of the underlying arterial disorder. Corrective surgery is the most effective therapy.

Pharmacologic

Topical Agents

Wet-to-dry saline compresses placed over the ulcer will aid in débridement of the lesion. (Dressings that have dried to the point of adhering to the ulcer should be resaturated before removal, to prevent tearing the new epithelium.) Thirty-minute whirlpool baths with **Hibiclens,** bid, used in conjunction with the saline solution compresses are the treatment of choice for wound débridement.

ISCHEMIC ULCER

- Will not heal until the underlying arterial insufficiency has been corrected; surgery is therefore indicated
- Can be improved by preventing secondary infection and chronic edema of the lower extremities
- Pain can be diminished by keeping the legs in a dependent position

Topical antibiotic ointment such as **Polysporin,** applied bid after the saline solution compresses, will help prevent secondary infection. **Duoderm** or **Vigilon** dressings applied directly to the wound after cleansing and débriding with hydrogen peroxide or normal saline solution create a moist environment that promotes wound healing. The dressing should extend at least 1 inch beyond the edges of the ulcer. **Metrogel** applied under the dressing helps prevent the development of anaerobic bacteria. The dressing may be left in place for 2 to 3 days but should be changed sooner if exudate leaks from around the edges. An **Unna boot** is also helpful therapy. It consists of zinc oxide paste applied directly to the wound, which is then wrapped with gauze and an elastic bandage. The dressing should stop just below the knee and should be changed no more than twice a week. Unna boot therapy should be continued for 2 weeks after the wound has healed to ensure adequate protection for the newly formed skin. Prolonged use of **neomycin** or **bacitracin** should be avoided since they can stimulate a contact dermatitis.

Systemic Agents

Antibiotics are indicated to treat secondary bacterial infections and should be selected on the basis of culture results. Common choices include **dicloxacillin** 250 mg PO q6h and **erythromycin** 250 to 500 mg PO q6h for patients allergic to penicillin. As a further adjunct to therapy **pentoxifylline (Trental)** 400 mg PO tid for a minimum of 6 to 8 weeks may encourage wound healing by stimulating blood flow to ischemic areas and modulating inflammatory mediators.

Indications for Referral

- Significant arterial insufficiency should be referred to a vascular surgeon for arteriographic studies and possible surgical correction.

Venous Stasis Ulcer

Overview

Pathophysiology

A venous stasis ulcer begins as the result of trauma to edematous skin and is the most common form of ulceration on the leg. The edema is caused by venous incompetence and poor lower extremity circulation. Other contributing factors include prolonged bed rest, malnutrition with hypoalbuminemia, thrombophlebitis, trauma to the limb, and severe congestive heart failure. Because of the edema and obstruction to normal blood flow, there is also reduced oxygenation of the skin, so healing occurs slowly. Even minor trauma can produce new ulcers.

Epidemiology

Venous statis ulcers are more common in persons after age 50, and in women more than men.

Assessment

Clinical Presentation

Venous stasis ulcers occur on the lower extremities, usually on the medial aspect above the ankle, and may vary in size from 2 cm to large enough to encircle the leg. They are irregularly shaped craters with rolled borders (see Figure 10-5). The border is pink if the ulcer is healing or boggy and dark if it is not healing. The center consists of granulation tissue; purulent material and crust may or may not be present. The surrounding skin is frequently edematous, indurated, and hyperpigmented. A "cobblestone" appearance is common. Although the ulcers themselves are frequently asymptomatic, a secondary infection may cause varying degrees of discomfort. Patients also frequently complain of a vague ache that is relieved by elevating the extremity. There may be pruritus (resulting from stasis dermatitis) surrounding the ulcer. When healing finally occurs, it is accompanied by scarring.

Diagnostics

- Venous stasis ulcers can be differentiated from other cutaneous ulcers on the basis of clinical presentation (location on the lower extremity), the presence of hyperpigmentation, and a history of predisposing conditions. A culture of the exudate will determine whether infection is present and will guide the choice of antibiotic. A skin biopsy should be performed on any ulcer that persists longer than 4 months, since malignant change can occur in chronic ulcers. A complete blood count and serum albumin levels should be obtained to ensure that the patient has adequate nutrition. Vitamin and zinc supplementation is also important, especially in the elderly patient.

Differential Diagnosis

- Contact dermatitis (no concurrent predisposing factors) (see Figure 7-2, *A*)

- Ischemic ulcers (usually located on pretibial area; surrounding skin is shiny and hairless) (see Figure 10-3)
- Neuropathic ulcers (predilection for weight-bearing areas of the feet)

Treatment

Nonpharmacologic

The **correction of any associated systemic disorders** is imperative. Circulation must also be improved; the **legs should be kept elevated above the level of the heart** as much as possible, and **constricting garments should be avoided. Pressure-graded support hose (Jobst, Medi, Juzo, or Sigvaris stockings) should be worn consistently** and should extend to midthigh. Additionally they should be classified as "Class II," thus providing 30- to 40-mmHg ankle pressure. (Support hose purchased in department stores do not provide graduated compression in sufficient strength.) Patients should be encouraged to **walk or flex their lower extremity muscles frequently,** to aid circulation and venous return. Prolonged standing or sitting with legs dependent should be avoided. **Moisturizers** should be used bid to prevent xerosis, fissuring, and the itch-scratch-itch cycle, which can predispose to infection.

Pharmacologic

Topical Agents

Wet-to-dry saline solution compresses placed over the ulcer will aid in débridement of the lesion. (Dressings that have dried to the point of adhering to the ulcer should be resaturated before removal, to prevent tearing of the new epithelium.) Thirty-minute whirlpool baths with **Hibiclens,** bid, used in conjunction with the saline solution compresses are the treatment of choice for wound débridement. Topical antibiotic ointment such as **Polysporin,** applied bid after the saline solution compresses, will help prevent secondary infection. **Duoderm** or **Vigilon** dressings applied directly to the wound after cleaning and débriding with hydrogen peroxide or normal saline solution create a moist environment that promotes wound healing. The dressing should extend at least 1 inch beyond the edges of the ulcer. **MetroGel** applied under the dressing helps prevent the development of anaerobic bacteria. The dressing may be left in place for 2 to 3 days but should be changed sooner if exudate leaks from around the edges. An **Unna boot** is also helpful therapy. It consists of zinc oxide paste applied directly to the wound, which is then wrapped with gauze and an elastic bandage.

VENOUS STASIS ULCER

- Will be less painful if legs are elevated above the heart as much as possible
- Can be minimized by avoiding constricting garments and prolonged sitting, wearing pressure-graded support hose consistently, and walking or flexing lower extremity muscles frequently
- Patients should take special precautions to protect legs from trauma

The dressing should stop just below the knee and should be changed no more than twice a week. Unna boot therapy should be continued for 2 weeks after the wound has healed to ensure adequate protection for the newly formed skin. Prolonged use of **neomycin** or **bacitracin** should be avoided since they can stimulate a contact dermatitis.

Systemic Agents

Antibiotics are indicated to treat secondary bacterial infections and should be selected on the basis of culture results. Common choices include **dicloxacillin** 250 mg PO q6h and **erythromycin** 250 to 500 mg PO q6h for patients allergic to penicillin. As a further adjunct to therapy **pentoxifylline (Trental)** 400 mg PO tid for a minimum of 6 to 8 weeks may encourage wound healing by stimulating blood flow to ischemic areas.

Indications for Referral

- Consultation with a dermatologist is appropriate if the ulcer shows no signs of healing after 3 to 4 weeks of therapy. Consider hyperbaric oxygen therapy.
- If the ulcer is very large, referral to a dermatologist or plastic surgeon is indicated for consideration of skin grafting.
- Evaluation with Doppler ultrasound or light reflection rheography will determine the extent of superficial and/or deep venous insufficiency.
- If varicose veins are present, they can be treated with surgical avulsion and/or sclerotherapy.

Oral Lesions

Figure 11-1 **ANGULAR CHEILITIS**

Erythematous and eroded skin occurs at the corners of the mouth

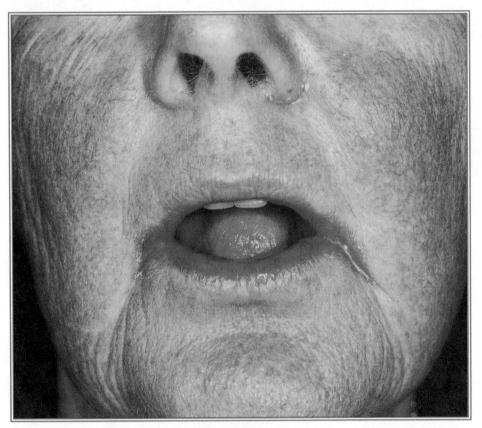

(From Habif TP: *Clinical dermatology,* ed 3, St Louis, 1996, Mosby.)

Figure 11-2 **APHTHOUS STOMATITIS**

Multiple small round, shallow ulcerations of grayish white appearance with surrounding erythema.

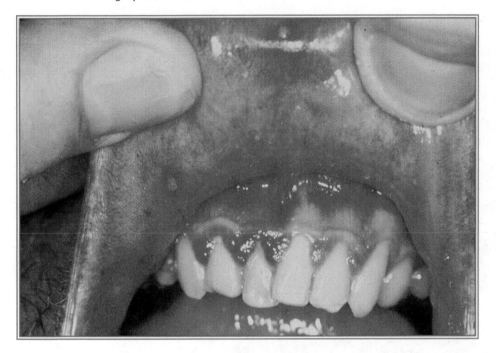

Figure 11-3 **HERPES SIMPLEX**

A, *Oral: Slightly crusted vesicular lesion on the upper lip.* **B,** *Genital: Small group of vesicles on an erythematous base.*

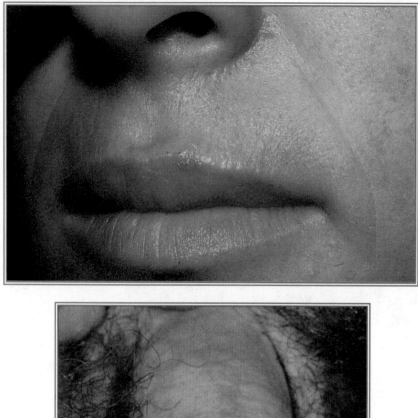

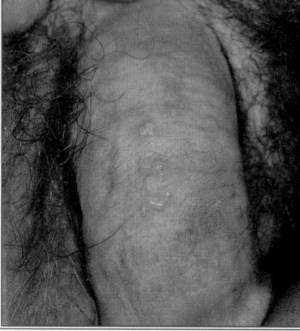

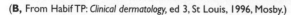

(**B,** From Habif TP: *Clinical dermatology,* ed 3, St Louis, 1996, Mosby.)

Figure 11-4 LEUKOPLAKIA

White plaques involve the lateral margins of the tongue.

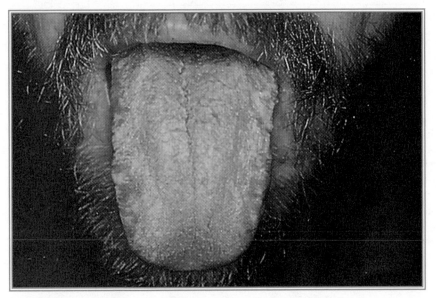

(From Goldstein BG, Goldstein AO: *Practical dermatology,* ed 2, St Louis, 1997, Mosby.)

Figure 11-5 ORAL CANDIDIASIS

Thickened white lesions on the tongue of a diabetic woman.

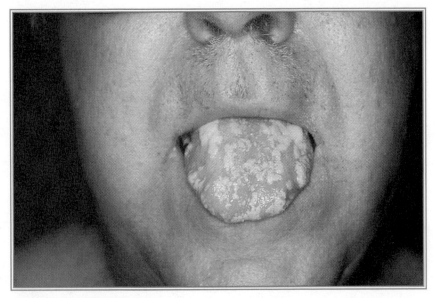

(Courtesy of Stacy R. Smith, MD.)

Table 11-1
Differential Diagnosis of Oral Lesions

DISORDER	TEXT	KEYS TO DIAGNOSIS
Angular cheilitis (perlèche)	Ch. 11, p. 411 (Figure 11-1)	Erythematous macerated, inflamed, cracked fissures at corners of mouth
Aphthous stomatitis (canker sore)	Ch. 11, p. 412 (Figure 11-2)	Ulcers of the movable oral mucosa; yellow base and erythematous margins
Herpes simplex	Ch. 2, p. 66 (Figure 11-3)	Grouped vesicles on an erythematous and edematous base; may be preceded by a prodrome of burning and tingling before eruption; occurs outside mouth, rather than on the mucosa
Leukoplakia	Ch. 11, p. 414 (Figure 11-4)	White well-defined plaque on oral mucosa; difficult to remove; bleeds if scraped off
Oral candidiasis (thrush)	Ch. 11, p. 416 (Figure 11-5)	White, cheesy plaque on oral mucus membranes and tongue; resembles curds of milk

Angular Cheilitis (Perlèche)

Overview

Pathophysiology
Angular cheilitis is a common disorder caused by age-related changes in skin and gum tissues. When the mouth closes such that a skin fold is created in the corners, saliva collects and predisposes to fissuring and a secondary yeast and/or bacterial infection. Aging causes wrinkling of the skin and narrowing of the oral palate with recession of the gums. Other contributing factors include iron or vitamin B deficiency.

Epidemiology
Patients at greatest risk are those with a tendency toward eczema whose mouth is anatomically abnormal, as a result of either a loss of teeth or the presence of braces or other oral devices. Consequently it is usually seen in the elderly (65% of geriatric wearers of full upper dentures suffer from perlèche) and in children with braces. Those who lick their lips frequently are also at risk. The disorder is particularly troublesome during winter months.

Assessment

Clinical Presentation
Lesions appear as erythematous macerated, inflamed, cracked, or crusted fissures at the corners of the mouth (see Figure 11-1). Chronic erythema and edema of the portion of the palate in contact with prosthetic appliances usually are present but symptomless. Scarring is possible with deeper infiltration. Patients describe the discomfort as dry or burning.

Diagnostics
- Culture results demonstrate colonies of *Candida albicans;* KOH scrapings show both budding spores and mycelial forms. The diagnosis is based on clinical presentation.

Differential Diagnosis
- The clinical presentation is distinctive. The differential diagnosis relates to possible causes of any secondary infection
- Candidiasis (satellite pustules are present, white exudate is easily scraped off, KOH finding is positive for pseudohyphae) (see Figure 4-7)
- Erythema multiforme (multiple acute ulcers, usually targetoid lesions elsewhere on skin) (see Figure 4-14)

ANGULAR CHELITIS (PERLÈCHE)

- Patients should avoid acidic foods and beverages to minimize discomfort
- Can be minimized or prevented by properly fitting dentures
- Patients should be reminded to avoid lip licking and to keep the corners of the mouth dry; corners may be coated with ointment for further protection

Treatment

Nonpharmacologic

Advise patient to avoid acidic foods and beverages (to prevent increased burning and discomfort). Avoid lip licking and keep the affected area well moisturized with protective ointments. If ill-fitting dentures or gum recession with crowded lower teeth is the cause, appropriate dental intervention is indicated.

Pharmacologic

Topical Agents

Hydrocortisone-iodoquinol (Vytone) is a combination low-potency steroid, antifungal, antibacterial agent that may be helpful when applied to the affected area bid. Once inflammation is controlled, treatment should be changed to an antiyeast agent such as **nystatin (Mycostatin) or ketoconazole (Nizoral),** also applied bid.

Systemic Agents

If the disorder does not respond to topical therapy, a secondary bacterial infection should be suspected. **Dicloxicillin** 250 mg PO qid for 10 days will reduce the bacteria. For penicillin-allergic patients, **erythromycin** 250 mg PO qid is an appropriate alternative.

Indications for Referral

- Referral to a dentist or orthodontist is indicated if any oral abnormality is present.

Aphthous Stomatitis (Canker Sore)

Overview

Pathophysiology

The exact cause is unknown, but precipitating factors include stress, trauma, allergies, and consumption of acidic foods and beverages. Deficiencies in folic acid, vitamin $B_{12,}$ and iron have been found in approximately 15% of patients with recurrent aphthous stomatitis.

Epidemiology

Aphthous stomatitis is a common disorder. Patients with altered immune systems and those with inflammatory bowel disease are considered to be at higher risk. Women are affected more often than men.

Assessment

Clinical Presentation

Round ulcerations of the movable oral mucosa (buccal, labial, or under surface of the tongue) are a hallmark of the disorder (see Figure 11-2). Ulcers characteristically have a yellowish base and erythematous margins. They may be singular or multiple, up to 1 cm in diameter. Recurrent ulcers are common, making the disorder a chronic one.

Lesions begin with a macular area of erythema. Ulceration develops after about 3 days, with epithelialization beginning 3 to 4 days later. Complete healing occurs within 2 weeks. There is no scarring and the lesions heal spontaneously with no other signs or symptoms.

Pain and discomfort may be moderate to severe, especially when multiple lesions are present. Eating may be painful and difficult.

Diagnostics

- The diagnosis is based on clinical presentation and history. A viral culture may be indicated to rule out herpes simplex.

Differential Diagnosis

- Traumatic oral ulcers (history of traumatic injury, chemical or thermal exposure, or ill-fitting dentures or orthodontic devices)
- Herpes simplex (multiple grouped vesicles, usually recurrent in the same location) (see Figure 2-10, *A*)
- Behçet's syndrome (the disorder begins with recurrent painful oral ulcers but progresses to include other symptoms, including ocular disorders, skin lesions, arthritis, thrombophlebitis, gastrointestinal [GI] manifestations, and generalized vasculitis)
- Oral erythema multiforme (lesions are more extensive and hemorrhagic, occurring on both oral mucosa and lips; systemic symptoms include various skin manifestations (target lesions, plaques, blisters, fever, and malaise) (see Figure 4-14)

Treatment

Nonpharmacologic

If the ulcer is due to a traumatic injury, prevention through education and appropriate dental or orthodontic intervention is indicated.

APHTHOUS STOMATITIS (CANKER SORE)

- If chronic, the presence of precipitating factors such as stress; trauma; consumption of acidic foods and beverages; folic, vitamin B_{12}, or iron deficiencies should be investigated and corrected
- Patients should be encouraged to follow up with internist if multiple metabolic imbalances are present
- Ulcers caused by traumatic injuries should be referred to the appropriate dentist or orthodontist

Pharmacologic

Topical Agents

Two percent **viscous lidocaine (Xylocaine)** used as a mouth-wash or applied directly on the ulcer q3h, may be helpful in reducing discomfort. **Zilactin** gel may be applied directly on the ulcer to form a protective coating that lasts for 4 to 6 hours. **Zilactin-B** includes **Benzocaine,** which provides additional anesthetic effect for maximum relief of pain. **Triamcinolone acetonide (Kenalog)** in dental paste **(Orabase)** also reduces discomfort and promotes healing. **Tetracycline** oral suspension (250 mg qid for 10 days) held in the mouth for 2 to 5 minutes before swallowing may hasten resolution of multiple oral lesions. (Children below age 12 should not be given oral tetracycline because of its effect on developing teeth enamel.) **Elixir of dexamethasone** 0.5 mg/5ml (1 tsp) to rinse and spit out, after meals and qhs for 5 days reduces inflammation.

Systemic Agents

If the patient is found to be deficient in either **folic acid, vitamin B₁₂,** or **iron,** systemic supplementation to increase serum levels to the normal range is appropriate. For severe ulceration **prednisone** 40 mg PO qAM tapered over 10 days is indicated.

Indications for Referral

- Consultation with a dentist or orthodontist is appropriate if the cause of the ulcer is ill-fitting oral appliances.
- Referral to an internist may be considered if multiple metabolic imbalances are discovered.
- Consultation with a dermatologist is appropriate if the disorder is severe enough to warrant consideration of systemic corticosteroids.

Leukoplakia

Overview

Pathophysiology

The exact cause is not always clear, but there is a strong association with chronic irritation, especially from smoking. The lesion itself is composed of atypical epidermal cells. Squamous cell carcinoma develops in 17% of all patients, with the greatest risk associated with lesions on the floor of the mouth and the undersurface of the tongue.

Epidemiology
The disorder is most common in males over age 50 who are chronic smokers.

Assessment

Clinical Presentation
A white well-defined plaque is evident on the oral mucosa, specifically the lips, gums, cheeks, and/or edges of the tongue (see Figure 11-4). Bleeding will result if the patch is scraped off. There are no concurrent systemic manifestations of disease, and the lesion itself is asymptomatic.

Diagnostics
• A biopsy of the oral mucosa is indicated to rule out the possibility of neoplasia. A KOH examination of scrapings will differentiate the disorder from oral candidiasis.

Differential Diagnosis
• Oral candidiasis (white exudate can be easily scraped off; KOH result is positive) (see Figure 11-5)
• Lichen planus (lacy-white appearance; difficult to distinguish from leukoplakia without a biopsy)
• Traumatic injuries (history of cheek biting, dentures, orthodontic appliances)
• Hairy leukoplakia (poorly demarcated lesion with white papillary projections ["hairs"] along the edges of the tongue in patients with acquired immunodeficiency syndrome [AIDS])

LEUKOPLAKIA

• Should be reevaluated annually to check for recurrences
• Patients should be advised to stop both smoking and chewing tobacco

Treatment

Nonpharmacologic
Cessation of smoking or chewing of tobacco is strongly advised. Surgical excision, destruction with laser, electrodesiccation, or freezing with liquid nitrogen to destroy abnormal cells is appropriate. Patients should be reevaluated annually to check for recurrences.

Pharmacologic

Topical Agents
None is indicated.

Systemic Agents
None is indicated.

Indications for Referral

- Referral to a dermatologist or oral surgeon may be appropriate, depending on the location of the lesion to be biopsied.
- Referral to a dermatologist is essential if the biopsy result is positive for cancerous cells.

Oral Candidiasis (Thrush)

Overview

Pathophysiology

Oral candidiasis results from an overgrowth of a normal inhabitant, *Candida albicans*. When conditions control or decrease the natural antagonists of *Candida* organisms, it replicates freely and disrupts the normal balance of organisms. In the newborn it can be transmitted during passage through the birth canal.

Epidemiology

Candidiasis is common in infants, debilitated patients, those receiving long-term broad-spectrum antibiotics, those receiving inhalant or systemic corticosteroid therapy, and those with depressed immune systems caused by either acquired immunodeficiency syndrome (AIDS) or cancer.

Assessment

Clinical Presentation

Oral mucus membranes and tongue become covered with a **white cheesy plaque** resembling curds of milk, which can be easily removed with a tongue blade (see Figure 11-5). The underlying mucosa is often inflamed and may bleed slightly. Patients are usually asymptomatic or have only mild discomfort. The disorder is not self-limiting and appropriate antiyeast treatments should be instituted.

Diagnostics

- KOH preparation of plaque scraping reveals pseudohyphae and/or spores.

- A biopsy is indicated if the KOH scraping result is negative, in order to rule out leukoplakia and lichen planus.

Differential Diagnosis
- Leukoplakia (white membrane is difficult to scrape away, causing bleeding) (see Figure 11-4)
- Lichen planus (difficult to distinguish without a biopsy)

Treatment

Nonpharmacologic
Cessation of antibiotics or corticosteroids is helpful, but risks and benefits must be carefully considered.

Pharmacologic

Topical Agents
Nystatin (Mycostatin) 5 ml (500,000 units) qid used as a mouth rinse is effective and very safe. The medication should be swished around the mouth for 5 minutes before it is swallowed. **Clotrimazole (Mycelex) buccal troches** 10 mg qid for 2 weeks are also effective.

Systemic Agents
Ketoconazole (Nizoral) 200 mg PO qd for 2 weeks may be effective in resistant cases of oral candidiasis. Alternatively **fluconazole (Diflucan)** 400 mg PO every week for 2 weeks may be helpful.

Indications for Referral

- A dermatologist should be consulted if the disorder is resistant to therapy.

ORAL CANDIDIASIS (THRUSH)

- Is not self-limiting, but requires antiyeast treatments
- Topical medications should be held in the mouth and swished around for 5 minutes (by the clock) before swallowing; the medication must be in contact with the yeast for maximum effectiveness

Vascular Lesions

Figure 12-1   **CAVERNOUS HEMANGIOMA**

Erythematous nodular lesion on the lateral aspect of the scalp.

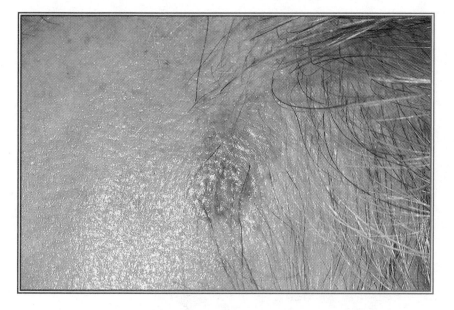

Figure 12-2   **CHERRY ANGIOMA**

Multiple erythematous papular lesions on the central chest.

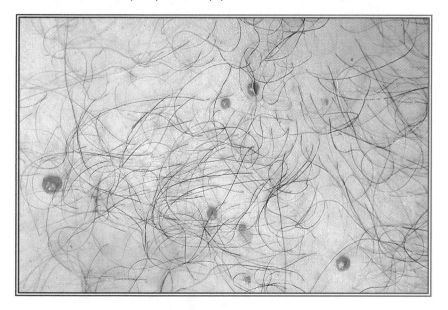

Figure 12-3   KAPOSI'S SARCOMA

Violaceous to erythematous nodules on an elderly male's leg.

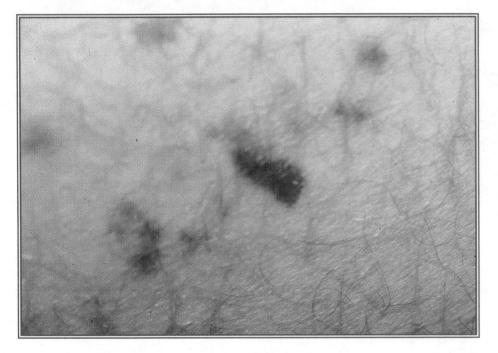

Figure 12-4   PORT WINE STAIN

Erythematous well-demarcated plaque on the lateral aspect of the face.

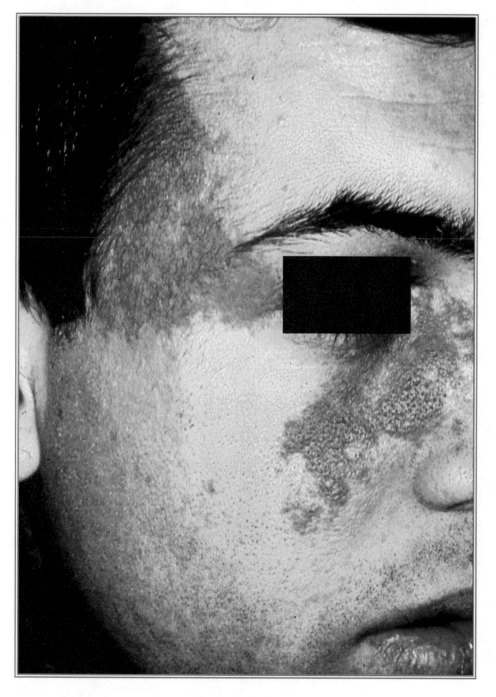

Figure 12-5 PYOGENIC GRANULOMA

Rapidly growing necrotic papule on the posterior aspect of the neck.

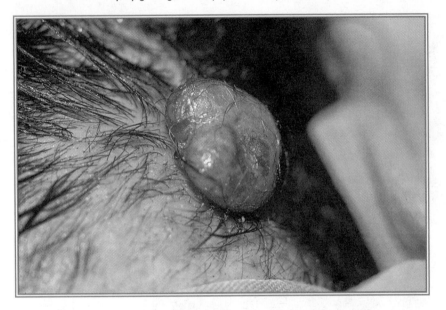

Figure 12-6 PURPURA

Erythematous to violaceous macule appearing after trauma to sun-damaged skin on the forearm of an elderly patient.

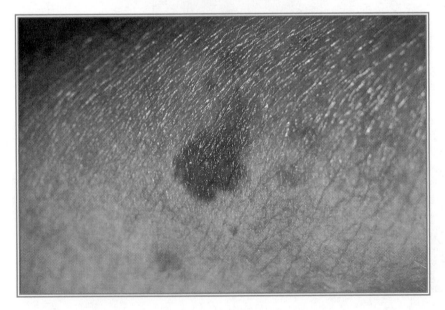

Figure 12-7   SPIDER ANGIOMA

Central red papule with radiating streaks on a young child's face

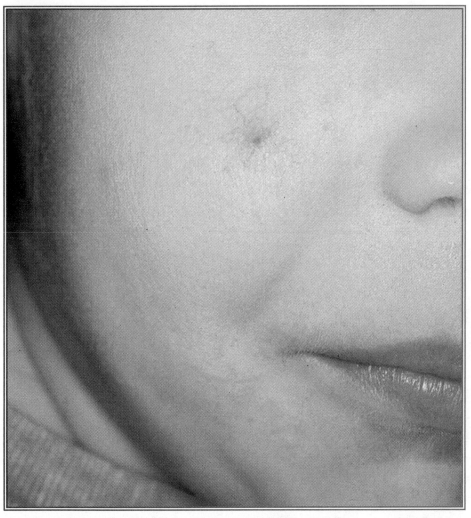

(Courtesy of Stacy R. Smith, MD.)

Figure 12-8   **STRAWBERRY ANGIOMA**

Enlarging erythematous nodule on the midcheek.

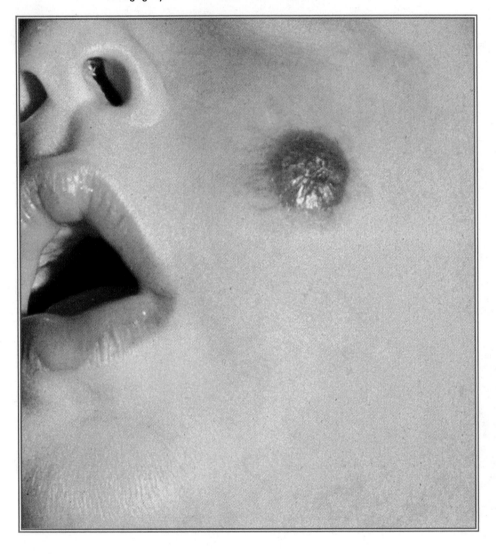

Figure 12-9 **TELANGIECTASIA**

Multiple dilated vessels on the cheek and nose of an elderly patient.

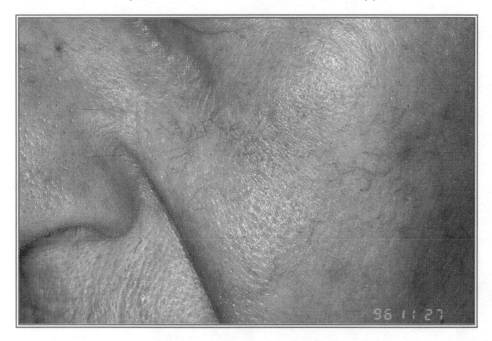

Figure 12-10   VENOUS LAKE

A violaceous papule on the lateral aspect of the nose.

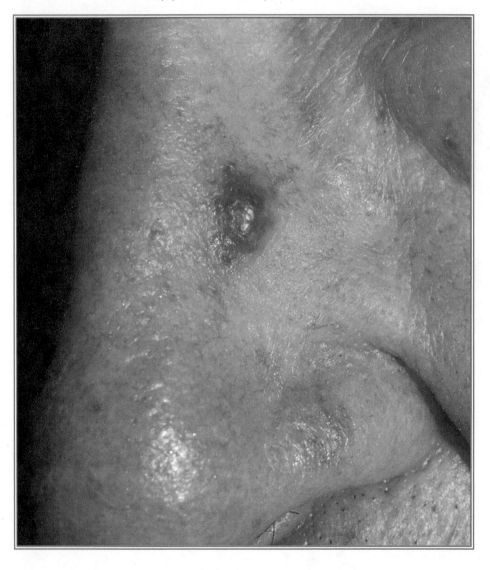

Table 12-1

Differential Diagnosis of Vascular Lesions

DISORDER	TEXT	KEYS TO DIAGNOSIS
Cavernous hemangioma	Ch. 12, p. 428 (Figure 12-1)	Skin-colored or reddish-blue slightly rounded mass with indistinct borders; present at or shortly after birth
Cherry angioma (De Morgan's spot)	Ch. 12, p. 429 (Figure 12-2)	Bright red to purple papule, usually on upper trunk; asymptomatic
Kaposi's sarcoma	Ch. 12, p. 431 (Figure 12-3)	Pink or reddish-purple macules that develop into plaques or nodules; occur mainly on upper half of the body; frequently affecting immunocompromised patients
Port wine stain (nevus flammeus)	Ch. 12, p. 432 (Figure 12-4)	Red-purple macule that appears at birth; usually occurs on face or neck
Pyogenic granuloma	Ch. 12, p. 434 (Figure 12-5)	Solitary, rapidly growing, dark-red papule with moist or scaly surface; usually on fingers, face, shoulders, feet; common in children, during pregnancy, or after trauma
Senile purpura (actinic purpura)	Ch. 12, p. 436 (Figure 12-6)	Purple macules on chronically sun-exposed skin in older adults; usually on arms and hands
Spider angioma (nevus araneus)	Ch. 12, p. 438 (Figure 12-7)	Small, bright-red dots with radiating telangiectasias, resembling a spider; common in children, pregnant women, and patients with liver disease
Strawberry hemangioma	Ch. 12, p. 439 (Figure 12-8)	Raised, red, soft compressible lesion with strawberry-like lobules; usually appears in first few weeks of life
Telangiectasia	Ch. 12, p. 441 (Figure 12-9)	Tiny, superficial, dilated blood vessels that appear as red wavy lines on the skin
Venous lake	Ch. 12, p. 442 (Figure 12-10)	Dark blue to black, slightly elevated, dome-shaped lesion; blanches with pressure; occurs on sun-exposed surfaces, especially the lower lip

Cavernous Hemangioma

Overview

Pathophysiology
Cavernous hemangiomas are congenital collections of dilated vessels that lie deep in the dermis.

Epidemiology
Cavernous hemangiomas develop in approximately 10% of infants: 20% are present at birth, and 90% occur during the first month of life. Sixty to seventy percent occur in females. There is an increased incidence in fetal alcohol syndrome.

Assessment

Clinical Presentation
The lesion presents at birth as a skin-colored or reddish-blue slightly rounded mass with indistinct borders (see Figure 12-1). The texture is described as similar to that of a "bag of worms." It enlarges for several months and then stabilizes. Regression may occur spontaneously but is usually incomplete. Thirty to sixty percent improve within 4 years, 90% within 9 years. A cavernous hemangioma may occur on any skin surface but has a predilection for the head and neck. Lesions range in size from 2 mm to 20 cm in diameter, with the majority 2 to 5 cm. Spontaneous or traumatic ulceration occurs in 20% of cases.

Diagnostics
- Diagnosis is based on the clinical appearance of the lesion.

Differential Diagnosis
- Port wine stain (macular rather than rounded; no ulceration or crusting) (see Figure 12-4)

Treatment

Nonpharmacologic
Usually no therapy is required if the lesion is small and does not grow significantly. Treatment with the pulsed dye laser or intense pulsed light (PhotoDerm VL) may hasten resolution and should occur as early as possible for best results.

CAVERNOUS HEMANGIOMA

- Is a cosmetic disorder only, without malignant potential
- May regress spontaneously, but incompletely

Pharmacologic

Topical Agents
If the lesion becomes secondarily infected due to ulceration, cultures should be obtained and the appropriate antibiotic therapy instituted.

Systemic Agents
Interferon or **corticosteroids** are indicated for large lesions or those affecting vital functions such as vision and nutrition. Because of the potential for side effects of prolonged therapy, patients should be referred to a dermatologist for institution of this treatment protocol.

Indications for Referral

- Consultation with a dermatologist is indicated if an arteriovenous fistula is suspected and surgical excision is a consideration.
- Referral to a dermatologist or laser surgeon is appropriate if lesions are ulcerated, large, impinging on vital structures, or rapidly growing.
- Dermatologists should be consulted for long-term therapy involving **interferon** or **corticosteroids.**

Cherry Angioma (De Morgan's Spots)

Overview

Pathophysiology
The exact cause of cherry angiomas is unknown. They are unrelated to systemic disease and are totally benign.

Epidemiology
The lesion appears in early adult life and increases in number with age. It occurs to some degree in most adults over age 30, making it the most common vascular malformation.

Assessment

Clinical Presentation
The lesion appears as a symptomless red macule that grows into a papule. It is bright red to purple, smooth, and less than 0.5 cm in

diameter (see Figure 12-2). It is most often located on the upper trunk. Because of the vascularity of the lesion, even slight trauma may produce bleeding. If this occurs and a black clot or scab forms, confusion with malignant melanoma may result. Lesions tend to enlarge very slowly.

Diagnostics

- In most cases the diagnosis is made on clinical presentation. If there is any concern that a less benign lesion is present, a skin biopsy should be performed.

Differential Diagnosis

- Malignant melanoma (more irregular borders, more varied pigmentation) (see Figure 5-27)
- Pyogenic granuloma (commonly follows trauma; predilection for fingers, face, and oral cavity) (see Figure 12-5)
- Spitz nevus (erythematous dome-shaped papule, usually in young children) (see Figure 5-37)

CHERRY ANGIOMA

- Is a cosmetic disorder only, without malignant potential
- Is the most common vascular lesion
- Development of additional lesions, especially in those above age 30 should be expected

Treatment

Nonpharmacologic

Treatment is for cosmetic reasons only. Electrodesiccation or curettage after cryotherapy is appropriate. A shave excision may be preferred for larger lesions. Various vascular-specific lasers and intense pulsed light **(PhotoDerm VL)** are the ideal modalities for treatment.

Pharmacologic

Topical Agents
None is indicated.

Systemic Agents
None is indicated.

Indications for Referral

- Referral to a dermatologist or laser surgeon may be appropriate if treatment with a laser is desired.

Kaposi's Sarcoma

Overview

Pathophysiology

Kaposi's sarcoma is not a true sarcoma, but rather a malignant tumor of vascular endothelial cells. There are two forms of the disorder: (1) a classic form that develops slowly and occurs in edematous extremities of elderly patients and (2) a fatal form that develops rapidly and occurs in patients who have acquired immunodeficiency syndrome (AIDS) or are immunocompromised. The exact cause of Kaposi's sarcoma is unknown, but one theory proposes that repeated infections stimulate the endothelial cells to change into a malignant form.

Epidemiology

Kaposi's sarcoma was initially identified in elderly men of Eastern European Jewish ancestry and black children in Africa. Since 1981 with the outbreak of AIDS, the disorder has become more closely identified with homosexual men infected with human immunodeficiency virus (HIV). The lesions of Kaposi's sarcoma are found in approximately 25% of men with AIDS, but are uncommon in women.

Assessment

Clinical Presentation

In the classic form lesions appear as blue-black plaques and nodules, localized to the feet and legs (see Figure 12-3). They progress slowly in a proximal direction. In immunocompromised patients lesions appear as pink or reddish purple macules that develop into plaques or nodules. They occur mainly on the upper half of the body rather than the legs. The most common sites of distribution are the face, arms, trunk, and mucus membranes. Lesions may be indolent or spread rapidly to involve internal organs such as the gastrointestinal tract and lungs, with fatal sequelae. In both forms of Kaposi's sarcoma the lesions themselves are predominantly asymptomatic.

Diagnostics

- In both forms of the disorder the diagnosis is suggested by clinical presentation and confirmed by skin biopsy.

Differential Diagnosis

- Purpura (no induration is present) (see Figure 12-6)
- Angiosarcoma (biopsy is necessary to confirm diagnosis)

KAPOSI'S SARCOMA

- Is closely associated with the aquired immunodeficiency syndrome (AIDS) virus, and as such is fatal

- May also occur in its classic form, on the extremities of elderly patients; in this case treatment may not be necessary as the lesions are asymptomatic

Treatment

Nonpharmacologic

In patients without AIDS treatment may not be required if the lesions are asymptomatic. In patients who have symptomatic lesions radiation therapy and chemotherapy are the usual treatments of choice. Vascular-specific lasers will also reduce the size of lesions.

Pharmacologic

Topical Agents
None is indicated.

Intralesional Agents
Vincristine or **bleomycin** is effective in some lesions, but patients should be referred to a dermatologist for treatment.

Systemic Agents
None is indicated.

Indications for Referral

- All patients with confirmed Kaposi's sarcoma should be referred to an oncologist.
- Treatment with intralesional agents or vascular lasers may require referral to a dermatologist, oncologist, or laser surgeon.

Port Wine Stain (Nevus Flammeus)

Overview

Pathophysiology

A port wine stain is a circumscribed developmental ectasia of dermal capillaries, arterioles, and venules. The exact cause is unknown, but may be a congenital weakness in the capillary walls, an increase in the number and size of the capillaries and/or deeper blood vessels, or an abnormality in arteriole vasodilatation.

Epidemiology

Port wine stains are present at birth on the posterior neck in 40% to 70% of infants. There is an equal sex distribution, and some evidence suggests an autosomal dominant inheritance. Port wine stains persisting into adulthood on other areas occur in 1% to 2% of the population.

Assessment

Clinical Presentation

Red-purple macules appear at birth and increase in size as the child grows. There is little fading. The color ranges from pale pink to deep red. They may occur on any area of the body but have a predilection for the face (especially the eyelids), nape of the neck, and midforehead (see Figure 12-4). Two types of lesions develop: (1) Medially located port wine stains appear faint red and present over the occipital scalp and nape of the neck or on the central face. These lesions remain flat throughout the patient's life and may fade with age. (2) Laterally located port wine stains are usually found on the face but may also occur on the extremities. They begin as red macules but become papular and deeper in color. They persist throughout life and may become even more prominent with age. All forms are usually asymptomatic but frequently become nodular with age and may become secondarily infected.

Diagnostics

* Diagnosis is made by clinical presentation. Diagnostic studies are usually not indicated, although a fast-growing lesion may require a biopsy to rule out the possibility of a malignant tumor.
* Occasionally angiography may be indicated to evaluate an underlying vascular malformation.

Differential Diagnosis

* Cavernous hemangioma (soft globular tumor with deeper tissue involvement) (see Figure 12-1)

PORT WINE STAIN

• Is a cosmetic disorder only, without malignant potential

• May be improved or eliminated with various treatments, including lasers

• In many cases can be visually eliminated with the application of cosmetics

Treatment

Treatment is not required unless the lesion is cosmetically unacceptable.

Nonpharmacologic

Regardless of treatment modality, serial photographs are essential in following the resolution of the lesion. Cosmetic cover-up with skin-colored preparations **(Covermark, Dermablend)** is appropriate. Laser therapy with a vascular-specific laser or intense pulsed light **(PhotoDerm VL)** is the best cosmetic treatment for vascular lesions.

Pharmacologic

Topical Agents
None is indicated.

Systemic Agents
None is indicated.

Indications for Referral

- Referral to a laser surgeon or dermatologist skilled in laser therapy is appropriate if the outcome of other treatment modalities is unsatisfactory.

Pyogenic Granuloma

Overview

Pathophysiology
The cause of pyogenic granulomas is unknown. They are not, however, pyogenic (caused by infection) as the name suggests. Histologically they are vascular malformations (angiomas) that may be the result of uncontrolled production of granulation tissue during the healing phase after trauma. Hormonal factors may play a role in their development, as may a defect in the surrounding vascular bed.

Epidemiology
Lesions usually occur in children and teenagers but may occur at any age. In adults they appear more frequently during pregnancy, and 50% of cases are preceded by trauma.

Assessment

Clinical Presentation
Pyogenic granulomas are asymptomatic solitary rapidly growing (up to 1.5 cm in diameter) dark-red papules that blanch under a glass slide (diascopy). Most are dome-shaped and smooth, but some are pedunculated (see Figure 12-5). They develop over the course of a few days to several weeks and bleed with minor trauma. Lesions are most common on the fingers, face, shoulders, feet, lips, and tongue. During pregnancy they may appear on the gingiva.

An epidermal collarette scale is usually present. Recurrence after treatment is not uncommon.

Diagnostics
- Diagnosis is made on clinical presentation. Because of their rapid growth and their similarity to malignant melanoma, lesions should undergo biopsy if any doubt exists as to their true identity.

Differential Diagnosis
- Malignant melanoma (more macular; no relation to previous trauma) (see Figure 5-27)
- Kaposi's sarcoma (multiple lesions; usually more purple and more macular) (see Figure 12-3)
- Keratoacanthoma (central keratotic dome-shaped core) (see Figure 5-23)
- Angioma (most common on trunk) (see Figure 12-2)

Treatment

Nonpharmacologic
Left untreated, most pyogenic granulomas undergo spontaneous resolution. To hasten resolution, a shave excision with electrodesiccation of the base is appropriate. Incomplete removal may lead to regrowth of the original lesion and/or multiple satellite lesions. Obliteration with a vascular-specific laser is also an alternative.

Pharmacologic

Topical Agents
None is indicated.

Systemic Agents
None is indicated.

PYOGENIC GRANULOMA

- *Usually undergoes spontaneous resolution without treatment*
- *Is a benign lesion, but necessitates biopsy to rule out malignant melanoma since both lesions display rapid growth characteristics*

Indications for Referral

- Consultation with a dermatologist is appropriate if malignant melanoma is possible.
- If the original lesion or satellite lesions recur after treatment, reexcision, and consultation with a dermatologist is indicated.

Senile Purpura (Actinic Purpura)

Overview

Pathophysiology

Senile purpura is caused by a leakage of blood into the skin resulting from trauma (even insignificant amounts) through weakened or abnormal blood vessels or coagulation abnormalities. On occasion it may occur spontaneously. Weakened vessel walls are caused by the normal aging process, exacerbated by chronic sun exposure.

Epidemiology

Senile or actinic purpura, as the name suggests, occurs in older individuals, particularly in areas of chronic sun exposure, and is a common problem.

Assessment

Clinical Presentation

Senile purpura is nonpalpable and asymptomatic. It is characterized by the presence of purple or yellow-brown macules, 0.5 to 5 cm in diameter, which occur predominantly on areas of the skin that are chronically sun-exposed (see Figure 12-6). Areas of predilection include the dorsal aspect of the hands and forearms, face, neck, and upper chest. The surrounding skin is frequently atrophic, wrinkled, and irregularly pigmented (dermatoheliosis). The macules do not blanch with pressure because the blood is not in the vessels but has leaked out into the surrounding tissues. A medication history frequently reveals the use of **aspirin, warfarin (Coumadin), nonsteroidal inflammatory drugs (NSAIDS),** and/or **steroids.** Corticosteroids increase the fragility of blood vessels, causing a variant of senile purpura known as *steroid purpura.* Mucosal bleeding (nosebleeds or bleeding during tooth brushing) may be reported by the patient. Lesions resolve spontaneously over several weeks but new ones continue to occur.

Diagnostics

• Diagnosis is usually made on the basis of clinical presentation. If an underlying coagulation defect is suspected, a complete blood count, platelet count, prothrombin time, partial thromboplastin time, and bleeding time are indicated.

Differential Diagnosis

• Steroid purpura (history reveals recent or concurrent use of topical or systemic corticosteroids)

- Ecchymosis (a thorough physical examination will reveal the distribution of lesions; patients who "bruise easily" have ecchymoses in both sun-exposed and non-sun-exposed areas; depending on the extent and distribution of lesions, consideration should be given to the possibility of elder abuse)
- Purpura pigmentosa chronica (chronic progressive purpura in which lesions appear primarily in areas of increased hydrostatic pressure [legs])

Treatment

Nonpharmacologic

No specific treatment is required. Prevention of trauma and avoidance of sun (or consistent use of sunscreen) are helpful in stabilizing the condition, but the damage already done is irreversible. Reassurance is always appropriate. Avoidance of topical and systemic corticosteroids is helpful when possible, but the risk/benefit ratio must be carefully determined.

Pharmacologic

Topical Agents

Some studies indicate the application of topical **vitamin K cream** bid hastens the resolution of purpuric lesions, but opinions vary and results are controversial. **Tretinoin (Retin-A, Renova, Avita)** applied qhs will thicken the superficial dermis and minimize purpura.

Systemic Agents

Good nutrition with **vitamin A and C supplementation** may be helpful.

SENILE PUPURA

- Is caused by an accumulation of years of sun exposure and the aging process
- Can be prevented from worsening by a conscientious effort to avoid continued sun exposure
- Can be minimized with the application of various topical products (vitamin K creams, cosmetics, self-tanners, etc.) and avoidance of trauma to the sun-damaged skin
- Lesions will resolve spontaneously, but new ones will occur
- Resolution can be enhanced through good nutrition with vitamin A and C supplementation

Indications for Referral

- Palpable purpura may indicate the development of vasculitis; the patient should be referred to a dermatologist.
- Unusually severe purpura coupled with abnormal lab test results (see Diagnostics) may indicate an underlying coagulation defect; the patient should be referred to a hematologist or internist.

Spider Angioma (Nevus Araneus)

Overview

Pathophysiology
The exact cause of spider angioma is unknown, but it is associated with pregnancy, cirrhosis, and the use of oral contraceptives.

Epidemiology
Spider angiomas are present in 15% to 25% of normal children and in 15% of normal adults. They occur in 60% of pregnant women and in more than 60% of patients with hepatic dysfunction. Lesions associated with estrogens or pregnancy usually regress upon estrogen withdrawal or delivery.

Assessment

Clinical Presentation
A small vascular lesion with a bright red central dot (arteriole) leading into radiating telangiectasias, the lesion resembles a spider (see Figure 12-7). It is found chiefly on the face, upper chest and upper back in adults. Lesions in children occur more frequently on the hands, forearms, or face. Occasionally the central dot is surrounded by a pale halo. Spider angiomas usually persist with age.

Diagnostics
- The diagnosis of a spider angioma can be made on clinical presentation. A distinguishing characteristic is the blanching of the central dot with pressure. Immediately upon release of the pressure the lesion returns to its normal bright red color.

Differential Diagnosis
- Telangiectatic mats (seen in scleroderma)

Treatment

As this lesion is primarily of cosmetic concern, no treatment is required unless the patient desires it.

Nonpharmacologic
Gentle electrodesiccation of the central arteriole leaves little scarring. (If the central arteriole is destroyed, the radiating capillaries will not fill.) Treatment with a vascular-specific laser or intense pulsed light **(PhotoDerm VL)** is an alternative.

SPIDER ANGIOMA

- Is a cosmetic disorder only, without malignant potential
- Can be easily treated and completely removed without disruption to the skin if the patient finds it cosmetically unacceptable

Pharmacologic

Topical Agents
None is indicated.

Systemic Agents
None is indicated.

 Indications for Referral

- Referral to a dermatologist or laser surgeon is appropriate if treatment with a laser or intense pulsed light is desired.

Strawberry Hemangioma

Overview

Pathophysiology
A strawberry hemangioma is a congenital lesion that results from an abnormal growth of vascular tissue. There may be a congenital weakness of the capillaries or an increase in their number and size. The exact cause is unknown.

Epidemiology
Lesions occur in 6% to 8% of children; the female/male ratio is 3 : 1.

Assessment

Clinical Presentation
The lesion is rarely present at birth or is very pale. It may first present as telangiectatic macules and be mistaken for a bruise, but within the first few weeks of life becomes a raised, red, soft, compressible lesion with strawberry-like lobules, about 2 to 3 cm in diameter (see Figure 12-8). Ulceration and crusting may occur. It may continue to grow for up to 1 year, then regress over the next 5 years. Complete resolution occurs in 95% of cases. The most common sites of predilection are the head, neck, and trunk.

Diagnostics
- Diagnosis is based on clinical appearance of the lesion.

Differential Diagnosis

- Pyogenic granuloma (has an epidermal collarette; not present at birth) (see Figure 12-5)
- Lymphangioma (clear, deep painless lesions that enlarge over time)
- Cavernous hemangioma (soft tumor with a texture similar to a "bag of worms"; deeper tissues are involved; persists longer) (see Figure 12-1)

Treatment

Nonpharmacologic

Treatment is not necessary unless the lesion is obstructing a vital organ or is rapidly enlarging. Vascular-specific laser or intense pulsed light **(PhotoDerm VL)** therapy may hasten resolution and should occur as early as possible for best results, especially if the lesion bleeds or ulcerates. Reassurance is indicated in all cases.

Pharmacologic

Topical Agents

Light cryotherapy may be beneficial for small lesions. If the lesion becomes secondarily infected as a result of ulceration, cultures should be obtained and the appropriate antibiotic therapy instituted.

Systemic Agents

Prednisone 2 to 3 mg/kg/day orally in divided doses bid for 4 weeks, followed by a single early morning dose tapered on an alternate day schedule for a few weeks and then discontinued, may be used for rapidly growing lesions or for those obstructing the pharynx or eye. Involution usually begins by the third week of treatment. Alternatively intralesional **triamcinolone (Kenalog)** 10 mg/ml every 1 to 4 weeks until lesion resolution occurs may be used. A second course of therapy may be given for recurrences.

> ## ✦ Indications for Referral
>
> - Consultation with a dermatologist or vascular surgeon is indicated if the lesion is obstructing the pharynx or eye.
> - Referral to a dermatologist for surgical excision is appropriate if the lesion does not regress by late childhood, and surgical excision is a consideration.
> - If the lesion becomes secondarily infected through ulceration, cultures should be obtained and the appropriate antibiotic therapy instituted.

STRAWBERRY HEMANGIOMA

- Regresses completely in 95% of cases, over a 5-year period
- Is a cosmetic defect only, without malignant potential
- Resolution can be hastened with appropriate laser therapy

Telangiectasia

Overview

Pathophysiology
The specific cause of telangiectasias is unknown, but they seem to be related to sun exposure or to underlying disease. However, the lesions themselves are only a cosmetic problem.

Epidemiology
Lesions are most frequently found in adults and those with actinic damage.

Assessment

Clinical Presentation
Telangiectasias are tiny superficial dilated blood vessels that appear as red, wavy lines in the skin (see Figure 12-9). Vessels may either be venules, capillaries, or arterioles, the diameter of which rarely exceeds 1 mm. They blanch when pressure is applied but are asymptomatic and rarely bleed. The most common site of predilection is the nasal alae, although the cheeks are also frequently affected. When numerous telangiectasias are present, they can produce a diffuse red color or appearance of a blush. On closer examination the individual dilated vessels can be discerned. The condition is chronic and does not resolve spontaneously.

Diagnostics
- The diagnosis is made on the basis of clinical presentation.
- Diascopy (applying pressure with a glass slide) reveals blanching.

Differential Diagnosis
- Telangiectatic mats (occur in scleroderma as part of the CREST [Calcinosis, Raynaud's phenomenon, Esophageal dysfunction, Sclerodactyly, Telangiectasia] syndrome)

Treatment

Nonpharmacologic
Treatment is not required unless the patient requests it for cosmetic reasons. Treatment with a vascular-specific laser or intense pulsed light **(PhotoDerm VL)** is most effective. Prevention, including the consistent use of sunscreens, is essential.

TELANGIECTASIA

- Is a cosmetic disorder without malignant potential
- Development is stimulated by chronic and prolonged sun exposure
- Further development can be reduced by a conscientious avoidance of the sun and use of sunscreens, and protective clothing
- Is a chronic condition that does not resolve spontaneously

Pharmacologic

Topical Agents
None is indicated.

Systemic Agents
None is indicated.

Indications for Referral

- Referral to a dermatologist or laser surgeon may be indicated.
- Referral to a rheumatologist may be indicated for treatment of underlying scleroderma.

Venous Lake

Overview

Pathophysiology
The exact cause of a venous lake is unknown, but a familial tendency is frequently identified. It is a totally benign lesion without malignant potential.

Epidemiology
Lesions most commonly occur in elderly patients.

Assessment

Clinical Presentation
Venous lakes are solitary dark-blue to black slightly elevated dome-shaped lesions, usually less than 1 cm in diameter (see Figure 12-10). They are easily compressed and blanch with pressure (diascopy). Lesions appear on sun-exposed surfaces such as the lip, ears, face, or neck. Because of the vascularity of the lesions, they may bleed easily after trauma but are otherwise asymptomatic. They will persist throughout life without treatment.

Diagnostics
- Diagnosis is based on clinical presentation, but if any doubt exists, skin biopsy is indicated.

Differential Diagnosis

- Malignant melanoma (does not disappear with compression) (see Figure 5-27)
- Blue nevus (does not disappear with compression and usually does not occur on face, ears, or lips) (see Figure 5-5)

Treatment

Nonpharmacologic

Because the disorder is a benign one, no treatment is necessary unless the patient requests it either for cosmetic reasons or because the lesion bleeds easily and is bothersome. Removal by electrodesiccation is effective, as is removal with vascular-specific lasers or intense pulsed light **(PhotoDerm VL).**

Pharmacologic

Topical Agents
None is indicated.

Systemic Agents
None is indicated.

Indications for Referral

- Referral to a dermatologist or laser surgeon is appropriate.

VENOUS LAKE

- Is a cosmetic disorder without malignant potential
- Does not require treatment unless desired by the patient for cosmetic reasons
- Can be cosmetically enhanced through the use of vascular lasers

Part III

Patient Education Materials

Acne Vulgaris

- The treatment of acne is slow. Be patient! It may take 6 to 8 weeks to show improvement.
- Your acne is caused by processes that occur under the skin; therefore it will not be improved by overwashing or scrubbing. It is not caused by dirtiness or by the foods you eat.
- Use the medications prescribed by your doctor exactly as ordered. Do not stop and start the medications as your acne gets better and worse.
- Acne is not just "something you have to go through." It can be treated!

If you have been prescribed **Retin-A, Renova,** or **Differin:**

- Start by using it every other night for a week, before increasing it to every night.
- Use it sparingly (a pea-sized amount is enough for your entire face).
- Use it all over your face. It is not just a "spot treatment."
- Use **Renova, Retin-A,** or **Avita** only at night. **Differin** may be used any time of day.
- Use it after you have washed your face and let it dry for a few minutes.
- Use a sunscreen in the morning when you will be outdoors, since you will be more likely to burn.
- The key to acne treatment is *prevention*. Continue to use these products after your skin is clear to keep it that way!

If you have been prescribed Accutane:

- Be responsible in taking it exactly as you have been told.
- Be sure to have your monthly lab work done *before* you run out of medication, to prevent lapses in treatment.
- Use two kinds of birth control. You absolutely *must not* become pregnant during treatment or for 1 month after you stop using **Accutane.**
- Avoid alcohol, Tylenol, and vitamin A supplements during treatment. You may take ibuprofen products for minor discomfort.
- Use sunscreen consistently. Remember: when you take these medications you will be more likely to burn.
- Report any headaches, visual changes, joint stiffness, or other side effects. Your dose may need to be adjusted.

To be reproduced for clinical use. Hooper: *Primary Dermatologic Care*, St Louis, 1999, Mosby.

Candidiasis

- Report any suspected pregnancy. The medication you have been prescribed may not be healthy for your baby.
- Check with your doctor before taking any antihistamines or antibiotics during your course of therapy.
- Lose weight if you are more than 20% over your ideal weight. Excess body fat causes the skin to fold over on itself and can create an environment that will prolong your condition or cause it to recur frequently.
- Try to keep your skin dry, especially during humid weather. Wear loose-fitting cotton clothing instead of nylon or polyester, which do not absorb moisture. Avoid nylon undergarments. Body powder such as **Zeasorb-AF** will help keep your skin dry.
- If the affected areas are moist or oozing, soak them several times a day with **Burow's solution** (available without a prescription) for 10 to 15 minutes and allow them to air dry. Repeated soakings will not only feel soothing, but also actually dry the lesions faster!
- If the corners of your mouth are cracked and red, be sure your dentures or orthodontic devices (if any) fit properly. Avoid licking your lips frequently.
- Housekeepers, launderers, barbers, and parents of young children must make an extra effort to keep their hands as dry as possible. A constant warm, moist environment between the fingers encourages the infection to develop and/or persist.
- Wear cotton-lined gloves when your hands are exposed to water, such as when washing dishes, clothes, or babies.

Folliculitis, Furuncles, and Carbuncles

- Good hygiene is essential in treating your condition. Wash the affected area(s) twice daily with an antibacterial soap such as **Lever 2000** or **Dial.**
- Change your razor blade daily when shaving infected areas. Use a spray shaving cream rather than a brush. If you use an electric shaver, wipe the cutting surface with alcohol after every shave.
- Do not share washcloths, towels, or bedding, and be sure to launder these items daily.
- Use all medications as prescribed.
- Avoid the use of products that irritate your skin.

To be reproduced for clinical use. Hooper: *Primary Dermatologic Care,* St Louis, 1999, Mosby.

Herpes Simplex (Fever Blisters, Cold Sores)

- The infection you have is one of the most common throughout the world, and you may never discover where or from whom you became infected.
- Some people who have frequent cold sores spread the virus even when they have no symptoms and don't know they are infected.
- There are basically two types of this disease. Type 1 usually causes cold sores around the mouth; type 2 usually causes them in the groin or genital area. These distinctions are not always clear, however.
- Some studies show that if you have type 1, you may have slight protection against development of type 2.
- Although it is very rare for herpes to develop in newborns, it is possible for you to infect your baby during birth even if you do *not* have lesions in the genital area. Be sure to tell your doctor that you have had herpes if you become pregnant.
- Although we don't understand exactly why it happens, we do know that stress, trauma, sunlight, fever, and menstrual periods frequently cause eruption of a cold sore.
- If you have had a herpes infection more than once, you probably noticed that the little blisters occurred in the same location. You probably also noticed that you "felt" it, even before you could see anything on your skin. This burning, tingling, or itching sensation you felt is called a *prodrome* and is an important sign. If you begin taking your medication at the very first sign of the prodrome, you may prevent or reduce the actual skin outbreak and amount of time you are contagious.
- The oral and/or topical medications you have been given are very safe and should be taken exactly as prescribed.
- Prevention is always the best treatment. Consistent application of sunscreens, use of condoms during sexual contact, and good hand washing will help prevent the spread of herpes simplex from—or to—you.

To be reproduced for clinical use. Hooper: *Primary Dermatologic Care*, St Louis, 1999, Mosby.

Pityriasis Rosea

- Pityriasis rosea is a skin disease that is not dangerous. It is usually mild; if you have it once, you will not get it again.
- Most cases (75%) occur between the ages of 10 and 35, with a peak incidence between 20 and 24. Eruptions occur most frequently in winter.
- Many patients have a personal or family history of asthma or atopic dermatitis.
- The first sign of the disease is a tawny or salmon-colored patch on the chest or back. One to two weeks later other smaller lesions appear and last for another 2 to 4 weeks, then fade gradually. The patches lie in a characteristic pattern that resembles a Christmas tree with drooping branches. In addition they usually have a faint white scale.
- Usually the only symptom is itching, which can be made worse by exercising or taking a hot bath. Patients do not report feeling sick.
- The actual cause of pityriasis rosea is not known. We do know what it is not: it is not caused by a fungus or bacteria, or by anything you ate or touched. More importantly it is not a sign of any kind of internal disease or disorder and is not contagious.
- The treatment consists mainly of controlling any itching until the disorder subsides. Sometimes antiitching lotions may be prescribed, but in other cases oral antihistamines will be ordered. Occasionally ultraviolet-A or ultraviolet-B light treatments may be prescribed by your doctor. These light treatments tend to have a drying effect and therefore speed up recovery.

There are usually no permanent marks or scars left after the disease fades.

To be reproduced for clinical use. Hooper: *Primary Dermatologic Care*, St Louis, 1999, Mosby.

Pruritic Disorders (Itching)

- Soaking the lesions with cool tap water, **Burow's solution,** or a mixture of vinegar and water (1:10) may be soothing and help relieve the itching.
- Try not to scratch! Scratching not only will spread the itching but can also lead to infection.
- Oral **antihistamines** are usually helpful in reducing the itch but can cause drowsiness. Be sure you don't drive or engage in activities that require alertness.
- Avoid the substance that you are allergic to! If you come in contact with it again, you may react even more quickly and strongly.

To be reproduced for clinical use. Hooper: *Primary Dermatologic Care,* St Louis, 1999, Mosby.

Pseudofolliculitis

- Stop shaving! If that is impossible, try to shave only every 2 to 3 days. Shaving acts to cut hairs at the skin surface and leave them with a sharp point, which can readily penetrate the skin as the hair grows and curves back around. Do not resume regular shaving until the inflammation is gone.
- If you *must* shave, it's better to use an electric shaver than a straight-edge blade.
- If you prefer a straight-edge blade, be sure your skin and beard are very wet.
- Use a shaving gel rather than a shaving cream, and use a single-edge blade instead of a double-edge blade. (The double-edge system will cut the hair below the skin surface and increase the chance of ingrown hairs.)
- Warm compresses with saline solution, tap water, or **Burow's solution** (no prescription needed) will help to remove crust, soothe the lesions, and soften the epidermis to allow easier release of ingrown hairs.
- Hair loops should be released but not plucked.
- Depilatory creams may be used as long as they don't irritate your skin.
- Applying a **1% hydrocortisone** cream once or twice a day may help reduce the inflammation.

To be reproduced for clinical use. Hooper: *Primary Dermatologic Care,* St Louis, 1999, Mosby.

Scabies

- You have been infected by a mite called *Sarcoptes scabiei humanis*. This infection does not mean you are dirty or live in unhealthy conditions. You may have simply been in close contact with someone who was infected.
- You were actually infected several days or weeks before you began itching, and you may continue itching for several days or weeks after you have been treated. This itching is caused by a sensitivity reaction your body has to the mite.
- You have been prescribed a small amount of cream or lotion to apply to your body *from the neck down* to destroy the mite. Over applying the medicine is dangerous and unnecessary. In fact, it may make the itching worse by irritating your skin.
- For the treatment to be most effective, all those who live with you and others who have been in close contact with you during the past month should be treated at the same time.
- Be sure to launder all clothing and bedding that you have worn or used during the past week.

If You Have Been Prescribed **Lindane (Kwell):**

- Apply 1 to 2 oz. of the cream or lotion to your entire body from the neck down, paying special attention to brushing it under your fingernails.
- Wash it off in 6 hours.
- Repeat the application in 1 week.
- Do *not* use on children below 5 years of age or if you are pregnant.

If You Have Been Prescribed **Crotamiton (Eurax):**

- Massage the lotion into all areas of your skin below your neck.
- Be sure to apply it in skin fold areas.
- Apply a second coat 24 hours later *without removing the first coat.*
- Bathe with soap and water 48 hours after the second application.

If You Have Been Prescribed A **Sulfur** Ointment:

- Apply the ointment from the neck down on 3 nights in a row.
- Wash it off with soap and water after day 4 of treatment.

If your condition does not improve within 3 weeks or if it worsens, please come into the office so we can more accurately evaluate your condition.

To be reproduced for clinical use. Hooper: *Primary Dermatologic Care*, St Louis, 1999, Mosby.

Seborrheic Dermatitis

- Seborrheic dermatitis is a chronic condition. Although there is no cure, it can be controlled.
- It is not contagious and cannot be spread by personal contact or by sharing of towels, bed linens, and so on.
- Although the exact cause is unknown, several factors may cause the condition to flare. Among them are stress, fatigue, infection, poor nutrition, and various medications. It is also common for it to worsen during the winter months.
- Eliminating aggravating factors may help reduce the frequency of flare-ups. As always prevention is the best treatment.
- In infancy the condition is frequently referred to as "cradle cap" and is usually outgrown during the first year of life.
- Infants with cradle cap may be treated by applying warm mineral oil to the scalp, followed in several hours by washing with **Dawn** liquid to remove the scale.
- Because the skin on your face and in your skin folds is very delicate, medications that you apply to those areas must be very gentle. Using the medications longer or more frequently than instructed may cause more problems than it helps.
- You may find that washing your face with a dandruff shampoo (especially if your eyelids are affected) is helpful.
- If your scalp is affected, be sure to shampoo frequently—daily is best. Massage the shampoo thoroughly into your scalp and leave it on for 10 to 15 minutes before rinsing.
- You may have better results by rotating your shampoos, rather than using the same one all the time. Some people change brands each time they buy a new bottle. Others keep two or three bottles in the shower and rotate them when they shampoo. You may need to experiment to find the routine that works best for you.
- If your chest or areas of your trunk are affected, as well as your face, you may be given two different medications. Be sure to use them only in the areas for which they were prescribed. If you run out of one, don't assume you can substitute the other, even though you are treating the same condition.
- It is very normal to feel frustrated and embarrassed during periods when your skin is "flaring." You may require a change in your medication or routine. Please come in to the office so we can more accurately evaluate your condition.

Tinea Cruris (Jock Itch)

- The scientific name for jock itch is tinea cruris. It is a fungal infection that can be cured with the proper combination of medicines and at-home treatments.
- Because a fungus likes to live where it is warm, dark, and moist, we must give it exactly the opposite conditions if we expect to treat it. (One of the reasons it grows so commonly in the groin area is that the conditions there are exactly what it likes.)
- One of the most important things you can do is to wear cotton underwear instead of nylon or polyester. Loose-fitting boxer shorts will allow more air circulation than tight-fitting jockey shorts.
- Change your clothes as soon as possible after a workout. Damp, snug athletic supporters, wet swimsuits, or nylon exercise clothing worn for long periods creates a perfect environment for fungus.
- Prevent chafing and friction from skin rubbing against skin or skin rubbing against clothing. Application of powder may help to smooth the skin and reduce friction.
- A fungus is also prone to develop in an area where skin touches skin— the *intertriginous areas*. People who are overweight tend to have more of these areas than other people. So here is another reason to lose that extra weight. Your heart will thank you, and so will your skin!

Tinea Pedis (Athlete's Foot)

- The scientific name for athlete's foot is *tinea pedis*. It is a fungal infection. In fact, it is the most common of all fungal infections, affecting about 7 of 10 people at some time during their lives.
- There are different types of athlete's foot. One type is dry, thick, and scaly and occurs along the sides of the foot and on the sole. The other type occurs between the toes and is wet, red, and sometimes associated with an unpleasant odor. Both types tend to itch.
- No matter what your specific symptoms are, *prevention* is the best treatment.
- Try to keep your feet as dry as possible, even changing socks during the day if they feel damp. Wearing cotton socks is helpful, too, because cotton will absorb more moisture (perspiration) than nylon or polyester.
- You may decide that sprinkling powder in your shoes or socks makes your feet feel drier. It's best to use an antifungal powder, such as **Zeasorb-AF.**
- Don't wear shoes at all if you don't have to. When you must wear shoes, try to select those that are well ventilated or will "breathe" as much as possible.
- If your feet are red and moist because of the fungus, try soaking them in **Burow's solution** four or five times a day. You can buy it at the drug store as a dry powder that you mix with water. Soaking your feet and then letting them air dry frequently throughout the day will actually make the lesions dry up faster.
- If your feet are dry and scaly, you must soften them by soaking them in water before applying creams or lotions. Apply the cream or lotion as soon as you pat your feet dry.
- Sometimes, because the skin is broken and moist, a bacterial infection will develop in addition to the fungal one. If that is your situation, you will also be given a prescription for an antibiotic. Be sure to follow the directions exactly.
- Because a fungal infection is somewhat contagious, it's best not to share socks or shoes. Unless you live alone, don't go barefoot around the house since other people may get it.
- Remember: keep your feet as clean and dry as possible. Wear sandals in the gym, in public showers, and around the pool.

Verrucae (Warts)

Warts are a very common skin disorder, so common, in fact, that almost 1 out of every 10 people has them. Although they can occur at any age, they are most common between the ages of 12 and 16.

Warts are caused by a virus, but because there are so many viruses, there are also many different types of warts.

Most warts will go away on their own, even without any treatment. Many of the treatments you can do at home, and it's important to do them properly. Read the guidelines and follow them carefully.

- **If your warts have been frozen with liquid nitrogen,** they will probably blister in a day or so. You should carefully remove the roof of the blister, *taking care not to contaminate other skin surfaces with the fluid, as you may spread the virus.* Keep the wound clean and covered. When it has healed, the wart should be smoother, flatter, and smaller than it was before treatment. It is very common, however, for a wart to need multiple freezings before it disappears completely.
- **If you use solutions or plasters at home,** follow these steps:

  1. Soak the wart in water for 10 minutes.
  2. File it down as much as you can with an emery board or pumice stone.
  3. Apply **petroleum jelly (Vaseline)** in a ring *around* the wart, to protect the normal skin.
  4. Apply 1 to 2 drops of solution (or the plaster) and allow it to dry.
  5. Cover the wart with adhesive tape and leave it in place for 24 hours.
  6. You may repeat the procedure every 24 hours, or until tenderness occurs.
  7. Combining at-home therapy with monthly office visits for freezing may help the wart resolve more quickly.

- **If you have plantar warts,** be sure to schedule your office visits when you won't have to be on your feet for the next few days. The wart itself is tender, but the treatment makes it even more so!
- **If you have genital warts,** be sure you use a condom when having sexual relations to prevent spreading the virus to your partner. If you are female, it is important to have annual gynecologic exams since you have a four times the normal risk of developing cervical cancer. If you are pregnant, you may infect your newborn during a vaginal delivery and may want to consider cesarean section.

In most cases the treatments described are successful in eliminating warts. However, it may seem that they are destined to be a part of your life forever. If that is the case, there are other avenues to be explored such as laser therapy, surgical excision, injections of chemotherapeutic agents, and various combinations of all.

To be reproduced for clinical use. Hooper: *Primary Dermatologic Care*, St Louis, 1999, Mosby.

Part IV

Directory of Support Groups

American Academy of Dermatology
930 N. Meacham Rd.
PO Box 4014
Schamburg, IL 60168-4014
Web sites: http://www.derm-infonet.com/SkinCa.html
http://www.derm-infonet.com/urticaria.html

American Cancer Society
1599 Clifton Road N.E.
Atlanta, GA 30329
1-800-ACS-2345
National Cancer Institute Hotline: 1-800-4-CANCER
Office of Cancer Communications
National Cancer Institute
Bldg. 31, Rm. 10A24
Bethesda, MD 20892

American Melanoma Foundation
UCSD Cancer Center
9500 Gilman Dr. 0658
La Jolla, CA 92093-0658
619-534-3840
Fax: 619-534-4628
Web sites: http://www.sonic.net/~jpat/getwell.html
http://cancer.med.upenn.edu/disease/melanoma

American Social Health Association
PO Box 13827
Research Triangle Park, NC 27709
919-361-8400
Fax: 919-361-8425
Web site: http://sunsite.unc.edu/ASHA

Bald-Headed Men of America
901 Arendell St.
Morehead City, NC 28557

Foundation for Ichthyosis and Related Skin Types (FIRST)
PO Box 669
Ardmore, PA 19003-0669
1-610-789-4366 or 1-800-545-3286

Lupus Foundation of America
1300 Piccard Dr. Ste.200
Rockville, MD 20850-303
301-670-9292 or 1-800-558-0121
Web site: http://www.lupus.org/lupus

National Alopecia Areata Foundation
710 C St. No.11
San Rafael, CA 94901
or
PO Box 150760
San Rafael, CA 94915-0760
415-456-4644
Fax: 415-456-4274
Web site: http://weber.u.washington.edu/~dvictor/alopecia.html

National Eczema Association for Science and Education
1221 S.W. Yamhill Ste.303
Portland, OR 97205
1-800-818-SKIN or 503-228-4430
Web site: http://www.hkma.com.hk/std/eczema.htm

National HIV/AIDS Hotline: 1-800-342-AIDS

National Institute on Aging Information Center
PO Box 8057
Gaithersburg, MD 20898-8057
1-800-222-2225

National Neurofibromatosis Foundation
95 Pine St. 16th Floor
New York, NY 10005
1-800-323-7938 or 212-344-6633
Fax: 212-747-0004
Web site: http://nf.org

National Psoriasis Foundation
6600 S.W. 92nd Ave. Ste.300
Portland, OR 97223-7195
503-244-7404
Fax: 503-245-0626
Web site: http://www.psoriasis.org

National Rosacea Society
800 S. Northwest Hwy, Ste.200
Barrington, IL 60010
847-382-8971
Web site: http://www.rosacea.org
E-mail: rosaceas@aol.com

National STD Hotline: 1-800-227-8922
Operators will answer questions regarding STDs from 8:00 AM to
11:00 PM EST

National Vitiligo Foundation
PO Box 6337
Tyler, TX 75711
903-531-0074
Web site: http://pegasus.uthct.edu/Vitiligo/index.html

Skin Cancer Foundation
245 Fifth Ave. Ste. 1403
New York, NY 10016
212-725-5176 or 1-800-SKIN-490
Web site: http://www.derm-infonet.com/Moles.html

Skin Cancer Foundation
PO Box 561
New York, NY 10156

United Scleroderma Foundation, Inc.
PO Box 399
734 East Lake Ave., Ste. 5
Watsonville, CA 95076
1-800-722-HOPE
Fax: 408-728-3328
Web site: http://www.scleroderm.org

Varicella Zoster Virus Research Foundation
40 East 72nd St.
New York, NY 10021
1-800-472-8478
Fax: 212-861-7033

Part V

Dermatopharmacology

Topical Therapy

In general 1 gram of a cream covers an area 10 cm by 10 cm, whereas 1 gram of an ointment covers a slightly larger area. When calculating the amount of a topical product to dispense, consider the following:

- Two grams is needed to cover both hands, the head, or the face.
- Three grams is needed to cover one arm or the anterior or posterior trunk.
- Four grams is needed to cover one leg.
- Thirty grams is needed to cover the entire body.

Vehicles

Water acts to cool or warm skin (depending on its temperature) and to macerate the superficial layer of skin. In so doing, it enhances penetration of any agent that is then applied. When the stratum corneum contains more than 10% water, it remains soft and pliable; when the water content drops below 10%, it becomes rough and may scale, crack, or become irritated. Repeated application of (or submersion in) water will enhance the drying effect.

Alcohol is used for cooling the skin, as an antiseptic, and as an astringent.

Propylene glycol is a solvent that readily absorbs water (hygroscopic) and, as such, has considerable moistening and softening action. It may burn or sting inflamed skin.

Zinc oxide and **talc** increase evaporation, reduce friction, and provide a cooling sensation. When mixed with ferric oxide, zinc obtains a pink color **(Calamine).** Talc may cause a severe granulomatous reaction when applied to open wounds.

Mineral oil, a mixture of high-molecular-weight petroleum hydrocarbons, is used as an emollient. There is no topical toxicity.

Ointments provide better penetration than creams and generally have fewer preservatives; thus they are tolerated better by patients with extremely sensitive skin.

Dry Dressings

Dry dressings promote formation of scabs, which act as a mechanical barrier to epithelialization and as such are to be prevented. Gauze may lead to disruption of the healing eschar. Telfa prevents the eschar from becoming incorporated into the dressing. Dressings should be changed every day or as needed. Antibiotic cream may be used to minimize the development of local microbial flora.

Unna Boots are for use on noninfected granulating ulcers. After cleaning the ulcer, an Unna Boot paste dressing is applied over a gauze-packed ulcer. An antibacterial ointment of choice (usually bacitracin, polymixin, or gentamycin sulfate) may be applied. A flesh-colored roll bandage impregnated with a paste of zinc oxide, calamine, glycerin, and gelatin is applied with greatest pressure at the ankle, diminishing as the roll moves upward. Each turn should overlap the preceding one. A double layer of tube gauze is then placed over the "boot" with tape securing the upper and lower ends. The dressing is changed at weekly intervals. The Unna Boot is ideal for stasis ulcers and stasis eczema with chronic venous insufficiency.

Occlusive Dressings

Duoderm (hydrocolloid occlusive dressing) is composed of gelatin, pectin, and various other components. It is applied over the ulcer and over 2 cm of normal surrounding skin and remains in place up to 7 days or until leakage occurs. Use of **metronidazole** gel under the Duoderm will help retard formation of anaerobic bacteria and the resultant odoriferous drainage. Removal of the dressing does not traumatize the epithelium.

Vapor-permeable membranes **(Vigilon, Op-Site, Tegaderm, Silon)** are elastic polyethylene films that allow passage of oxygen, carbon dioxide, and water vapor, while impeding the movement of proteins and bacteria. Dressings should only be changed if leakage of exudate occurs, or if the ulcer is covered with eschar or necrotic debris. Advantages include decreased pain, visibility of signs of infection, ability to shower with the dressing in place, and superior cosmetic healing. The average duration of healing is usually decreased by half.

Wet Dressings

Wet dressings cool, soothe, and dry skin or wounds through the evaporation of water. The cooling effect that occurs during the repeated application of wet dressings leads to vasoconstriction. When covered with plastic or other occlusive product, wet dressings macerate and soften the skin surface. They should be left in place for $\frac{1}{2}$ to 2 hours (and are changed every 5 to 15 minutes), tid to qid. Six to eight layers of soft gauze soaked in the desired solution should be applied to prevent rapid drying.

A 5% aluminum acetate solution **(Burow's solution)** is moderately bacteriostatic, especially for gram-positive organisms. It does not stain and is soothing. A 15% acetic acid solution is effective for wounds infected with *Pseudomonas aeruginosa*.

Lotions

A lotion is a suspension of powder in a liquid medium and is used for subacute inflammations to provide a protective, cooling effect. The addition of alcohol produces a drying effect. Menthol, phenol, and camphor produce antipruritic action.

Emollients

Emollients soften skin by forming an occlusive oil film on the stratum corneum. This film prevents evaporation of the water that diffuses to the surface from the underlying layers of skin.

Alpha-Keri Bath Oil deposits a thin film of oil over the skin. It does not need to be used with soap because of its inherent cleansing properties. A 10- to 20-minute soak is adequate.

Ureacin lotion/cream contains 10%, 20%, or 40% urea in a vegetable oil base. Urea acts to increase the water binding capacity of the stratum corneum.

Lac-Hydrin 12% cream/lotion contains lactic acid, which is an effective humectant in the skin and helps reduce excessive epidermal keratinization, not only leaving the skin smoother, but also enhancing penetration of the hydrating component (water).

Antiacne Preparations

Benzoyl peroxide has broad-spectrum antimicrobial activity that persists for 48 hours on skin. It is a bacteriostatic agent against *Propionibacterium acnes*, decreasing the inflammation of lesions. It also has a keratolytic effect, and possible sebum-suppressing action. In general gels are more effective than creams or lotions because they have greater follicular penetration. Products with 10% **benzoyl peroxide** are not necessarily more effective than those with lower percentages, but may be more irritating to the skin. **Benzoyl peroxide** should be rubbed into the lesions qd or bid. The amount and the frequency of application should be limited initially, then gradually increased as tolerance permits.

Retinoic acid/tretinoin (Retin-A) increases cell turnover, preventing keratinous plugs and comedone formation. Dosage should begin with a low concentration cream, used qhs (the active ingredient is inactivated by sunlight) on dry skin (to prevent excessive penetration). Improvement is seen in 75% of patients within 3 months. It should not be used on eczematous skin or on the nose, around the eyes, or on mucus membranes. Skin may take up to 2 weeks to become acclimated to retinoic acid.

Toxicity: Acne may be aggravated during the first 2 to 4 weeks of therapy. Skin irritation increases with exposure to cold, low humidity, and exposure to sunlight (phototoxicity).

Tretinoin (Avita) cream has a specialized topical delivery system to decrease the irritability of **Retin-A** while providing increased penetration.

Salicyclic acid is present in many acne preparations. A 0.5% to 3% solution promotes desquamation by its effect on the surface squamous cells; a 5% to 10% solution is both comedolytic and keratinolytic. **Salicyclic acid** is most commonly used as a surface cleanser without notable toxicity.

Sulfur medications have both a keratolytic and a drying action to help lesions heal, but do not prevent new lesion formation. The bacteriostatic action occurs when **sulfur** comes in contact with the epidermal cells or microorganisms on the epidermis. The medication should be applied bid to lesions and has minimal if any toxicity.

Antibacterial Agents

Bacitracin inhibits bacterial wall synthesis and is active against many gram-positive cocci and bacilli. It is not active against

Pseudomonas or *Candida* organisms. It may be applied qd or bid. There is no toxicity with topical use.

Clindamycin phosphate (Cleocin-T) suppresses protein synthesis of bacterial ribosomes, although only 1% to 3% of the medication is absorbed topically. The antiinflammatory effects that occur also play an important role in the treatment of acne.

Erythromycin 2% is a 2% erythromycin solution in acetone, alcohol, and polyethylene glycol. It suppresses protein synthesis of bacterial ribosomes but is much more effective against gram-positive cocci than is **Clindamycin.** It is not effective against most aerobic gram-negative bacilli.

Polymyxin (Polysporin) is a mixture of polymyxin B sulfate and bacitracin zinc in white petrolatum. It alters the membrane permeability of the bacterial cells and is primarily effective against gram-negative bacteria. It can be applied as needed since there is almost complete lack of absorption. **Neosporin** is similar to polysporin but includes neomycin sulfate, the addition of which results in a higher rate of topical allergic reactions.

Povidone-iodine (Betadine) is lethal to microflora, microzoa, and viruses. The solution will decrease the usual cutaneous bacterial population by about 85% for 1 hour after application. As a preparation for surgery the skin should be scrubbed with the **Betadine** cleansing solution for 15 seconds. The ointment can be applied postoperatively qd.

Antifungal Agents

Ciclopirox (Loprox) interferes with fungal energy metabolism and is effective against a wide variety of fungi, yeasts, and bacteria. It should be applied bid and is generally nonirritating and nonsensitizing. It also demonstrates good penetration of nail keratin.

Clotrimazole (Lotrimin, Mycelex) inhibits the growth of fungi and yeasts by altering cell wall permeability. The drug remains in the stratum corneum for up to 96 hours after a single application. There is a 59% to 70% cure rate reported when it is applied to the affected area bid. Toxic reactions are rare.

Econazole nitrate (Spectazole) is similar to clotrimazole in that it interferes with fungal cell membrane synthesis, but is more effective against coexistent gram-positive bacteria than other antifungal agents.

Miconazole nitrate (Monistat) may be fungicidal or fungistatic, depending on the concentration. There is also a broad spectrum of bactericidal activity against many forms of gram-positive bacteria. A 75% to 100% cure rate has been reported. **Monistat** is applied bid for 2 to 4 weeks.

Nystatin (Mycostatin) acts by disrupting the membrane permeability of fungal cells. It is effective against all *Candida* species and many fungi. It can be used bid for 2 weeks as a powder, cream, or lotion. Orally it can be used tid to eliminate gastrointestinal colonization.

Selenium sulfide (Selsun) is effective against dandruff and acts as an antifungal treatment against tinea versicolor. It should be applied to the scalp or to the skin one to three times weekly. Treatment is enhanced if **Selsun** is left on for 10 minutes before being washed off.

Tolnaftate (Tinactin), a fungistatic rather than fungicidal agent, is available over the counter. It is active against specific species only and should be applied bid for 2 to 3 weeks. There is a 73% to 93% cure rate reported.

Undecylenic acid (Desenex, Cruex) may help as a fungistatic powder, although a cure rate of only 50% to 88% has been reported. It is available over the counter.

Antiinflammatory Agents

Corticosteroids produce a vasoconstrictive action on dilated vessels by inhibiting the inflammatory response, regardless of the inciting event or agent. Therapy is only palliative, however, as the causative agent or event remains. Tolerance to vasoconstrictive actions may develop within a week of application, with responsiveness returning after a 4-day absence. Occlusion increases absorption 10- to 100-fold. Hydration of the skin before application increases penetration 5-fold. Use should be limited to bid application. The total amount of a moderate to potent steroid should be limited to 45 g weekly in an adult. Less than 15 g weekly of a low-potency to midpotency steroid should be used in a child.

Toxicity: Skin atrophy, telangiectasias, striae, and purpura evolve with continued use of high-potency preparations, especially on the face or flexural areas. Striae may not be reversible. Atrophy resolves after 6 months of discontinuing steroids. A rosacealike eruption may occur with the use of fluorinated steroids applied to the face, resulting in persistent erythema, telangiectasias, papules, and pustules. Systemic effects are rare and occur only with prolonged use of high-potency preparations on denuded skin or with occlusive dressings. A rebound phenomenon or possible pustular flare in psoriasis may occur when more than 45 g of potent agents is used per week.

Antineoplastic Agents

5-Fluorouracil (5-FU) (Efudex) blocks the deoxyribonucleic acid (DNA) synthesis of cells. Combined with **Retin-A,** it is useful on the arms and hands when applied qd or bid for 4 to 6 weeks. Concurrent avoidance of sun exposure is required. The nasolabial folds should be avoided since an accumulation of **5-FU** will produce irritation. Erythema occurs in 3 to 7 days and increases until scaling, tenderness, erosions, and superficial ulcerations occur in the areas of keratoses. Therapy is discontinued after the inflammatory reaction occurs but treatment may be repeated in 3 to 4 years. Only 6% of the ointment is absorbed systemically. Hyperpigmentation, burning, and contact dermatitis may occur, especially after sun exposure.

Bleaching Agents

Hydroquinone (Eldopaque, Eldoquin, Solaquin, Neostrata Bleaching Cream/Gel, Melanex, Lustra) acts by inhibiting melanin synthesis, leading to depigmentation. The changes are reversible when the medication is discontinued. It should be applied to the affected area qd to bid for 4 to 6 weeks. Efficacy increases when it is combined with 0.05% **retinoic acid.** Concomitant use of sunscreen is essential.

Scabicides and Pediculicides

Lindane (Kwell) produces seizures in the parasites *Sarcoptes scabiei, Pediculos capitis, Phthirus pubis,* and their ova. It should be rubbed into the affected area, left on for 6 to 24 hours (cure rates appear constant throughout), and then washed off. The treatment should be repeated in 1 week.

Toxicity: Irritant contact dermatitis may develop with prolonged use. Convulsion may result from extensive cutaneous absorption. Severe irritation occurs with contact to eyes or mucus membranes.

Sunscreens

Highly alcoholic vehicles should not be used with eczematous or inflamed skin. All products should be applied 1 to 2 hours before exposure and hourly thereafter, especially during swimming or heavy sweating.

Chemical sunscreens act by absorbing ultraviolet B (UVB) and/or UVA light. **Para-aminobenzoic acid (PABA)** effectively absorbs UVB light but is the most common cause of contact dermatitis from sunscreens.

Physical sunscreens act by reflecting light radiation. Examples include **zinc oxide** and **titanium dioxide.**

Systemic Therapy

Antibacterial Agents

Erythromycin is a macrolide, effective against most gram-positive bacteria and some gram-negative. It is not effective against enterobacterium or *Pseudomonas aeruginosa.* Gastrointestinal (GI) upset is common, especially with larger doses. It may also increase serum levels of **warfarin** and **digoxin.** No teratogenic effects appear to occur, even with large doses.

Tetracycline has a wide range of antimicrobial activity against gram-positive and gram-negative bacteria, as well as rickettsiae and *Mycoplasma* and *Chlamydia* organisms. *Proteus vulgaris* and *Pseudomonas aeruginosa* are resistant. The medication is best absorbed on an empty stomach. Absorption is significantly impaired by milk, aluminum hydroxide, calcium and magnesium salts, iron, sodium bicarbonate, and zinc tablets. **Minocycline (Minocin)** is a tetracycline derivative that is less affected by food and dairy products.

Toxicity: All tetracyclines may produce dose-related gastrointestinal upset. Phototoxicity is common. Children below the age of 12 should not receive **tetracycline** because of the increased possibility of discoloring the permanent teeth. Pregnant women are particularly susceptible to severe tetracycline-induced hepatic damage. **Minocycline** may produce dizziness, ataxia, nausea, and vomiting during the first few doses. Other cutaneous reactions are rare.

Antifungal Agents

Fluconazole (Diflucan) is an effective agent against *Candida* spp. and dermatophyte fungal infections. It appears to be safer than **ketoconazole,** but the price is significantly higher.

Griseofulvin (Fulvicin) disrupts the DNA synthesis of fungal cells. It is taken up by and released from keratinocytes in the stratum corneum and is also secreted in sweat and deposited on the skin surface. It is *ineffective* against *Candida* organisms. Absorption is enhanced after a high-fat meal. The microcrystalline form should be administered at 500 mg qd or bid until the infected structures are physically and microscopically normal. With the ultramicrocrystalline form 250 to 500 mg should be given qd or bid. Children should be given 5 mg/kg body weight in single or divided doses.

Ketoconazole (Nizoral) demonstrates a broad spectrum of activity against yeasts and fungi. It is rapidly absorbed after oral administration with meals. Absorption is decreased with concomitant administration of **cimetidine** or **antacids.** Because of its high cost **ketoconazole** is the treatment of choice only for **griseofulvin-**

resistant disorders or for short-term therapy (such as for tinea versicolor).

Toxicity: Liver function tests (LFTs) should be monitored every month.

Terbinafine (Lamisil) is extremely effective against dermato-phytes and is available in both oral and topical forms. There are no adverse interactions with other medications, and it is not necessary to check laboratory test values.

Antihistamines

Hydroxyzine (Atarax) is an extremely safe antihistamine that di-minishes the perception of itching. It blocks the local effects of his-tamine, thus reversing some urticarial reactions. As such, it helps treat urticaria, not merely reduce symptoms. Drowsiness and dry-ness of the mouth occur commonly. Caution should be exercised if it is used during the first trimester of pregnancy to prevent fetal abnormalities.

Diphenhydramine (Benadryl) is also sedating and has a similar mechanism of action and dosage to **Atarax.** It is available over the counter.

Loratadine (Claritin) is a nonsedating antihistamine that is ad-ministered qd. It is frequently prescribed for morning dosing, in conjunction with a sedating antihistamine administered at bedtime.

Cimetidine (Tagamet) and **ranitidine (Zantac)** are H_2 antago-nists usually prescribed for the treatment of ulcerative GI disorders but may be helpful for the resolution of urticaria as well. For partic-ularly recalcitrant urticaria, they may be used in conjunction with H_1 antagonists **(diphenhydramine, loratadine, hydroxyzine).**

Antiinflammatory Agents

Prednisolone (Prednisone) dosages depend on the disease being treated. (Specific recommendations are made in the treatment sec-tion for each disease.) The entire daily dose should be given at 8:00 AM to produce the least suppressive effect on the body. An al-ternate-day dose may be preferred for long-term use (greater than 14 days) to minimize the development of a cushingoid appearance, hypertension, growth failure, and infection. The 24- to 36-hour half-life of **prednisolone** makes it ideal for qod therapy, and no ta-pering is needed if used for less than 3 weeks.

Antiviral Agents

Acyclovir (Zovirax) is effective against herpes simplex types I and II, varicella zoster, Epstein-Barr virus, and cytomegalovirus.

Treatment should begin as soon as prodromal symptoms or vesicles are noticed, at least within 48 hours of the onset of lesions. Oral administration is well tolerated with few side effects.

Famciclovir (Famvir) and **valacyclovir (Valtrex)** are newer-generation antiviral agents that some studies have shown to be more effective than **acyclovir.** The cost of the newer medications may be prohibitive, however.

Part VI

Dermatologic Surgery Techniques

Acne Surgery

Comedome extraction is effective in preventing pustules and removing blackheads and whiteheads. Pricking the center of the lesion with a lancet may be helpful in encouraging expulsion with minimal discomfort. The aperture of the comedone extractor is placed so that the dark area (or white head) is near the edge of the opening. Downward and lateral pressure will result in expulsion of the follicular plug.

Milia are extracted as described previously.

Pustules heal more quickly if they are opened and drained. Unfortunately such treatment may increase the risk of "ice-pick" scarring if excessive trauma is used to dislodge the contents of the follicle. The lesions are usually opened with a #11 blade or lancet, and the contents evacuated with gentle pressure.

Cysts are opened with a #11 blade and the contents evacuated with gentle pressure. The cyst wall is teased loose with a hemostat or curette. The opening should be of minimal size to reduce scarring.

Hypertrophic scars and *keloids* may be treated with cryotherapy, the pulse dye laser, intralesional corticosteroids (triamcinolone acetonide [Kenalog] 10 to 40 mg/ml every month), or a combination of treatments.

"Ice-pick scars" may be treated with a 2-mm punch biopsy followed by laser resurfacing.

Cryosurgery

The extent and intensity of freezing are determined by the duration of time that skin is in contact with the freezing agent, as well as the amount of pressure applied. The resultant depth of tissue necrosis is approximately 0.5 mm with sprays, 1 mm with solid carbon dioxide, and 1.5 to 2 mm with liquid nitrogen applied with a cotton-tipped applicator. Repeated applications will produce deeper damage with any of the techniques.

The lesion is frozen such that an area approximately double the apparent size of the lesion is frozen in cycles with a slow, visible thaw time. Common warts usually require 20 to 30 seconds of freezing when located on the dorsum of hands, and 40 to 60 seconds on palmar or plantar surfaces. Shortly after freezing erythema and urticaria result from histamine release and blood vessel damage. On thicker skin this reaction appears later and is less severe.

Epidermal regeneration is well under way within 3 days after superficial freezing. Scarring is uncommon as the full thickness of skin is not destroyed. Large blood vessels are resistant to cryogenic injury.

Lesions responding best to freezing include the following:

- Verruca vulgaris with a cure rate of approximately 60% after one treatment and 80% after two treatments. A 30- to 90-second freeze time is usually required.
- Keratoacanthomas and seborrheic keratoses may be frozen entirely or frozen and removed with curettage to provide both diagnosis and cure. Thaw times of 30 to 45 seconds are adequate. An interval of 8 to 12 weeks is used for repeated therapy if needed. A 98.5% cure rate in lesions up to 2.5 cm in diameter has been reported.
- Keloids may be frozen with subsequent softening, allowing better penetration with intralesional steroids.
- Other disorders that respond well include molluscum, angiomas, dermatofibromas, and lentigines.

Complications include temporary stinging and burning of the treatment site, urticaria and edema (occasionally exaggerated on the periorbital, lateral forehead and anterior scalp), and ulceration in thin or devitalized skin (with possible resultant scarring). Temporary hypopigmentation usually occurs because melanocytes are damaged to a greater extent than keratinocytes. Anesthesia or paresthesia may occur, especially when nerves lie superficially.

Curettement

A curetting ring of 3.5 mm allows sufficient tissue for microscopy for basal cell carcinoma, squamous cell carcinoma, actinic or seborrheic keratoses, verrucae, and Bowen's disease.

The curetting ring's cutting edge is applied to the skin surface and scraped across the lesion repeatedly. The tissue sample is removed from the curette by inversion and shaking in the fixative solution.

This technique is best reserved for friable tissue only, as the cutting edge is not sharp enough for normal skin. Curettage to delineate the extent of the lesion (friable tissue) may be followed by shave excision to ensure complete removal of the lesion.

Electrocautery

The electrocautery procedure uses resistance to the flow of electrical current to generate heat, which in turn causes tissue destruction. Verruca vulgaris may be cauterized with subsequent curettage of adjacent tissue. Additional cauterization may be used to control bleeding. For old or deeply embedded lesions two treatments 7 to 10 days apart may be necessary. Vascular lesions are ideally treated with this technique since the hemostatic effect of cautery encourages simple and rapid removal.

The area to be destroyed is anesthetized with a local anesthetic solution, usually without **epinephrine** (which is unnecessary because of the hemostatic effect of cautery). An anesthetic zone of approximately 1 cm surrounding the lesion should be obtained in order to prevent discomfort from the heat of the cautery. Curettage is used to remove carbonized tissue and to delineate pathologic tissue.

Punch Biopsy

Punches are circular cutting blades varying in diameter from 1 mm to 1.2 cm, in increments of 0.25 to 0.5 mm. A cylindrical sample of tissue from the epidermis to the underlying fat is obtained through this procedure. A disadvantage is that the full-thickness dermal wound must be sutured and may heal with scarring.

After the skin is cleansed with alcohol and injected with **lidocaine** (with or without **epinephrine**), the skin is stretched perpendicular to the skin wrinkle lines. This stretching changes the circular defect to an elliptical shape. The punch is pressed gently against the skin surface and rotated clockwise and counterclockwise until a small "give" is felt as the cutting edge transverses the reticular dermis. The instrument is then withdrawn. If the tissue sample is retained in the wound, it may be gently removed with forceps. The wound can be closed with one or two sutures or allowed to heal by primary intension.

Shave Biopsy

The shave biopsy procedure removes a portion of epidermis and underlying papillary dermis to obtain biopsy specimens and remove superficial tumors or papules. The advantage is minimal scarring with a very shallow depression and rapid epithelialization.

After the lesion is cleansed with alcohol and anesthetized with a local injection of **lidocaine** (with or without **epinephrine**), a #15 blade (or one-half of a razor blade) is used gently to saw under the lesion. The blade must be kept parallel to the skin surface to ensure removal of the lesion without leaving a depressed scar.

Lesions suitable for this technique include seborrheic keratoses, verrucae planae, benign nevi, squamous papillomas, and benign keratoses. Color differences in the biopsy site may be noticed if the specimen was taken from a telangiectatic area, because of lack of re-formation of telangiectasias from the biopsied site.

Index